Medicinal Chemistry

Medicinal Chemistry

Phoebe Gates

NY RESEARCH
P R E S S

New York

Published by NY Research Press
118-35 Queens Blvd., Suite 400,
Forest Hills, NY 11375, USA
www.nyresearchpress.com

Medicinal Chemistry
Phoebe Gates

International Standard Book Number: 978-1-63238-789-9 (Hardback)

Cataloging-in-Publication Data

Medicinal chemistry / Phoebe Gates.
    p. cm.
Includes bibliographical references and index.
ISBN 978-1-63238-789-9
1. Pharmaceutical chemistry. 2. Chemistry. I. Gates, Phoebe.
RS403 .M43 2020
615.19--dc23

TABLE OF CONTENTS

Permissions

Index

PREFACE

This book aims to help a broader range of students by exploring a wide variety of significant topics related to this discipline. It will help students in achieving a higher level of understanding of the subject and excel in their respective fields. This book would not have been possible without the unwavered support of my senior professors who took out the time to provide me feedback and help me with the process. I would also like to thank my family for their patience and support.

Medicinal chemistry deals with the design, chemical synthesis and development of pharmaceutical agents for the market. It makes use of principles from numerous sciences such as synthetic organic chemistry, pharmacology and other biological fields. The organic compounds which are used as medicines are classified into small organic molecules and biologics. This field also studies the inorganic and organometallic compounds which are used as drugs. Medicinal chemistry plays an important role in studying the chemical aspects of identification and synthetic alteration of new chemical entities to make them suitable for therapeutic agents. This book presents the complex subject of medicinal chemistry in the most comprehensible and easy to understand language. While understanding the long-term perspectives of the topics, it makes an effort in highlighting their impact as a modern tool for the growth of the discipline. Those in search of information to further their knowledge will be greatly assisted by this book.

A brief overview of the book contents is provided below:

Chapter – Introduction

Medicinal chemistry is a field of chemistry that is concerned with the design, chemical synthesis and development of pharmaceutical agents and bio-active molecules. This is an introductory chapter which will introduce briefly all the significant aspects of medicinal chemistry such as common types of drugs.

Chapter – Sub-disciplines of Medicinal Chemistry

Medicinal chemistry is sub-divided into various disciplines. Some of them are pharmacokinetics, pharmacodynamics, pharmacology, pharmacognosy and pharmacometrics. The topics elaborated in this chapter will help in gaining a better perspective about these sub-disciplines of medicinal chemistry as well as their importance.

Chapter – Compounds used in Medicinal Chemistry

Some of the major compounds used in medicinal chemistry are inorganic compounds and organic carbamates. The chemical compounds that lack carbon-hydrogen bonds are known as inorganic compounds. Organic carbamates are the organic compounds which are derived from carbamic acid. The diverse uses of these compounds in medicinal chemistry have been thoroughly discussed in this chapter.

Chapter – Classification of Medicinal Drugs

Drugs are broadly classified on the basis of their chemical makeup and their effects. Some of the common types of drugs are analgesics, antibiotics, antiviral drugs, antiseptics and tranquilizers. The chapter closely examines these classes of drugs to provide an extensive understanding of the subject.

Chapter – Drug Discovery, Design and Development

Drug discovery refers to the process by which new candidate medications are discovered. The inventive process of finding new medications based on the knowledge of a biological target is referred to as drug design. Drug development is the process of bringing new pharmaceutical drugs to the market. The topics elaborated in this chapter will help in gaining a better perspective about drug discovery, design and development.

Phoebe Gates

Introduction

1

- **Medicinal Chemistry of Herbs**
- **Medication**

Medicinal chemistry is a field of chemistry that is concerned with the design, chemical synthesis and development of pharmaceutical agents and bio-active molecules. This is an introductory chapter which will introduce briefly all the significant aspects of medicinal chemistry such as common types of drugs.

Medicinal chemistry is a discipline that encloses the design, development, and synthesis of pharmaceutical drugs. The discipline combines expertise from chemistry, especially synthetic organic chemistry, pharmacology, and other biological sciences. It is also part of medicinal chemistry the evaluation of the properties of existing drugs.

The use of plants, minerals, and animal parts as medicines has been recorded since the most ancient civilizations. With the evolution of the knowledge the means for drug discovery also evolved. New molecules with potential pharmaceutical interest, "hits', are natural products, or compounds generated by computational chemistry, or compounds from a screening of chemical libraries, from combinatorial chemistry, and from pharmaceutical biotechnology. The "hit" compound is improved for its pharmacologic, pharmacodynamic and pharmacokinetic properties by chemical or functional group modifications, transforming it into a lead compound. A lead compound should have a known structure and a known mechanism of action. The lead compound is further optimized to be a drug candidate that is safe to use in human clinical trials.

Drug Discovery

Natural Products

Natural products have been major sources of lead compounds in the discovery of new drugs for the treatment of infectious diseases, lipid disorders, neurological diseases, cardiovascular and metabolic diseases, immunological, inflammatory and related diseases, and oncologic diseases. From the pharmaceutical entities approved worldwide between 1981 and 2006, 5.7% were natural products and 27.6% were natural-product derived molecules, whereas from 2005 to 2010, seven natural products and 12 natural product derivatives were approved for use in clinical practice. Traditional medicine, however, can also produce false leads, as reviewed recently for curcumin.

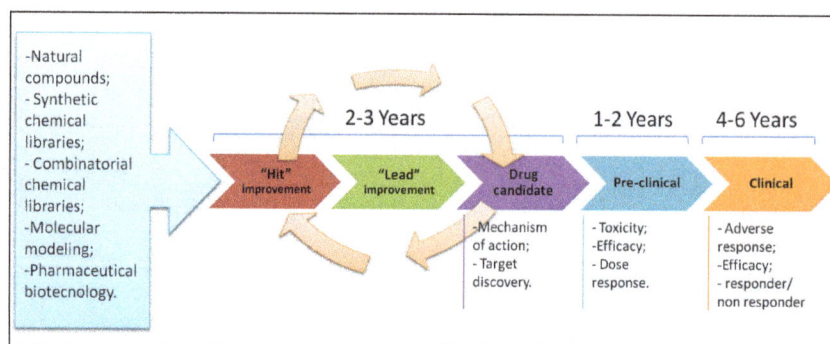

A time frame for drug discovery.

Selection of an Organism

Natural compounds have high chemical diversity. They come from different organisms. The choice of plants, microorganisms, fungi or other organisms for investigation for new compounds tend to be based on random screening, selection of specific taxonomic groups, a chemotaxonomic group of secondary metabolites like alkaloids, database surveillance of a species collection, or ethnomedical approach. Several drugs trace their origin to ethnobotanical use.

Table: Examples of natural products and natural product derivatives currently in clinical use.

Disease area	Generic name (Trade name)	Lead compound	Year
Antibacterial	Doripenem (Finibax/Doribax)	Thienamycin	2005
Antiparasitic	Fumagillin (Flisint)	Fumagillin	2005
Oncology	Romidepsin (Istodax)	Romidepsin	2009
Alzheimer's disease	Galantamine (Reminyl)	Galantamine	2002
Immunosuppression	Mycophenolate sodium (Myfortic)	Mycophenolic acid	2003
Dyslipidemia	Rosuvastatin (Crestor)	Mevastatin	2003
Pain	Capsaicin (Istodax)	Capsaicin	2009
Diabetes	Exenatide (Byetta)	Exenatide	2006

Sample Collection

0.3 to 1 Kg of dried plant or 1 Kg of wet weight of marine samples should be collected from different parts of the organism. If the sample needs to be re-collected, it should be performed in the same localization and at the same time during the day, since different habitats can lead to different secondary metabolites. Of importance is also the deposit of a representative voucher specimen in a central repository, for later access . Besides plants, in the last decade the interest in fungi, cyanobacteria of marine origin and the evolution of the "genome mining" techniques for culturing microorganisms in the laboratory led to the discovery of new natural products.

Extraction

The extraction protocols differ from laboratory to laboratory. The initial extraction of plants usually is done with a polar solvent, like methanol or ethanol. It is then subject to a defatting process through partition with a nonpolar solvent, such as hexane or petroleum ether. The extract is partitioned between a semipolar solvent, such as chloroform or dichloromethane, and a polar aqueous solvent. Marine and aquatic organisms are extracted fresh with methanol or dichloromethane. Vegetable tannins have to be removed from the extracts. Their presence can lead to protein precipitation and enzyme inhibition, interfering with the biologic assays.

Purification and Isolation

Separation of the active compound is done using several chromatographic techniques. High pressure liquid chromatography (HPLC) and its coupling with high-throughput screening (HST) assays simplify the purification and isolation of active compounds. The compounds are identified by nuclear magnetic resonance (NMR) and mass spectrometry (MS). These techniques, when coupled with liquid chromatography (LC), allow simultaneous purification and structure elucidation of biologically active compounds. Purification and isolation of the active compound are measured by biologic assays. HTS assays can evaluate a large number of extracts or compounds in a cell-based or non-cell-based context.

The major challenge in natural compounds development is to obtain significant amounts for further development. Re-collection of the species of origin, or plant tissue culture, or cultivation and fermentation in large scale for microbes of terrestrial origin can produce the compounds in large scale. The natural compounds can also be synthesized. For example, Kawano S et al. achieved the total synthesis of one of halichondrins, a group of structurally complex natural products isolated from various marine sponges, and addressed the issue of limited material supply .

Computational Chemistry

Molecular modeling, or more generally, computational chemistry, has become a well-established part of drug development. Molecular modeling searches new molecules, based on a theoretical platform or by screening a library. Crystallographic and/or NMR information on receptors and specific targets, such as that of cystic fibrosis transmembrane conductance regulator (CFTR) , allows through molecular modeling techniques, the design of new molecules for the target. Other approaches use known active molecules as a target, and design new molecules or search the libraries for similar molecules.

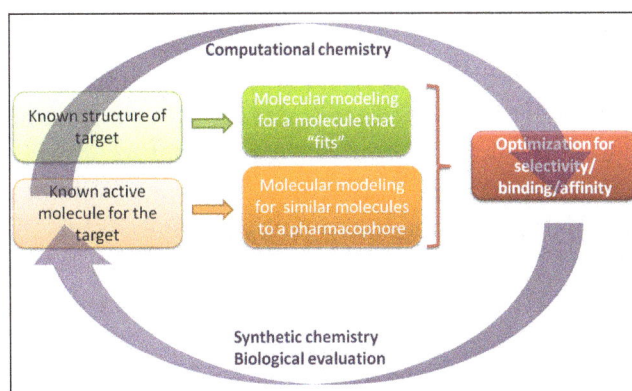

Computational chemistry approaches for the development of new drugs.

The found "hit" molecules can either be synthesized in the laboratory or purchased. After evaluation and structure-activity-relationship (SAR) disclosure, new studies of molecular modeling can be performed to find a more active molecule or to optimize the found molecule.

Computational chemistry is based on the visualization and manipulation of three-dimensional molecular models. Rotation of bonds, structure building, molecular mechanisms and/or dynamics, conformational analysis, electronic properties, molecular surface displays and calculation of various physical properties are possible through molecular modeling. The techniques used are molecular mechanisms and molecular dynamics simulations, Monte Carlo techniques, ligand docking, and virtual screening methods.

The current state-of-the art systems allow working with more than 20 molecules and thousands of molecular surface points in real time. Each molecule can be color labeled and controlled in three dimensions, where the intramolecular distances and the noncontiguous dihedral angles can be adjusted and monitored. Shape, charge and hydrophobicity of the atoms in the molecule can also be simulated. The electrostatic potential gradient or electrical field can also be displayed graphically using short vectors. Molecular modeling requires make-bond, break-bond, fuse rings, delete-atom, add-atom, add-hydrogens, invert chiral center, etc. These operations should allow a refined structure for a selected target.

Several systems were developed for storing and retrieving the information generated by molecular modeling. The number of new molecules generated by molecular modeling can number thousands for a target, making the synthesis and biological evaluation of all these new molecules a challenge. The development of virtual screenings allowed to overcome the previous problem. After virtual screening evaluation only the molecules with the required biological activity would be synthesized or purchased for further biological evaluation.

Chemical Databases

An abundance of compounds is synthesized and biologically evaluated, almost daily. In the past years around 2000-3000 compounds were published in the main medicinal chemistry journals.

PubChem, CheMBL and BindingBD are public databases of compounds and their bioactivity. Other databases such as ChemBank and IUPHARDB are also available.

The National Institute of Health (NIH) founded in 2004 PubChem database, a public library containing more than 33 million compounds. The main purpose of this database is to collect and disseminate information on the biological activities of small molecules. It started by collecting the bioassays performed in NIH, today it accepts data from other sources such as depositions. PubChem does not include information extracted from literature, however the incorporation of data from CheMBL and BindingBD allows the access to several sets of curated literature data. As of August 20, 2018, the database contains 96,479,457 compounds, 247,255,508 substances, 1,252,901 bioassays, 3,151,922 tested compounds, 5,264,801 tested substances, 172 RNAi bioassays, 237,061,979 bioactivities, 10,859 protein targets and 58,009 gene targets.

Database name	Number of compounds
PubChem	96 million
CheMBL	1.82 million

BindingBD	0.65 million
ChemSpider	67 million
DrugBank	11682
SwissADME	

CheMBL was initiated with a set of commercial products, it became public in January of 2010. This library captures data from the literature in medicinal chemistry. In the scope of this database are protein-ligand affinities and cell-based data. More recently ChEMBL incorporated therapeutic proteins and other drug types besides the data on small molecules. ChEMBL24_1 release contains 2,275,906 compound records, 1,828,820 compounds (of which 1,820,035 have mol files), 15,207,914 activities, 1,060,283 assays, 12,091 targets, and 69,861 documents, as of August 20, 2018.

BindingBD originated in an academic environment, in the late 1990s. This database initially focused on small molecules with reported biological activity. BindingBD focuses on the assay conditions and factors reported to influence the outcome of the assay, such as pH, temperature and substrates. Virtual screening can be performed directly using the BindingBD website tools. As of August 20, 2018, BindingDB contains 1,454,892 binding data, for 7,082 protein targets and 652,068 small molecules.

With the increasing number of compounds being published every year, the importance of chemical libraries with free access in drug discovery is critical.

Combinatorial Chemistry

Combinatorial chemistry is defined as the laboratory synthesis or computational aided design of a large number of molecules, starting from one scaffold. The scaffold should have diverse points for modification, through combination with know molecules or molecules derived from a molecular modeling study. Combinatorial chemistry has been used to optimize a lead compound.

One of the best approaches in combinatorial chemistry is to use a central scaffold with several substituents, which can be independently modified. This approach increases the possibility of finding a "hit" molecule, since the synthesized molecules have a higher molecular diversity.

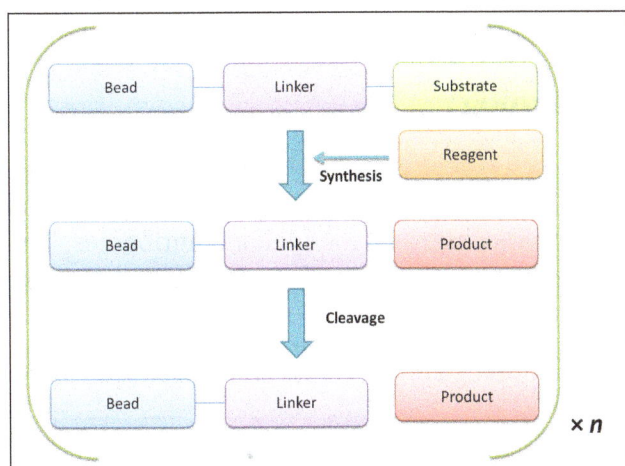

Simplified scheme of combinatorial chemistry.

Parallel synthesis, a method of combinatorial chemistry, allows the formation of a large set of compounds. The formed mixture can be tested for biological activity. If the mixture does not have activity it can be archived and later tested for other biological activities. When the mixture turns out to be active, the challenge becomes the isolation of the active compound. One of the disadvantages of synthesized molecules in combinatory chemistry is that it has poor diversity, compared to natural compounds.

The majority of the combinatorial synthesis is performed through solid phase techniques. The starting material is bound, directly or through a linker, to a bead. The reagents are added and the product is formed. This procedure can be repeated several times using the previously formed product as a starting material. The product can be removed from the bead or directly tested with the bead attached, for biologic activity. The bead reduces side reactions and formation of by-products. The linkers should be resistant to reaction conditions and easily removed after synthesis.

The simple techniques of combinatorial chemistry allow the synthesis of one product per vessel. More complex methods, such as mixed combinatorial synthesis, allow the synthesis of complex mixtures. Manual techniques for the synthesis of one compound per vessel, such as the Houghton's tea bag procedure, are still used. Automated parallel synthesis is currently the most used method.

The synthesis of large quantities of diverse compounds often makes use of the mix and split technique. In this method, the first mixture of compounds synthesized is divided in n parts, the n parts are again subject to a new modification, synthesizing z new mixtures (z = n × number of different modifications). This procedure can be repeated until the number of desired modifications is reached. The mixtures can be tested before a new modification is performed. This will exclude mixtures where no biological activity is observed, avoiding further modification.

When a mixture is biologically active, micromanipulation, recursive deconvolution and sequential release techniques can be used to separate the active(s) compound(s). Identification and structural elucidation are performed after isolation of the active(s) compound(s).

The evaluation of the libraries generated by combinatorial chemistry is usually made by HTS . Screening methods using fluorescence and chemoluminescence are being developed; which allow the simultaneous identification of the active compounds.

Pharmaceutical Biotechnology

Pharmaceutical biotechnology is a recent area of medicinal chemistry, producing new therapeutic and diagnostic products. The common products are peptides and protein, hormones of different origins, and enzymes, including vaccines and monoclonal antibodies. The discovery of new drugs in pharmaceutical biotechnology is made through genomics, transcriptomics, proteomics, pharmacogenomics and metabolics.

Table: Some examples of biotechnological pharmaceutical products currently in clinical use.

Disease area	Generic name (Trade name)	Type of bioproduct
Type II diabetes	Exenatide (Byetta)	Peptide

Oncology (Prostate cancer)	Degarelix (Firmagon)	Peptide
Osteoporosis	Teriparatide (Forteo)	Hormone
Type I diabetes	Glucagon (GlucaGen)	Hormone
Hepatitis C	Consensus Interferon (IFN Alfacon-1)	Enzyme
Rheumatic arthritis	Anakinra (Kineret)	Enzyme
Polio	Polio (Ipol)	Vaccine
Measles	Rubella (Meruvax)	Vaccine
Lupus	Belimumab (Benlysta)	Monoclonal antibody
Asthma	Omalizumab (Xolair)	Monoclonal antibody

Lead Optimization

The optimization of a lead compound can be made after a "hit" compound is found through biological evaluation. The optimization aims to improve the absorption, distribution, metabolism and excretion of the drug (ADME properties), reduction of the toxicity, and improvement of the efficacy.

The optimization can be made through chemical synthesis, computational chemistry or/and combinatorial chemistry. These should take into account the SAR studies and the preliminary mechanism of action. Lead optimization can direct the research to the synthesis of a new pharmacophore or a more active molecule. The techniques used for lead optimization overlap with drug discovery.

A lead compound can be modified through its functional groups to achieve better absorption, to avoid enzymatic degradation and to improve the excretion profile. The improvement of absorption can be done by the synthesis of a pro-drug. To avoid enzymatic degradation the target group can be modified to block the action of a key metabolic enzyme. The excretion profile can be improved through chemical modification of the lead compound in order to reduce the binding to albumin, for example. Organic synthesis can also improve the pharmacologic properties of a lead molecule, by increasing the bioactivity and reducing side effects.

The lead compound can be modified by combination with a series of molecules from chemical libraries or from molecular modeling. This can be achieved through the previously described combinatorial chemistry techniques. This procedure is especially useful in leads with different functional groups, which can be independently modified through mix and split techniques. Modifications performed by combinatorial chemistry can improve the ADME properties, and increase the specificity and efficacy of the lead molecule.

Computational modulation of a lead molecule can increase the specificity when the structural 3D image of the target is available, fitting the molecule for the target. The use of computational chemistry to produce almost perfect fits for a target also reduces the probability of side effects and toxicity. Computational chemistry is also useful to create and screening virtually lead compounds with better absorption properties and less metabolic degradation.

Natural compounds can be subject to the lead optimization, with chemical modifications, formulation optimization, and pharmacokinetics improvement. It is relevant to refer that some important SAR conclusions can be achieved by the observation of the biological activity of the compounds isolated in parallel with the lead compound.

The compounds selected from molecular modeling and screening of chemical and combinatorial libraries can be subject to optimization by the described techniques. This aims to improve the pharmacokinetic and pharmacologic properties of the compounds. The SAR between the different compounds can also be drawn in this phase.

Studies around a potential drug candidate can always return to the development of the lead molecule at any giving point of the pre and clinical studies. The interaction of diverse fields such as chemistry, biology, biochemistry, pharmacology, and medicine contribute to successful drug design.

Medicinal Chemistry of Herbs

Herbs contain numerous phytochemicals. Some of these may be pharmacologically active. Herbs are any phytogenic (derived from plants) substances used in food, cosmetics, cooking, and medicine. With the increase in popularity of 'alternative medicine', many herbal mixtures and concoctions have become available. These usually contain an herb as an ingredient. These mixtures are said to treat certain medical conditions.

Advertisers often falsely market 'herbal remedies' as "nondrugs" and "free from chemicals". This is obviously not the case. Herbs are plant-derived drugs. One must also be wary as there is a lot of pseudoscience in this area. While many of these concoctions do contain pharmacologically active compounds, the placebo effect is often observed.

Despite this, some herbs do contain phytochemicals that have observable benecial biological effects. As stated earlier, these herbs contain numerous different phytochemicals. Identifying the active principles is a challenge. In some cases, these phytochemicals undergo drug-drug interactions with prescribed drugs. It is generally thought that the constituents of herbs work synergistically. The individual constituents may be identied through spectroscopic and chromatographic techniques. Studying the medicinal chemistry of herbs and their constituents is a challenging task.

The individual constituents of herbs may serve as useful lead compounds. Many herbs also contain toxic compounds.

Camomile

Camomile (or chamomile) is an interesting case. The herbal product is derived from the daisy-like plants, matricaria chamomilla and chamaemelum nobile. The two plants have highly similar activities. The active principles of the plants are found in the oil. Bisabolol is the compound mostly responsible for the effect of camomile. Bisabolol has been observed to exhibit antiinammatory effects.

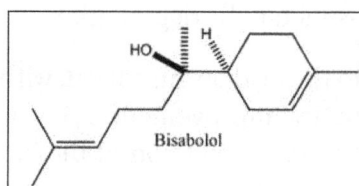
Bisabolol

Other phytochemicals found in camomile includes luteolin, apigenin, chamazulene, and angelic acid. Luteolin and apigenin have anti-inammatory activity comparable to that of indomethacin. Chamazulene is the compound responsible for the light blue colour of the essential oil. This compound is known to possess anti-allergenic and anti-inammatory effects.

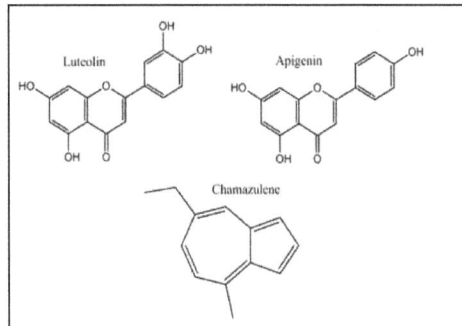

Saint John's Wort

Saint John's Wort (Hypericum perforatum), a notable drug in pharmacology, is indigenous to Europe but has been introduced to numerous temperate regions on Earth. The plant grows in the wild and is typically found in meadows. The herb is commonly employed to treat conditions such as depression and anxiety. The herb also has a mild sedative effect. Saint John's Wort is generally believed to be effective in the treatment of mild depression. However, it was shown that Saint John's Wort is ineffective in the treatment of major depressive disorder. Saint John's Wort contains many phytochemicals. A select few are shown below (Hypericin, Norathyriol & Kaempferol). The herb is also associated with phototoxic side effects. Some of the phytochemicals found in the herb are photosensitisers.

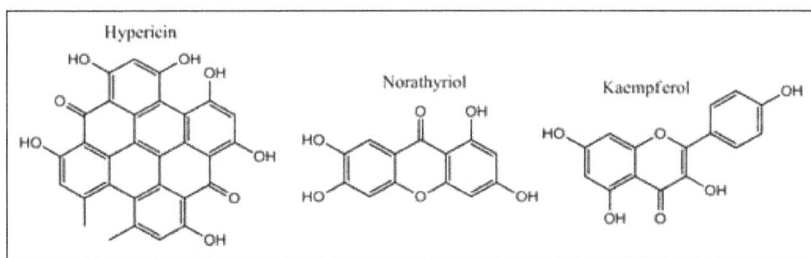

Garlic

Garlic (Allium sativum) is one of the most widely used herbal substances used in cooking and in medicine. The plant has been used in herbal medicine for a long time and is widely studied. Many of garlic's phytochemicals are organosulfur compounds. One of the most notable ones is the cysteine derivative, alliin. Alliin contains a sulfoxide functional group.

Just like onions (Allium cepa), garlic releases alliinase enzymes when their tissue is damaged. These enzymes catalyse the conversion of alliin to allicin. Allicin is the organosulfur compound mainly responsible for the distinct odour of garlic. Allicin is known to have some antiprotozoal, antifungal, antibacterial, and antiviral activity. Garlic is claimed to treat numerous medical conditions. However, some of the claims lack concrete scientic evidence.

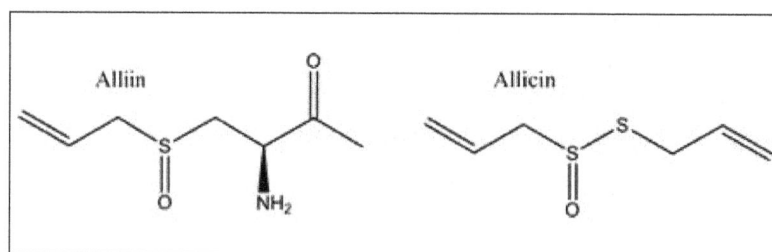

Aloe Vera

The aloe vera plant, colloquially known as 'the wand of heaven', is an example of a plant used in herbal medicine. The plant is popular in alternative medicine. While many proponents of alternative medicine claim that the aloe vera plant has medicinal properties, currently there is little scientic evidence to support these claims. The leaves of the plant contain compounds such as anthrones, anthraquinones, and acetylated mannans. Many of its phytochemicals are currently being investigated to show if they truly possess pharmacology activity.

Foxglove

Foxgloves are Eurasian plants of the genus Digitalis. Herbal preparations of foxglove were formerly used by herbalists to treat heart conditions. The use has ended because of the narrow therapeutic index of the preparations. The cardiac glycoside, digoxin is one of the active principles extracted from certain species of Digitalis.

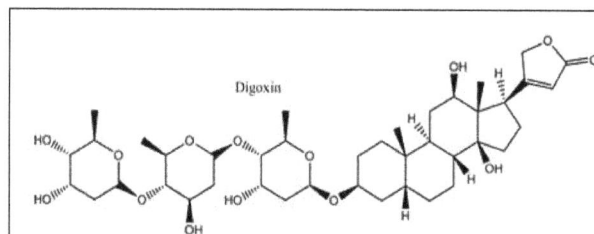

Liquorice

Liquorice is the herbal product derived from the root of the plant, glycyrrhiza glabra. The plant is a perennial shrub found in the Mediterranean region and some parts of Asia. Liquorice has been documented in ancient Chinese writings and was actively used in the Roman Empire. The herb contains compounds such as sugars and triterpenoids. Glycyrrhizin is a steroidal triterpene glycoside. The root of the plant contains up to 9% of this phytochemical.

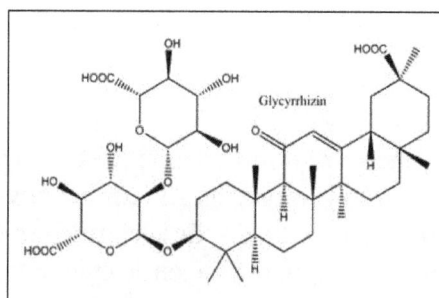

The compound is converted in the body to a pharmacologically active compound, glycyrrhetic acid by intestinal ora. To some extent, both glycyrrhizin and glycyrrhetic acid exhibit anti-inammatory activity. Glycyrrhizin is also thought to cause gastric mucus secretion. This is thought to be the origin of liquorice's antiulcer properties. This phytochemical has demonstrated antiviral activity during in vitro and in vivo studies. Glycyrrhizin has been used as an anti-hepatitis C drug in Japan.

Valerian

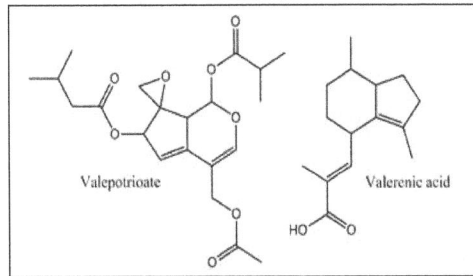

Valerian (Valeriana ofcinalis) is a perennial angiosperm that has a characteristic sweet odour. The plant is native to Europe and certain parts of Asia but has been introduced and cultivated in North America. The herb is known to have sedative effects. It is currently unclear which compounds are responsible for the sedative effects but it is thought that the active principles interact with the GABAergic neurotransmitter system. Some of the compounds present in valerian include valepotrioate and valerenic acid.

Ginseng

Ginseng can be derived from the dried root of panax quinquefolius (Western Ginseng) or panax ginseng (Asian Ginseng). These two highly similar species produce unique phytochemicals of the genus Panax. These compounds are known as ginsenosides. Some of the ginsenosides have been successfully isolated, puried, and studied. Interestingly, it was found that two of them have opposing pharmacological effects. Ginsenoside Rg-1 is a CNS stimulant whereas ginsenoside Rb-1 was discovered to be a CNS depressant.

Ginseng is regarded by some as a cognitive enhancer. However, studies conducted comparing ginseng with placebo showed statistically insignicant improvement. Some also regard the herb as an aphrodisiac, stimulant, or a cure for sexual dysfunction in men.

Vervain

Verbena (commonly known as vervain) is a genus of perennial or annual angiosperms used as herbs. Monoterpenes and sesquiterpenes are some of the main phytochemicals. There are claims that vervain is useful in the control of cancers. However, there is no scientic evidence to prove these claims.

Wolfsbane

Wolfsbane plants (genus Aconitum) are herbaceous plants mostly found in mountainous regions of the northern hemisphere. Most species of wolfsbane are toxic. For instance, the roots of aconitum ferox contain an acetylcholinesterase inhibitor, pseudaconitine (nepaline). Despite this, wolfsbane is used in herbal mixtures.

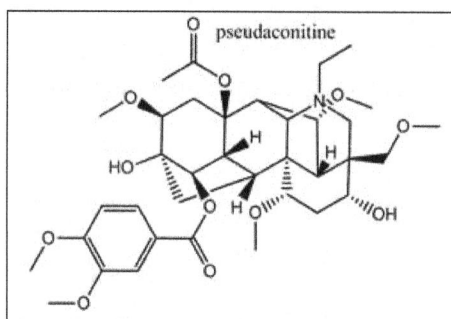

Feverfew

Feverfew (Tanacetum parthenium) is a perenial herb native to the Balkan Peninsula, the Caucasus, and Anatolia. Cultivation of the herb has spread to certain parts of South America, Europe and North America. The herb has been used since ancient times to alleviate fever, migraine, and arthritis. However, scientic studies suggest that this is due to the placebo effect.

Feverfew is thought to inhibit prostaglandin synthesis through a COX-independent mechanism. Parthenolide is generally regarded as the main active constituent of feverfew. Another phytochemical found in feverfew is the pentacyclic compound, canin.

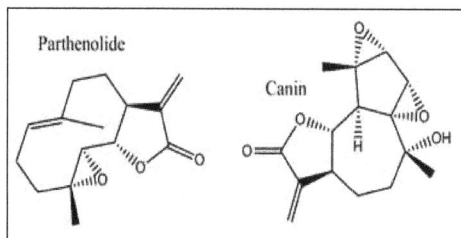

Rhubarb

Rhubarb roots (rheum rhabarbarum) are commonly used in Chinese herbal medicine as a laxative. The root is rich in cathartic and laxative anthraquinones such as rhein and emodin. These molecules were used as lead compounds for the development and design of the laxative, dantron.

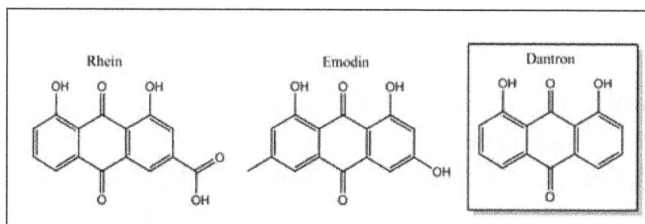

The natural products found in herbs are highly diverse. Some of them may have benecial effects while some of them are dangerous to humans. Often the combination of the phytochemicals found in herbs work synergistically. As shown above, there is still much that is not known about the chemical and pharmacological properties of herbal preparations. There is a need to know which compounds are responsible for the observed effects and if they demonstrate synergy. There is also a need to show whether or not certain herbs truly have benecial effects.

Medication

A medication (also referred to as medicine, pharmaceutical drug, or simply drug) is a drug used to diagnose, cure, treat, or prevent disease. Drug therapy (pharmacotherapy) is an important part of the medical field and relies on the science of pharmacology for continual advancement and on pharmacy for appropriate management.

Drugs are classified in various ways. One of the key divisions is by level of control, which distinguishes prescription drugs (those that a pharmacist dispenses only on the order of a physician, physician assistant, or qualified nurse) from over-the-counter drugs (those that consumers can order for themselves). Another key distinction is between traditional small-molecule drugs, usually derived from chemical synthesis, and biopharmaceuticals, which include recombinant proteins, vaccines, blood products used therapeutically (such as IVIG), gene therapy, monoclonal antibodies and cell therapy (for instance, stem-cell therapies). Other ways to classify medicines are by mode of action, route of administration, biological system affected, or therapeutic effects. An elaborate and widely used classification system is the Anatomical Therapeutic Chemical Classification System (ATC system). The World Health Organization keeps a list of essential medicines.

Drug discovery and drug development are complex and expensive endeavors undertaken by pharmaceutical companies, academic scientists, and governments. As a result of this complex path from discovery to commercialization, partnering has become a standard practice for advancing drug candidates through development pipelines. Governments generally regulate what drugs can be marketed, how drugs are marketed, and in some jurisdictions, drug pricing. Controversies have arisen over drug pricing and disposal of used drugs.

Usage

Drug use among elderly Americans has been studied; in a group of 2377 people with average age of 71 surveyed between 2005 and 2006, 84% took at least one prescription drug, 44% took at least one over-the-counter (OTC) drug, and 52% took at least one dietary supplement; in a group of 2245 elderly Americans (average age of 71) surveyed over the period 2010 – 2011, those percentages were 88%, 38%, and 64%.

Classification

One of the key classifications is between traditional small molecule drugs; usually derived from chemical synthesis, and biologic medical products; which include recombinant proteins, vaccines, blood products used therapeutically (such as IVIG), gene therapy, and cell therapy (for instance, stem cell therapies).

Pharmaceuticals or drugs or medicines are classified in various other groups besides their origin on the basis of pharmacological properties like mode of action and their pharmacological action or activity, such as by chemical properties, mode or route of administration, biological system affected, or therapeutic effects. An elaborate and widely used classification system is the Anatomical Therapeutic Chemical Classification System (ATC system). The World Health Organization keeps a list of essential medicines.

A sampling of classes of medicine includes:

- Antipyretics: reducing fever (pyrexia/pyresis).

- Analgesics: reducing pain (painkillers).

- Antimalarial drugs: treating malaria.

- Antibiotics: inhibiting germ growth.

- Antiseptics: prevention of germ growth near burns, cuts and wounds.

- Mood stabilizers: lithium and valpromide.

- Hormone replacements: Premarin.

- Oral contraceptives: Enovid, "biphasic" pill, and "triphasic" pill.

- Stimulants: methylphenidate, amphetamine.

- Tranquilizers: meprobamate, chlorpromazine, reserpine, chlordiazepoxide, diazepam, and alprazolam.

- Statins: lovastatin, pravastatin, and simvastatin.

Pharmaceuticals may also be described as "specialty", independent of other classifications, which is an ill-defined class of drugs that might be difficult to administer, require special handling during administration, require patient monitoring during and immediately after administration, have particular regulatory requirements restricting their use, and are generally expensive relative to other drugs.

Types of Medicines

For the Digestive System

- Upper digestive tract: antacids, reflux suppressants, antiflatulents, antidopaminergics, proton pump inhibitors (PPIs), H_2-receptor antagonists, cytoprotectants, prostaglandin analogues.

- Lower digestive tract: laxatives, antispasmodics, antidiarrhoeals, bile acid sequestrants, opioid.

For the Cardiovascular System

- General: β-receptor blockers ("beta blockers"), calcium channel blockers, diuretics, cardiac glycosides, antiarrhythmics, nitrate, antianginals, vasoconstrictors, vasodilators.

- Affecting blood pressure/(antihypertensive drugs): ACE inhibitors, angiotensin receptor blockers, beta-blockers, α blockers, calcium channel blockers, thiazide diuretics, loop diuretics, aldosterone inhibitors.

- Coagulation: anticoagulants, heparin, antiplatelet drugs, fibrinolytics, anti-hemophilic factors, haemostatic drugs.

- HMG-CoA reductase inhibitors (statins) for lowering LDL cholesterol inhibitors: hypolipidaemic agents.

For the Central Nervous System

Drugs affecting the central nervous system include: Psychedelics, hypnotics, anaesthetics, antipsychotics, eugeroics, antidepressants (including tricyclic antidepressants, monoamine oxidase inhibitors, lithium salts, and selective serotonin reuptake inhibitors (SSRIs)), antiemetics, Anticonvulsants/antiepileptics, anxiolytics, barbiturates, movement disorder (e.g., Parkinson's disease) drugs, stimulants (including amphetamines), benzodiazepines, cyclopyrrolones, dopamine antagonists, antihistamines, cholinergics, anticholinergics, emetics, cannabinoids, and 5-HT (serotonin) antagonists.

For Pain

The main classes of painkillers are NSAIDs, opioids and Local anesthetics.

For Consciousness (Anesthetic Drugs)

Some anesthetics include Benzodiazepines and Barbiturates.

For musculo-skeletal Disorders

The main categories of drugs for musculoskeletal disorders are: NSAIDs (including COX-2 selective inhibitors), muscle relaxants, neuromuscular drugs, and anticholinesterases.

For the Eye

- General: adrenergic neurone blocker, astringent.

- Diagnostic: topical anesthetics, sympathomimetics, parasympatholytics, mydriatics, cycloplegics.

- Antibacterial: antibiotics, topical antibiotics, sulfa drugs, aminoglycosides, fluoroquinolones.

- Antiviral drug.

- Anti-fungal: imidazoles, polyenes.

- Anti-inflammatory: NSAIDs, corticosteroids.

- Anti-allergy: mast cell inhibitors.

- Anti-glaucoma: adrenergic agonists, beta-blockers, carbonic anhydrase inhibitors/hyper-osmotics, cholinergics, miotics, parasympathomimetics, prostaglandin agonists/prostaglandin inhibitors. nitroglycerin.

For the Ear, Nose and Oropharynx

Antibiotics, sympathomimetics, antihistamines, anticholinergics, NSAIDs, corticosteroids, antiseptics, local anesthetics, antifungals, cerumenolytic.

For the Respiratory System

Bronchodilators, antitussives, mucolytics, decongestants inhaled and systemic corticosteroids, Beta2-adrenergic agonists, anticholinergics, Mast cell stabilizers, Leukotriene antagonists.

For Endocrine Problems

Androgens, antiandrogens, estrogens, gonadotropin, corticosteroids, human growth hormone, insulin, antidiabetics (sulfonylureas, biguanides/metformin, thiazolidinediones, insulin), thyroid hormones, antithyroid drugs, calcitonin, diphosponate, vasopressin analogues.

For the Reproductive System or Urinary System

Antifungal, alkalinizing agents, quinolones, antibiotics, cholinergics, anticholinergics, antispasmodics, 5-alpha reductase inhibitor, selective alpha-1 blockers, sildenafils, fertility medications.

For Contraception

- Hormonal contraception
- Ormeloxifene
- Spermicide

For Obstetrics and Gynecology

NSAIDs, anticholinergics, haemostatic drugs, antifibrinolytics, Hormone Replacement Therapy (HRT), bone regulators, beta-receptor agonists, follicle stimulating hormone, luteinising hormone, LHRH gamolenic acid, gonadotropin release inhibitor, progestogen, dopamine agonists, oestrogen, prostaglandins, gonadorelin, clomiphene, tamoxifen, Diethylstilbestrol.

For the skin

Emollients, anti-pruritics, antifungals, disinfectants, scabicides, pediculicides, tar products, vitamin A derivatives, vitamin D analogues, keratolytics, abrasives, systemic antibiotics, topical antibiotics, hormones, desloughing agents, exudate absorbents, fibrinolytics, proteolytics, sunscreens, antiperspirants, corticosteroids, immune modulators.

For Infections and Infestations

Antibiotics, antifungals, antileprotics, antituberculous drugs, antimalarials, anthelmintics, amoebicides, antivirals, antiprotozoals, probiotics, prebiotics, antitoxins and antivenoms.

For the Immune System

Vaccines, immunoglobulins, immunosuppressants, interferons, monoclonal antibodies.

For Allergic Disorders

Anti-allergics, antihistamines, NSAIDs, Corticosteroids.

For Nutrition

Tonics, electrolytes and mineral preparations (including iron preparations and magnesium preparations), parenteral nutritions, vitamins, anti-obesity drugs, anabolic drugs, haematopoietic drugs, food product drugs.

For Neoplastic Disorders

Cytotoxic drugs, therapeutic antibodies, sex hormones, aromatase inhibitors, somatostatin inhibitors, recombinant interleukins, G-CSF, erythropoietin.

For Diagnostics

Contrast media.

For Euthanasia

A euthanaticum is used for euthanasia and physician-assisted suicide. Euthanasia is not permitted by law in many countries, and consequently medicines will not be licensed for this use in those countries.

Administration

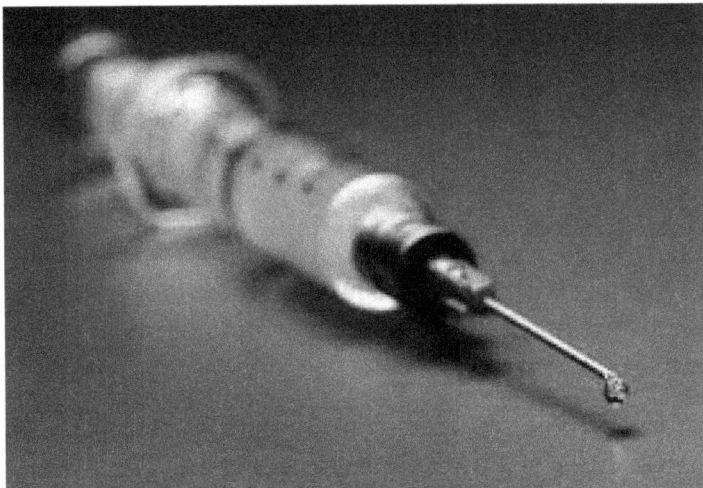

Administration is the process by which a patient takes a medicine. There are three major categories of drug administration; enteral (by mouth), parenteral (into the blood stream), and other (which includes giving a drug through intranasal, topical, inhalation, and rectal means).

It can be performed in various dosage forms such as pills, tablets, or capsules. The drug may contain a single or multiple active ingredients.

There are many variations in the routes of administration, including intravenous (into the blood through a vein) and oral administration (through the mouth).

They can be administered all at once as a bolus, at frequent intervals or continuously. Frequencies are often abbreviated from Latin, such as *every 8 hours* reading Q8H from *Quaque VIII Hora*.

Development

Drug development is the process of bringing a new drug to the market once a lead compound has been identified through the process of drug discovery. It includes pre-clinical research (microorganisms/animals) and clinical trials (on humans) and may include the step of obtaining regulatory approval to market the drug.

Common Types of Drugs

There are a wide variety of addictive substances that exist, but the most common types are classified under six main categories: alcohol, benzodiazepines, illicit drugs, opiates, sleeping pills and stimulants.

Alcohol

Alcohol is a legal controlled substance that slows down the body's vital functions when consumed in excess. Its many forms include beer, wine and liquor. Some of the physical effects of heavy alcohol consumption are slurred speech, loss of coordination and slowed reaction time. Psychological effects include inhibiting judgment and lowering a person's ability to think rationally. Typically, drinking alcohol in moderation does not signify a problem. However, consuming more than four alcoholic beverages per day for men – or more than three per day for women – can indicate an alcohol use disorder (AUD).

Typically, drinking alcohol in moderation does not signify a problem. However, consuming more than four alcoholic beverages per day for men – or more than three per day for women – can indicate an alcohol use disorder (AUD).

Topics on Alcohol Addiction

- Symptoms and Warning Signs: Alcoholism can stem from consumption and experimentation during a person's teen years. Knowing the symptoms and warning signs to look for can help determine if an addiction is present.

- Withdrawal and Detox: When an individual develops a tolerance to alcohol over time, they can experience withdrawal symptoms when stopping use. The symptoms of withdrawal are impacted by the amount, frequency and duration of alcohol abuse.

- Treatment and Rehab: There are many treatment options available to help a person overcome the toxic cycle of alcohol abuse. It's important to recover from alcoholism under the supervision of medical professionals.

- High-Functioning Alcoholics: A high-functioning alcoholic is a person who is able to manage their everyday responsibilities despite an underlying problem with alcohol abuse. It is particularly difficult to identify the signs of a high-functioning alcoholic, and he or she might deny their struggle if confronted.

- Drunk Driving: Choosing to drive while intoxicated is often a telltale sign of alcohol abuse. Sadly, getting behind the wheel after drinking can prove to be a deadly mistake. Over 30 percent of all car crashes in 2014 were caused by drunk driving.

- Is There a Cure for Alcoholism?: While there is no cure for alcoholism, people can overcome an alcohol addiction by attending a treatment program. Treatment for alcohol abuse can help a person maintain their sobriety and manage alcohol cravings.

- Alcohol and the Liver: Chronic drinking can increase a person's risk of developing liver disease. Those who struggle with excessive alcohol consumption will need treatment in order to avoid major health complications later in life.

- Genetics of Alcoholism: Individuals with a family history of alcoholism have a higher risk of incurring alcohol abuse patterns at some point in their life. Research shows that genetics make up 40 to 60 percent of a person's likelihood of developing an alcohol addiction.

Benzodiazepines

Benzodiazepines, or benzos, include pharmaceutical drugs used to treat a wide array of mental disorders, including severe anxiety and panic attacks. People can build a tolerance to benzos if they are consumed for an extended period of time, which can lead to dependency.

Some people choose to take benzos with alcohol, which strengthens its effects and can lead to overdose. Withdrawal from benzos can include dangerous symptoms such as Grand Mal seizures, so it's always recommended to detox from these drugs under medical supervision.

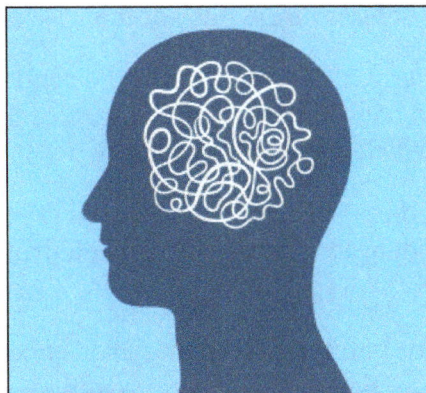

Comprehensive treatment for a benzodiazepine addiction typically includes cognitive behavioral therapy, support groups and medications to help reduce cravings.

Types of Benzodiazepines

- Ativan: Ativan, the brand name for the drug lorazepam, is an intermediate-acting benzodiazepine used to treat anxiety disorders, depression and panic attacks. Ativan is extremely potent when compared to other benzos. Because of this, people who consume Ativan have a high risk of developing an abuse disorder.

- Halcion: Halcion is prescribed to treat anxiety and insomnia. As a short-acting medication, Halcion is processed through the body faster than other benzos. As a result, people may be inclined to increase their dose in order to keep experiencing a high, which can lead to an addiction.

- Klonopin: Klonopin has a high potential for abuse and addiction – even when prescribed to treat a medical condition. Klonopin is a long-acting benzo, meaning that it takes longer to feel its full effects. Once Klonopin leaves the body, a person can experience severe and potentially life-threatening symptoms of withdrawal.

- Librium: Librium is typically used to treat a wide array of anxiety disorders. It is often abused due to the calming effects this drug produces. Because Librium has a low potency when compared to other benzos, many people consume it in combination with other substances to achieve a greater high.

- Xanax: With over 44 million scripts written every year, Xanax is the most prescribed medication in the country. It is highly addictive when taken in high doses or over an extended period of time. A person struggling with Xanax addiction will typically exhibit symptoms of fatigue and loss of motivation.

- Valium: Valium is the brand name for diazepam, which is used to treat muscle spasms and seizures. When prescribed, it's meant to be taken on a daily basis. However, people who start taking more Valium than recommended are at risk of addiction.

Illicit Drugs

Illicit drugs include powerfully addictive and illegal substances such as heroin and meth. The nature of these substances is vastly different from one another.

For example, marijuana's short-term effects slow down the central nervous system and interfere with a person's reaction time and concentration. In contrast, cocaine puts brain functioning into hyper speed, resulting in increased alertness and anxiety.

Even just a single use of some of these substances can spawn devastating patterns of abuse. Once a physical or psychological dependence is formed, using illicit drugs takes priority over everything else in a person's life.

People looking to quit a dangerous habit of consuming illicit substances should seek professional guidance to aid in their recovery. A licensed inpatient treatment center can provide everything a person needs to achieve and maintain sobriety, from medical detox services to therapy and 12-step programs.

Types of Illicit Drugs

- Cocaine: A stimulant with effects similar to excessive amounts of caffeine, cocaine is most often snorted in powder form. This illicit drug is highly addictive and continued abuse can cause severe weight loss and damage to the nasal passages.

- Crack Cocaine: The more potent, freebase form of cocaine, crack cocaine is usually smoked through a short pipe that often causes blisters and burns on the mouth and hands. An addiction to crack cocaine can develop in as little as one use.

- Ecstasy: Ecstasy is often consumed by young adults attending parties or raves. It is a stimulant with potentially hallucinogenic effects. Many forms of ecstasy on the black market are cut with much more dangerous substances, such as heroin and LSD.

- Hallucinogens: Hallucinogens are mind-altering, psychoactive substances with a high potential for abuse. These substances are often taken by people looking to distort their perception of reality. Hallucinogens are also sometimes used to self-medicate a mental disorder, such as depression. However, taking hallucinogens for self-medication purposes can make an underlying condition even worse.

- Heroin: One of the most addictive substances on earth, heroin is a synthetic derivative of morphine. Heroin comes as either a powder or a sticky gel, known as black tar heroin. Long-term abuse of heroin can cause abscesses and scabs on the skin, in addition to psychological and internal damage.

- Inhalants: Inhalants are categorized by their method of administration and include many household objects that can be abused for a brief high. Commonly abused inhalants are nail polish remover, paint thinner, gasoline and lighter fluid. Long-term use of inhalants can cause severe damage including muscle deterioration and psychological disturbances.

- Ketamine: Ketamine is primarily used as an anesthetic for animals undergoing surgery, but is often abused recreationally among teens and college students. Not only is it incredibly addictive, but it has also been used as a date rape drug. Because it is odorless and tasteless, it cannot be detected when mixed in a beverage.

- Marijuana: As one of the most commonly abused illicit substances, marijuana comes from the cannabis plant and is usually dried out, rolled up and smoked. More commonly known as "weed" or "pot", marijuana is gaining legal recognition in some states. However, continued abuse of marijuana can cause diminished brain function and lung damage.

- Meth: A deadly and addictive substance, methamphetamine (or meth) is a substance that can be made from easily obtained items, such as lithium batteries and drain cleaner. As a result, manufacturing meth is extremely dangerous. Continued abuse of meth can cause tooth decay and the appearance of accelerated aging.

- Synthetic Marijuana: Also known as Spice or K2, synthetic marijuana is a manufactured substance that contains an ingredient similar to tetrahydrocannabinol (THC) – the active ingredient in marijuana. Because synthetic marijuana can be purchased legally, many people believe it is a safer alternative to marijuana. However, synthetic marijuana is dangerously addictive and can produce psychoactive effects that are just as strong as its natural counterpart.

Opiates

Opiates encompass prescription drugs that are used to treat acute and chronic pain. While they can be effective when taken as directed, opiates pose a major risk of addiction among their users.

An opiate addiction often manifests itself within a person's drug-seeking behavior. This can involve visiting multiple doctors in order to obtain more prescriptions – otherwise known as "doctor shopping." If drugs cannot be obtained through various doctor visits, some people turn to heroin use as a cheaper, easier-to-get alternative.

Withdrawal from opiates can be agonizing and should never be attempted alone. Medically-assisted detox is the safest way to endure the withdrawal process. After detox, it is highly recommended to enter an inpatient addiction treatment program to ensure the lowest chances of relapse.

Types of Opiates

- Codeine: Codeine is most often found in over-the-counter and prescription-grade cough medicines. Because of its easy accessibility, many people don't perceive codeine to be as dangerous as other opiates. In some cases, codeine can act as a gateway drug to harder substances down the road, such as morphine or oxycodone.

- Demerol: Demerol is a highly potent opiate with growing rates of addiction. While a prescription of Demerol is legal, it is rarely prescribed outside of intensive hospital care. It has similar effects of other opiates like morphine, putting users in a "dreamlike" state when abused.

- Dilaudid: As one of the more powerful opiates, Dilaudid is mainly prescribed to patients diagnosed with cancer or serious injuries. It is abused for its intense calming and euphoric effects; however, Dilaudid comes with a high risk of overdose, which can be fatal.

- Fentanyl: Fentanyl is known to be up to 100 times stronger than morphine and is used primarily to treat pain after surgery. Recreational use of fentanyl is especially dangerous when combined with other opiates or heroin. Fentanyl causes the respiratory system to slow down, leading to overdose and potentially even death.

- Hydrocodone: Hydrocodone is commonly prescribed for pain relief following oral surgery. However, taking this opiate without a prescription is illegal and constitutes abuse. Abusing hydrocodone over an extended period of time, or in large amounts, can evolve into an addiction.

- Methadone: Methadone is widely known for its common use of treating a heroin use disorder. Despite its intended legal use, methadone is still an extremely potent opiate with highly addictive qualities. Methadone should only be taken under the careful supervision of a physician.

- Morphine: Morphine is primarily prescribed to hospital patients recovering from surgery or diagnosed with cancer. However, a black market for morphine exists due to its intensely pleasurable effects. A person suffering from an addiction to morphine may compulsively seek out and abuse the substance – despite legal ramifications.

- Oxycodone: Oxycodone is a powerful painkiller and one of the most abused prescription medications in the United States. Many people unknowingly kickstart an addiction by taking their regularly prescribed dose. Once a tolerance is established, using or obtaining oxycodone may be prioritized over personal obligations and social activities.

- Propoxyphene: Propoxyphene, otherwise known as Darvon or Darvocet, was once prescribed for moderate pain relief. The FDA banned propoxyphene in 2010 after recognizing its lethal side effects. Users who abuse propoxyphene experience a rush of euphoria, followed by heavy sedation.

- Tramadol: Tramadol is used to treat moderate pain from medical conditions such as fibromyalgia. It is perceived to be less addictive than other opiates, and is therefore commonly prescribed by doctors. As with any other opiate prescription, the risk of addiction is still at large.

Sleeping Pills

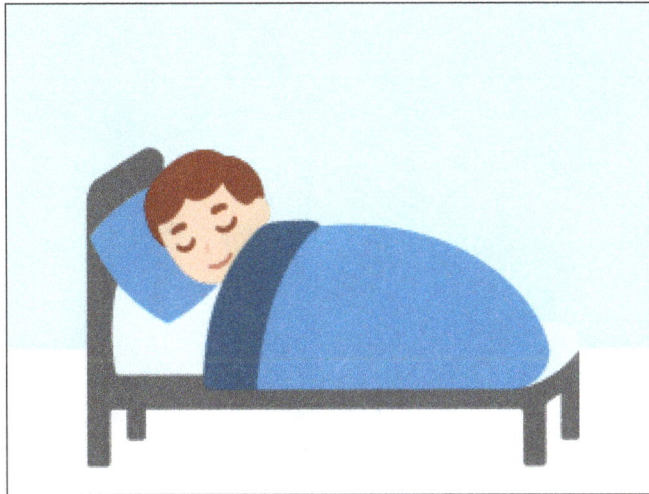

Sleeping pills fall under a category of prescription medications known as sedative-hypnotics. Many individuals assume they cannot develop a sleeping pill addiction; however, becoming addicted is easier than most may think.

A dependency on sleeping pills often begins forming when a person increases their prescribed dose without consulting their physician first. They may believe that taking more pills will improve their quality of sleep. Over time, a person will feel the need to take larger amounts each time in order to fall asleep, which often leads to an overwhelming addiction.

When a person who is dependent on sleeping pills tries to quit cold turkey, their body may experience withdrawal. Symptoms of withdrawal can be uncomfortable, so it is best to go through the process at a medical detox center. Further treatment at an inpatient rehab center or outpatient program can address the psychological impact of an addiction to sleeping pills.

Types of Sleeping Pills

- Ambien: Ambien is generally prescribed for short-term insomnia. Most cases of Ambien dependence start when a person takes more than their recommended dosage to fall asleep faster. An addiction to Ambien can form in as little as a few weeks.

- Amytal: Amytal is the brand name for the barbiturate amobarbital. Because of its level of potency, Amytal is used as a pre-anesthetic for surgeries and to treat chronic sleep disorders. It produces effects that feel similar to alcohol intoxication, which causes users to abuse the medication and subsequently become addicted.

- Lunesta: Many people mistakenly believe that Lunesta is a non-habit forming medication. However, Lunesta is a highly potent sleeping pill that can cause a spiraling addiction. Some people who develop a Lunesta dependency will mix the medication with other substances in order to increase its sedative effects.

- Sonata: Sonata is a fast-acting sleeping pill that remains in the body for about an hour. This makes Sonata a prime target for accidental abuse, as people might take too much in order to help them sleep. While Sonata isn't as potent as other sleeping pills, its long-term use can lead to an addiction.

Stimulants

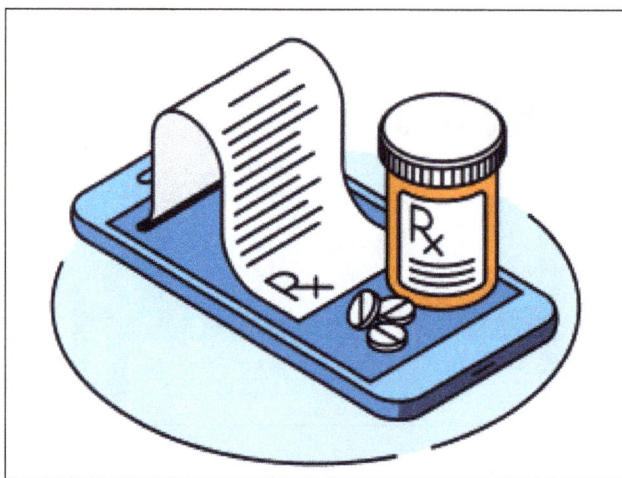

Prescription stimulants include amphetamines and methylphenidates. Typically, stimulants are used to treat mental disorders like attention deficit hyperactivity disorder (ADHD). They are generally used to enhance performance, rather than to achieve a high.

Stimulants work by activating the central nervous system, inciting feelings of excitement and increasing physical and cognitive function. When a person uses these substances, they feel a rush of intense pleasure caused by a surge of dopamine. A tolerance can build up over time from frequent stimulant use, which can signify the early stages of an abuse disorder.

In order to overcome an addiction to stimulants, detox at a treatment center may be required before transitioning into therapy and group support.

Types of Stimulants

- Adderall: Adderall is the most commonly prescribed stimulant for treating symptoms of ADHD. People who habitually use Adderall to increase their productivity and improve their mental focus have the highest risk of becoming addicted.

- Antidepressants: Unlike other addictive prescription medications, antidepressants don't produce a "high" or cause intense cravings. In fact, people who have clinical depression typically won't feel its full effects for over a month. The true danger lies in other substances a person chooses to abuse while taking antidepressants, such as alcohol or benzodiazepines.

- Concerta: Concerta is a prescription stimulant similar to cocaine. People who develop a dependence on Concerta will feel strong compulsions to seek out the drug in any way they can. Individuals who cannot obtain more of the drug may experience withdrawal symptoms, which are sometimes referred to as the "Concerta crash."

- Dexedrine: Dexedrine is an amphetamine with a high potential for abuse and addiction. After repeated use of Dexedrine, the brain cannot function normally without the drug. Side effects of Dexedrine include insomnia, blurred vision and dizziness.

- Diet Pills: Diet pills include a number of over-the-counter and prescription supplements designed to help users lose weight. Aside from their appetite-suppressant effects, diet pills can cause elevated energy levels and feelings of euphoria, which increase the likelihood of abuse and dependency.

- Ritalin: As a central nervous system stimulant, Ritalin increases alertness and concentration. It is effective in treating ADHD among children; however, Ritalin also comes with a high potential for abuse. Those with other types of mental disorders, such as bipolar, run the risk of experiencing negative side effects from using the drug.

- Anabolic Steroids: Anabolic steroids are synthetic substances that mimic the male hormone testosterone. They are commonly abused by people wanting to increase athletic performance. While they don't produce the same euphoric "high" as other addictive substances, frequent use of anabolic steroids can lead to an addiction.

References

- Medicinal-Chemistry, method: labome.com, Retrieved 28 August, 2019

- Spatz I, mcgee N (25 November 2013). "Specialty Pharmaceuticals". Health Policy Briefs. Health Affairs. What's The Background?. Retrieved 28 August 2015

- Medicinal-chemistry-of-herbs: pharmafactz.com, Retrieved 30 January, 2019

- Kesselheim, Aaron S.; Avorn, Jerry; Sarpatwari, Ameet (23 August 2016). "The High Cost of Prescription Drugs in the United States". JAMA. 316 (8): 858–71. doi:10.1001/jama.2016.11237. PMID 27552619

- Drugs: addictioncenter.com, Retrieved 29 January, 2019

Sub-disciplines of Medicinal Chemistry 2

- **Pharmacokinetics**
- **Pharmacodynamics**
- **Pharmacology**
- **Pharmacognosy**
- **Pharmacometrics**

Medicinal chemistry is sub-divided into various disciplines. Some of them are pharmacokinetics, pharmacodynamics, pharmacology, pharmacognosy and pharmacometrics. The topics elaborated in this chapter will help in gaining a better perspective about these sub-disciplines of medicinal chemistry as well as their importance.

Medicinal chemistry has its roots in several branches of chemistry and biology. However, essentially it concerns with the understanding of mechanisms of action of drugs. It attempts to establish relationship between structure and function (activity) and to link biodynamic behaviour with chemical reactivity and physical properties. Rightly, therefore, medicinal chemistry is also called therapeutic chemistry, pharmaceutical chemistry, pharmacochemistry etc.. Emphasis is laid on drugs, nevertheless, the interests of the medicinal chemist does not stop at drugs and include bioactive compounds in general. It encompasses discovery, development, identification and interpretation of mode of action at the molecular level. This is also concerned with study, identification, and synthesis of the metabolic products of drugs and related compounds. Besides this, medicinal chemistry also involves the isolation, characterization and synthesis of compounds that can be used in medicine for the prevention, treatment and cure of disease.

With the advent of greater understanding of physiological mechanisms it has become possible to take a more mechanistic approach to research and start from a rationally argued hypothesis to design drugs. The target disease selected for study are generally those prevalent in western society and progress depends largely upon the current state of understanding of physiology in relation to diseases.

A logical approach to the study of drugs and their activities is the recognition of the basic principles behind the biochemical events leading to drug actions. Biochemical pathways of action for drugs are gradually being elaborated, and a rapidly increasing amount of biochemical information about drug action is now found in the literature. An amazing amount of insight into the behaviour of drugs at the macromolecular level has been developed, and there is much direct and indirect evidence supporting these biochemical postulations of drug action. A review of the historical development of our knowledge of enzymes and related aspects of interest to medicinal chemists, including enzyme activities and structure, and the effect of drugs on these activities and structure, and the effect of drugs on these activities, might provide a logical introduction to this volume. The effect of drugs on enzyme systems has occupied the greatest share of attention the medicinal chemist has devoted to interaction of drugs with cellular macromolecules.

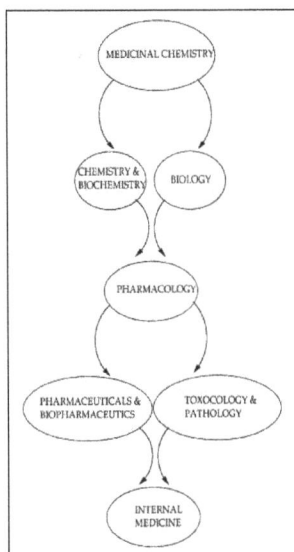

Shows the ramifications of medicinal chemistry in different branches of other sciences.

Pharmacokinetics

Pharmacokinetics sometimes abbreviated as PK, is a branch of pharmacology dedicated to determine the fate of substances administered to a living organism. The substances of interest include any chemical xenobiotic such as: pharmaceutical drugs, pesticides, food additives, cosmetics, etc. It attempts to analyze chemical metabolism and to discover the fate of a chemical from the moment that it is administered up to the point at which it is completely eliminated from the body. Pharmacokinetics is the study of how an organism affects a drug, whereas pharmacodynamics (PD) is the study of how the drug affects the organism. Both together influence dosing, benefit, and adverse effects, as seen in PK/PD models.

Pharmacokinetics describes how the body affects a specific xenobiotic/chemical after administration through the mechanisms of absorption and distribution, as well as the metabolic changes of the substance in the body (e.g. by metabolic enzymes such as cytochrome P450 or glucuronosyltransferase enzymes), and the effects and routes of excretion of the metabolites of the drug. Pharmacokinetic properties of chemicals are affected by the route of administration and the dose of administered drug. These may affect the absorption rate.

Models have been developed to simplify conceptualization of the many processes that take place in the interaction between an organism and a chemical substance. One of these, the multi-compartmental model, is the most commonly used approximations to reality; however, the complexity involved in adding parameters with that modelling approach means that *monocompartmental models* and above all *two compartmental models* are the most-frequently used. The various compartments that the model is divided into are commonly referred to as the ADME scheme (also referred to as LADME if liberation is included as a separate step from absorption):

- Liberation – The process of release of a drug from the pharmaceutical formulation.

- Absorption – The process of a substance entering the blood circulation.

- Distribution – The dispersion or dissemination of substances throughout the fluids and tissues of the body.

- Metabolism (or biotransformation, or inactivation) – The recognition by the organism that a foreign substance is present and the irreversible transformation of parent compounds into daughter metabolites.

- Excretion – The removal of the substances from the body. In rare cases, some drugs irreversibly accumulate in body tissue.

The two phases of metabolism and excretion can also be grouped together under the title elimination. The study of these distinct phases involves the use and manipulation of basic concepts in order to understand the process dynamics. For this reason in order to fully comprehend the *kinetics* of a drug it is necessary to have detailed knowledge of a number of factors such as: the properties of the substances that act as excipients, the characteristics of the appropriate biological membranes and the way that substances can cross them, or the characteristics of the enzyme reactions that inactivate the drug.

All these concepts can be represented through mathematical formulas that have a corresponding graphical representation. The use of these models allows an understanding of the characteristics of a molecule, as well as how a particular drug will behave given information regarding some of its basic characteristics such as its acid dissociation constant (pKa), bioavailability and solubility, absorption capacity and distribution in the organism.

The model outputs for a drug can be used in industry (for example, in calculating bioequivalence when designing generic drugs) or in the clinical application of pharmacokinetic concepts. Clinical pharmacokinetics provides many performance guidelines for effective and efficient use of drugs for human-health professionals and in veterinary medicine.

Pharmacokinetic Models

Pharmacokinetic modelling is performed by noncompartmental or compartmental methods. Noncompartmental methods estimate the exposure to a drug by estimating the area under the curve of a concentration-time graph. Compartmental methods estimate the concentration-time graph using kinetic models. Noncompartmental methods are often more versatile in that they do not assume any specific compartmental model and produce accurate results also acceptable for bioequivalence studies. The final outcome of the transformations that a drug undergoes in an organism and the rules that determine this fate depend on a number of interrelated factors. A number of functional models have been developed in order to simplify the study of pharmacokinetics. These models are based on a consideration of an organism as a number of related compartments. The simplest idea is to think of an organism as only one homogenous compartment. This *monocompartmental model* presupposes that blood plasma concentrations of the drug are a true reflection of the drug's concentration in other fluids or tissues and that the elimination of the drug is directly proportional to the drug's concentration in the organism (first order kinetics).

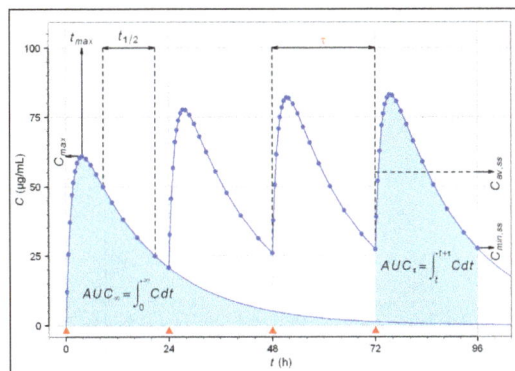

The time course of drug plasma concentrations over 96 hours following oral administrations every 24 hours. Note that in steady state and in linear pharmacokinetics AUCτ=AUC∞. Steady state is reached after about 5 × 12 = 60 hours. The graph depicts a typical time course of drug plasma concentration and illustrates main pharmacokinetic metrics.

However, these models do not always truly reflect the real situation within an organism. For example, not all body tissues have the same blood supply, so the distribution of the drug will be slower in these tissues than in others with a better blood supply. In addition, there are some tissues (such as the brain tissue) that present a real barrier to the distribution of drugs, that can be breached with greater or lesser ease depending on the drug's characteristics. If these relative conditions for the different tissue types are considered along with the rate of elimination, the organism can be considered to be acting like two compartments: one that we can call the *central compartment* that has a more rapid distribution, comprising organs and systems with a well-developed blood supply; and a *peripheral compartment* made up of organs with a lower blood flow. Other tissues, such as the brain, can occupy a variable position depending on a drug's ability to cross the barrier that separates the organ from the blood supply.

This *two compartment model* will vary depending on which compartment elimination occurs in. The most common situation is that elimination occurs in the central compartment as the liver and kidneys are organs with a good blood supply. However, in some situations it may be that elimination occurs in the peripheral compartment or even in both. This can mean that there are three possible variations in the two compartment model, which still do not cover all possibilities.

This model may not be applicable in situations where some of the enzymes responsible for metabolizing the drug become saturated, or where an active elimination mechanism is present that is independent of the drug's plasma concentration. In the real world each tissue will have its own distribution characteristics and none of them will be strictly linear. If we label the drug's volume of distribution within the organism Vd_F and its volume of distribution in a tissue Vd_T the former will be described by an equation that takes into account all the tissues that act in different ways, that is:

$$Vd_F = Vd_{T1} + Vd_{T2} + Vd_{T3} + \cdots + Vd_{Tn}$$

This represents the *multi-compartment model* with a number of curves that express complicated equations in order to obtain an overall curve. A number of computer programs have been developed to plot these equations. However complicated and precise this model may be, it still does not truly represent reality despite the effort involved in obtaining various distribution values for a drug. This is because the concept of distribution volume is a relative concept that is not a true reflection of reality. The choice of model therefore comes down to deciding which one offers the lowest margin of error for the drug involved.

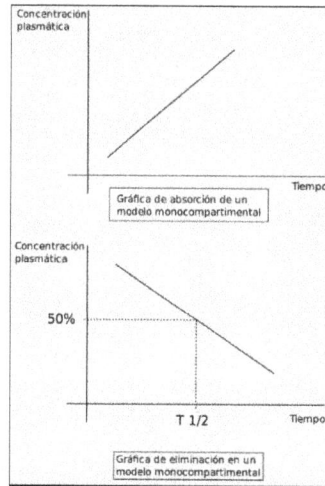

Graph representing the monocompartmental action model.

Noncompartmental Analysis

Noncompartmental PK analysis is highly dependent on estimation of total drug exposure. Total drug exposure is most often estimated by area under the curve (AUC) methods, with the trapezoidal rule (numerical integration) the most common method. Due to the dependence on the length of x in the trapezoidal rule, the area estimation is highly dependent on the blood/plasma sampling schedule. That is, the closer time points are, the closer the trapezoids reflect the actual shape of the concentration-time curve.

Compartmental Analysis

Compartmental PK analysis uses kinetic models to describe and predict the concentration-time curve. PK compartmental models are often similar to kinetic models used in other scientific disciplines such as chemical kinetics and thermodynamics. The advantage of compartmental over some noncompartmental analyses is the ability to predict the concentration at any time. The disadvantage is the difficulty in developing and validating the proper model. Compartment-free modelling based on curve stripping does not suffer this limitation. The simplest PK compartmental model is the one-compartmental PK model with IV bolus administration and first-order elimination. The most complex PK models (called PBPK models) rely on the use of physiological information to ease development and validation.

Single-compartment Model

Linear pharmacokinetics is so-called because the graph of the relationship between the various factors involved (dose, blood plasma concentrations, elimination, etc.) gives a straight line or an approximation to one. For drugs to be effective they need to be able to move rapidly from blood plasma to other body fluids and tissues.

The change in concentration over time can be expressed as $C = C_{initial} \times e^{-k_{el} \times t}$.

Multi-compartmental Models

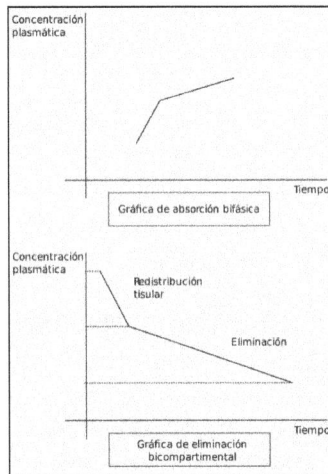

Concentración plasmática

Tiempo

Gráfica de absorción bifásica

Concentración plasmática

Redistribución tisular

Eliminación

Tiempo

Gráfica de eliminación bicompartimental

Graphs for absorption and elimination for a non-linear pharmacokinetic model.

The graph for the non-linear relationship between the various factors is represented by a curve; the relationships between the factors can then be found by calculating the dimensions of different areas under the curve. The models used in *non-linear pharmacokinetics* are largely based on Michaelis–Menten kinetics. A reaction's factors of non-linearity include the following:

- Multiphasic absorption: Drugs injected intravenously are removed from the plasma through two primary mechanisms: (1) Distribution to body tissues and (2) metabolism + excretion of the drugs. The resulting decrease of the drug's plasma concentration follows a biphasic pattern.

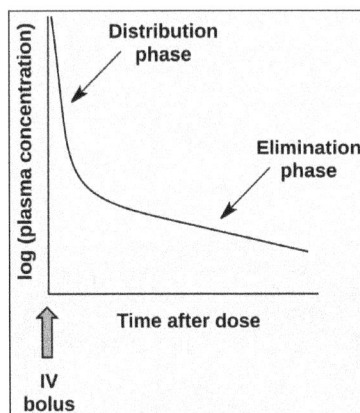

Plasma drug concentration vs time after an IV dose.

- Alpha phase: An initial phase of rapid decrease in plasma concentration. The decrease is primarily attributed to drug distribution from the central compartment (circulation) into the peripheral compartments (body tissues). This phase ends when a pseudo-equilibrium of drug concentration is established between the central and peripheral compartments.

- ○ Beta phase: A phase of gradual decrease in plasma concentration after the alpha phase. The decrease is primarily attributed to drug metabolism and excretion.

- ○ Additional phases (gamma, delta, etc.) are sometimes seen.

- A drug's characteristics make a clear distinction between tissues with high and low blood flow.

- Enzymatic saturation: When the dose of a drug whose elimination depends on biotransformation is increased above a certain threshold the enzymes responsible for its metabolism become saturated. The drug's plasma concentration will then increase disproportionately and its elimination will no longer be constant.

- Induction or enzymatic inhibition: Some drugs have the capacity to inhibit or stimulate their own metabolism, in negative or positive feedback reactions. As occurs with fluvoxamine, fluoxetine and phenytoin. As larger doses of these pharmaceuticals are administered the plasma concentrations of the unmetabolized drug increases and the elimination half-life increases. It is therefore necessary to adjust the dose or other treatment parameters when a high dosage is required.

- The kidneys can also establish active elimination mechanisms for some drugs, independent of plasma concentrations.

It can therefore be seen that non-linearity can occur because of reasons that affect the entire pharmacokinetic sequence: absorption, distribution, metabolism and elimination.

Variable Volume in Time Models

Variable volume pharmacokinetic models can be drug centered models that imply a volume of drug distribution to be that volume in which the drug is distributed at that elapsed time following drug administration. Another possibility occurs when the body volume is changing in time, which would occur, for example, during dialysis when the volume in which a drug can be distributed is itself changing in time.

Bioavailability

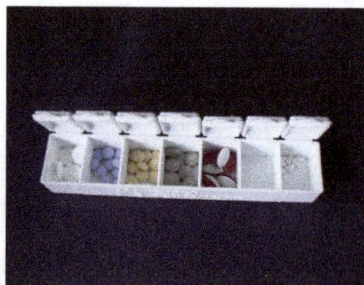

Different forms of tablets, which will have different pharmacokinetic behaviours after their administration.

At a practical level, a drug's bioavailability can be defined as the proportion of the drug that reaches its site of action. From this perspective the intravenous administration of a drug provides the greatest possible bioavailability, and this method is considered to yield a bioavailability of 1 (or 100%). Bioavailability of other delivery methods is compared with that of intravenous injection ("absolute bioavailability") or to a standard value related to other delivery methods in a particular study ("relative bioavailability").

$$B_A = \frac{[ABC]_P \cdot D_{IV}}{[ABC]_{IV} \cdot D_P}$$

$$B_R = \frac{[ABC]_A \cdot \text{dose}_B}{[ABC]_B \cdot \text{dose}_A}$$

Once a drug's bioavailability has been established it is possible to calculate the changes that need to be made to its dosage in order to reach the required blood plasma levels. Bioavailability is therefore a mathematical factor for each individual drug that influences the administered dose. It is possible to calculate the amount of a drug in the blood plasma that has a real potential to bring about its effect using the formula:

$$De = B \cdot Da$$

where De is the effective dose, B bioavailability and Da the administered dose.

Therefore, if a drug has a bioavailability of 0.8 (or 80%) and it is administered in a dose of 100 mg, the equation will demonstrate the following:

$$De = 0.8 \times 100 \text{ mg} = 80 \text{ mg}$$

That is the 100 mg administered represents a blood plasma concentration of 80 mg that has the capacity to have a pharmaceutical effect.

This concept depends on a series of factors inherent to each drug, such as:

- Pharmaceutical form
- Chemical form
- Route of administration
- Stability
- Metabolism

These concepts, can be mathematically quantified and integrated to obtain an overall mathematical equation:

$$De = Q \cdot Da \cdot B$$

where Q is the drug's purity.

$$Va = \frac{Da \cdot B \cdot Q}{\tau}$$

where Va is the drug's rate of administration and τ is the rate at which the absorbed drug reaches the circulatory system.

Finally, using the Henderson-Hasselbalch equation, and knowing the drug's pKa (pH at which there is an equilibrium between its ionized and non ionized molecules), it is possible to calculate the non ionized concentration of the drug and therefore the concentration that will be subject to absorption:

$$pH = pKa + \log\frac{B}{A}$$

When two drugs have the same bioavailability, they are said to be biological equivalents or bioequivalents. This concept of bioequivalence is important because it is currently used as a yardstick in the authorization of generic drugs in many countries.

LADME

A number of phases occur once the drug enters into contact with the organism, these are described using the acronym LADME:

- Liberation of the active substance from the delivery system,

- Absorption of the active substance by the organism,

- Distribution through the blood plasma and different body tissues,

- Metabolism that is inactivation of the xenobiotic substance, and finally

- Excretion or elimination of the substance or the products of its metabolism.

Some textbooks combine the first two phases as the drug is often administered in an active form, which means that there is no liberation phase. Others include a phase that combines distribution, metabolism and excretion into a disposition phase. Other authors include the drug's toxicological aspect in what is known as *ADME-Tox* or *ADMET*.

Each of the phases is subject to physico-chemical interactions between a drug and an organism, which can be expressed mathematically. Pharmacokinetics is therefore based on mathematical equations that allow the prediction of a drug's behavior and which place great emphasis on the relationships between drug plasma concentrations and the time elapsed since the drug's administration.

Analysis

Bioanalytical Methods

Bioanalytical methods are necessary to construct a concentration-time profile. Chemical techniques are employed to measure the concentration of drugs in biological matrix, most often plasma. Proper bioanalytical methods should be selective and sensitive. For example, microscale thermophoresis can be used to quantify how the biological matrix/liquid affects the affinity of a drug to its target.

Mass Spectrometry

Pharmacokinetics is often studied using mass spectrometry because of the complex nature of the matrix (often plasma or urine) and the need for high sensitivity to observe concentrations after a low dose and a long time period. The most common instrumentation used in this application is LC-MS with a triple quadrupole mass spectrometer. Tandem mass spectrometry is usually employed for added specificity. Standard curves and internal standards are used for quantitation of usually a single pharmaceutical in the samples. The samples represent different time points as a pharmaceutical is administered and then metabolized or cleared from the body. Blank samples taken before administration are important in determining background and ensuring data integrity with such complex sample matrices. Much attention is paid to the linearity of the standard curve; however it is common to use curve fitting with more complex functions such as quadratics since the response of most mass spectrometers is not linear across large concentration ranges.

There is currently considerable interest in the use of very high sensitivity mass spectrometry for microdosing studies, which are seen as a promising alternative to animal experimentation.

Population Pharmacokinetics

Population pharmacokinetics is the study of the sources and correlates of variability in drug concentrations among individuals who are the target patient population receiving clinically relevant doses of a drug of interest. Certain patient demographic, pathophysiological, and therapeutical features, such as body weight, excretory and metabolic functions, and the presence of other therapies, can regularly alter dose-concentration relationships. For example, steady-state concentrations of drugs eliminated mostly by the kidney are usually greater in patients suffering from renal failure than they are in patients with normal renal function receiving the same drug dosage. Population pharmacokinetics seeks to identify the measurable pathophysiologic factors that cause changes in the dose-concentration relationship and the extent of these changes so that, if such changes are associated with clinically significant shifts in the therapeutic index, dosage can be appropriately modified. An advantage of population pharmacokinetic modelling is its ability to analyse sparse data sets (sometimes only one concentration measurement per patient is available).

Clinical Pharmacokinetics

Drugs where pharmacokinetic monitoring is recommended			
Antiepileptic medication	Cardioactive medication	Immunosuppressor medication	Antibiotic medication
• Phenytoin • Carbamazepine • Valproic acid • Lamotrigine • Ethosuximide • Phenobarbital • Primidone	• Digoxin • Lidocaine	• Ciclosporin • Tacrolimus • Sirolimus • Everolimus • Mycophenolate	• Gentamicin • Tobramycin • Amikacin • Vancomycin
Bronchodilator medication	Cytostatic medication	Antiviral (HIV) medication	Coagulation factors

• Theophylline	• Methotrexate	• + Efavirenz	• Factor VIII,
	• 5-Fluorouracil	• Tenofovir	• Factor IX,
	• Irinotecan	• Ritonavir	• Factor VIIa,
			• Factor XI

Clinical pharmacokinetics (arising from the clinical use of population pharmacokinetics) is the direct application to a therapeutic situation of knowledge regarding a drug's pharmacokinetics and the characteristics of a population that a patient belongs to (or can be ascribed to).

An example is the relaunch of the use of ciclosporin as an immunosuppressor to facilitate organ transplant. The drug's therapeutic properties were initially demonstrated, but it was almost never used after it was found to cause nephrotoxicity in a number of patients. However, it was then realized that it was possible to individualize a patient's dose of ciclosporin by analysing the patients plasmatic concentrations (pharmacokinetic monitoring). This practice has allowed this drug to be used again and has facilitated a great number of organ transplants.

Clinical monitoring is usually carried out by determination of plasma concentrations as this data is usually the easiest to obtain and the most reliable. The main reasons for determining a drug's plasma concentration include:

- Narrow therapeutic range (difference between toxic and therapeutic concentrations).

- High toxicity.

- High risk to life.

Importance of Pharmacokinetics Testing before Beginning Clinical Trials

Researchers and pharmaceuticals in the midst of designing a stronger pre-clinical study will need to understand the ways pharmacokinetics testing can play a role in their trials. Pharmacokinetics is a science that studies how certain substances affect a living organism when administered.

This particular science determines what happens to a drug from the time it is administered throughout its circulation within the body and to the moment when it is ultimately eliminated from the body. The fate of any drug may change based on the site of administration, formulation and dosage.

There are several different models that are used to understand the concepts of pharmacokinetics testing along with the processes that take place. The multi-compartment model is a commonly used mathematical standard and illustrates how certain materials or energies move throughout a system.

The European Medicines Agency released a guideline discussing safety issues within pharmacology studies. The brief discussed the importance of ensuring medications are safe to use in humans by analyzing the drug's effects on cardiovascular, central nervous, and respiratory systems in animal models first.

The guideline recommends researchers to conduct in vivo testing along with standard toxicity studies to ensure their drug development efforts are safe and to reduce animal use within pre-clinical trials. These tests determine the overall effects of the medication when compared to its desired therapeutic target. Safety pharmacology studies can also be included in future clinical drug development.

There are specific studies that need to be conducted before researchers move forward with human clinical trials. These include in vitro metabolic and plasma protein binding trials on animals as well as systemic exposure data in repeated-dose toxicity studies.

Some of the most important pharmacokinetic properties to understand during pre-clinical testing include distribution, absorption, metabolism, and excretion. All species and in vitro biochemical data regarding drug reactions will need to be reported and analyzed before proceeding with human clinical trials.

Afterward, animal metabolites data can be compared to the statistics of human metabolites and then it can be determined whether further testing is necessary. Additionally, the EMA brief explains that for drugs with an administration dose of less than 10 milligrams, it may be necessary to test a greater amount of the drug material to learn of any adverse reactions.

Acute toxicity studies are also important to conduct, but lethality should not be the expected endpoint for such tests, according to the EMA guidelines. Pharmacokinetic testing can ensure that drugs do not fail during clinical trials for reasons that could have been predicted and avoided.

Pharmacodynamics

Pharmacodynamics (PD) is the study of the biochemical and physiologic effects of drugs (especially pharmaceutical drugs). The effects can include those manifested within animals (including humans), microorganisms, or combinations of organisms (for example, infection). Pharmacodynamics is the study of how a drug affects an organism, whereas pharmacokinetics is the study of how the organism affects the drug. Both together influence dosing, benefit, and adverse effects. Pharmacodynamics is sometimes abbreviated as PD and pharmacokinetics as PK, especially in combined reference (for example, when speaking of PK/PD models).

Pharmacodynamics places particular emphasis on dose–response relationships, that is, the relationships between drug concentration and effect. One dominant example is drug-receptor interactions as modeled by:

$$L + R \rightleftharpoons LR$$

where L, R, and LR represent ligand (drug), receptor, and ligand-receptor complex concentrations, respectively. This equation represents a simplified model of reaction dynamics that can be studied mathematically through tools such as free energy maps.

Effects on the Body

The majority of drugs either:

- Mimic or inhibit normal physiological/biochemical processes or inhibit pathological processes in animals.

- Inhibit vital processes of endo- or ectoparasites and microbial organisms.

There are 7 main drug actions:

- Stimulating action through direct receptor agonism and downstream effects.

- Depressing action through direct receptor agonism and downstream effects (ex.: inverse agonist).

- Blocking/antagonizing action (as with silent antagonists), the drug binds the receptor but does not activate it.

- Stabilizing action, the drug seems to act neither as a stimulant or as a depressant (ex.: some drugs possess receptor activity that allows them to stabilize general receptor activation, like buprenorphine in opioid dependent individuals or aripiprazole in schizophrenia, all depending on the dose and the recipient).

- Exchanging/replacing substances or accumulating them to form a reserve (ex.: glycogen storage).

- Direct beneficial chemical reaction as in free radical scavenging.

- Direct harmful chemical reaction which might result in damage or destruction of the cells, through induced toxic or lethal damage (cytotoxicity or irritation).

Desired Activity

The desired activity of a drug is mainly due to successful targeting of one of the following:

- Cellular membrane disruption.

- Chemical reaction with downstream effects.

- Interaction with enzyme proteins.

- Interaction with structural proteins.

- Interaction with carrier proteins.

- Interaction with ion channels.

- Ligand binding to receptors:

  ○ Hormone receptors.

  ○ Neuromodulator receptors.

  ○ Neurotransmitter receptors.

General anesthetics were once thought to work by disordering the neural membranes, thereby altering the Na^+ influx. Antacids and chelating agents combine chemically in the body. Enzyme-substrate binding is a way to alter the production or metabolism of key endogenous chemicals, for example aspirin irreversibly inhibits the enzyme prostaglandin synthetase (cyclooxygenase) thereby preventing inflammatory response. Colchicine, a drug for gout, interferes with the function of the structural protein tubulin, while Digitalis, a drug still used in heart failure, inhibits the activity of the carrier molecule, Na-K-ATPase pump. The widest class of drugs act as ligands which bind to receptors which determine cellular effects. Upon drug binding, receptors can elicit their normal action (agonist), blocked action (antagonist), or even action opposite to normal (inverse agonist).

In principle, a pharmacologist would aim for a target plasma concentration of the drug for a desired level of response. In reality, there are many factors affecting this goal. Pharmacokinetic factors determine peak concentrations, and concentrations cannot be maintained with absolute consistency because of metabolic breakdown and excretory clearance. Genetic factors may exist which would alter metabolism or drug action itself, and a patient's immediate status may also affect indicated dosage.

Undesirable Effects

Undesirable effects of a drug include:

- Increased probability of cell mutation (carcinogenic activity).
- A multitude of simultaneous assorted actions which may be deleterious.
- Interaction (additive, multiplicative, or metabolic).
- Induced physiological damage, or abnormal chronic conditions.

Therapeutic Window

The therapeutic window is the amount of a medication between the amount that gives an effect (effective dose) and the amount that gives more adverse effects than desired effects. For instance, medication with a small pharmaceutical window must be administered with care and control, e.g. by frequently measuring blood concentration of the drug, since it easily loses effects or gives adverse effects.

Duration of Action

The *duration of action* of a drug is the length of time that particular drug is effective. Duration of action is a function of several parameters including plasma half-life, the time to equilibrate between plasma and target compartments, and the off rate of the drug from its biological target.

Receptor Binding and Effect

The binding of ligands (drug) to receptors is governed by the law of mass action which relates the large-scale status to the rate of numerous molecular processes. The rates of formation and un-formation can be used to determine the equilibrium concentration of bound receptors. The equilibrium dissociation constant is defined by:

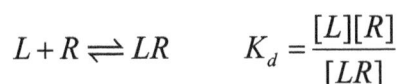

$$L + R \rightleftharpoons LR \qquad K_d = \frac{[L][R]}{[LR]}$$

where L=ligand, R=receptor, square brackets [] denote concentration. The fraction of bound receptors is,

$$p_{LR} = \frac{[LR]}{[R]+[LR]} = \frac{1}{1+\dfrac{K_d}{[L]}}$$

Where p_{LR} is the fraction of receptor bound by the ligand.

This expression is one way to consider the effect of a drug, in which the response is related to the fraction of bound receptors. The fraction of bound receptors is known as occupancy. The relationship between occupancy and pharmacological response is usually non-linear. This explains the so-called *receptor reserve* phenomenon i.e. the concentration producing 50% occupancy is typically higher than the concentration producing 50% of maximum response. More precisely, receptor reserve refers to a phenomenon whereby stimulation of only a fraction of the whole receptor population apparently elicits the maximal effect achievable in a particular tissue.

The simplest interpretation of receptor reserve is that it is a model that states there are excess receptors on the cell surface than what is necessary for full effect. Taking a more sophisticated approach, receptor reserve is an integrative measure of the response-inducing capacity of an agonist (in some receptor models it is termed intrinsic efficacy or intrinsic activity) and of the signal amplification capacity of the corresponding receptor (and its downstream signaling pathways). Thus, the existence (and magnitude) of receptor reserve depends on the agonist (efficacy), tissue (signal amplification ability) and measured effect (pathways activated to cause signal amplification). As receptor reserve is very sensitive to agonist's intrinsic efficacy, it is usually defined only for full (high-efficacy) agonists.

Often the response is determined as a function of log[L] to consider many orders of magnitude of concentration. However, there is no biological or physical theory which relates effects to the log of concentration. It is just convenient for graphing purposes. It is useful to note that 50% of the receptors are bound when $[L]=K_d$.

The graph shown represents the conc-response for two hypothetical receptor agonists, plotted in a semi-log fashion. The curve toward the left represents a higher potency (potency arrow does not indicate direction of increase) since lower concentrations are needed for a given response. The effect increases as a function of concentration.

Multicellular Pharmacodynamics

The concept of pharmacodynamics has been expanded to include Multicellular Pharmacodynamics (MCPD). MCPD is the study of the static and dynamic properties and relationships between a set of drugs and a dynamic and diverse multicellular four-dimensional organization. It is the study of the workings of a drug on a minimal multicellular system (mMCS), both in vivo and in silico. Networked Multicellular Pharmacodynamics (Net-MCPD) further extends the concept of MCPD to model regulatory genomic networks together with signal transduction pathways, as part of a complex of interacting components in the cell.

Toxicodynamics

Pharmacokinetics and pharmacodynamics are termed toxicokinetics and toxicodynamics in the field of ecotoxicology. Here, the focus is on toxic effects on a wide range of organisms. The corresponding models are called toxicokinetic-toxicodynamic models.

Pharmacology

Pharmacology is the branch of biology concerned with the study of drug or medication action, where a drug can be broadly defined as any man-made, natural, or endogenous (from within the body) molecule which exerts a biochemical or physiological effect on the cell, tissue, organ, or organism (sometimes the word pharmacon is used as a term to encompass these endogenous and exogenous bioactive species). More specifically, it is the study of the interactions that occur between a living organism and chemicals that affect normal or abnormal biochemical function. If substances have medicinal properties, they are considered pharmaceuticals.

The field encompasses drug composition and properties, synthesis and drug design, molecular and cellular mechanisms, organ/systems mechanisms, signal transduction/cellular communication, molecular diagnostics, interactions, chemical biology, therapy, and medical applications and antipathogenic capabilities. The two main areas of pharmacology are pharmacodynamics and pharmacokinetics. Pharmacodynamics studies the effects of a drug on biological systems, and pharmacokinetics studies the effects of biological systems on a drug. In broad terms, pharmacodynamics discusses the chemicals with biological receptors, and pharmacokinetics discusses the absorption, distribution, metabolism, and excretion (ADME) of chemicals from the biological systems. Pharmacology is not synonymous with pharmacy and the two terms are frequently confused. Pharmacology, a biomedical science, deals with the research, discovery, and characterization of chemicals which show biological effects and the elucidation of cellular and organismal function in relation to these chemicals. In contrast, pharmacy, a health services profession, is concerned with application of the principles learned from pharmacology in its clinical settings; whether it be in a dispensing or clinical care role. In either field, the primary contrast between the two are their distinctions between direct-patient care, for pharmacy practice, and the science-oriented research field, driven by pharmacology.

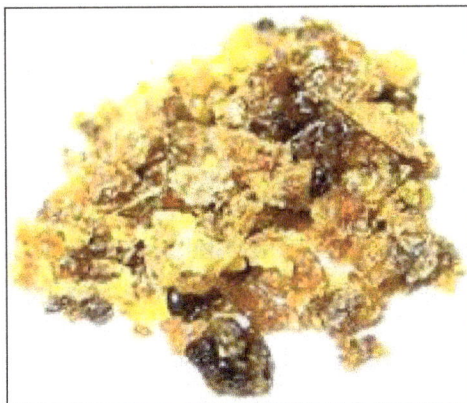

Naturally derived opium from opium poppies has been used as a drug since before 1100 BCE.

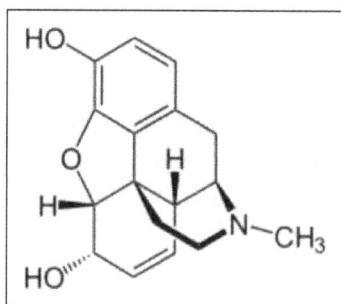

Opium's major active constituent, morphine, was first isolated in 1804 and is now known to act as an opioid agonist.

The origins of clinical pharmacology date back to the Middle Ages, with pharmacognosy and Avicenna's *The Canon of Medicine*, Peter of Spain's *Commentary on Isaac*, and John of St Amand's *Commentary on the Antedotary of Nicholas*. Early pharmacology focused on herbalism and natural substances, mainly plant extracts. Medicines were compiled in books called pharmacopoeias. Crude drugs have been used since prehistory as a preparation of substances from natural sources. However, the active ingredient of crude drugs are not purified and the substance is adulterated with other substances.

Traditional medicine varies between cultures and may be specific to a particular culture, such as in traditional Chinese, Mongolian, Tibetan and Korean medicine. However much of this has since been regarded as pseudoscience. Pharmacological substances known as entheogens may have spiritual and religious use and historical context.

In the 17th century, the English Physician Nicholas Culpeper translated and used pharmacological texts. Culpepper detailed plants and the conditions they could treat. In the 18th century, much of clinical pharmacology was established by the work of William Withering. Pharmacology as a scientific discipline did not further advance until the mid-19th century amid the great biomedical resurgence of that period. Before the second half of the nineteenth century, the remarkable potency and specificity of the actions of drugs such as morphine, quinine and digitalis were explained vaguely and with reference to extraordinary chemical powers and affinities to certain organs or tissues. The first pharmacology department was set up by Rudolf Buchheim in 1847, in recognition of the need to understand how therapeutic drugs and poisons produced their effects. Subsequently, the first pharmacology department in England was set up in 1905 at University College London.

Pharmacology developed in the 19th century as a biomedical science that applied the principles of scientific experimentation to therapeutic contexts. The advancement of research techniques propelled pharmacological research and understanding. The development of the organ bath preparation, where tissue samples are connected to recording devices, such as a myograph, and physiological responses are recorded after drug application, allowed analysis of drugs' effects on tissues. The development of the ligand binding assay in 1945 allowed quantification of the binding affinity of drugs at chemical targets. Modern pharmacologists use techniques from genetics, molecular biology, biochemistry, and other advanced tools to transform information about molecular mechanisms and targets into therapies directed against disease, defects or pathogens, and create methods for preventative care, diagnostics, and ultimately personalized medicine.

Divisions

The discipline of pharmacology can be divided into many sub disciplines each with a specific focus.

Systems of the Body

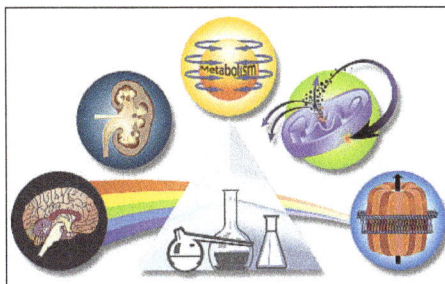

A variety of topics involved with pharmacology, including neuropharmacology, renal pharmacology, human metabolism, intracellular metabolism, and intracellular regulation.

Pharmacology can also focus on specific systems comprising the body. Divisions related to bodily systems study the effects of drugs in different systems of the body. These include neuropharmacology, in the central and peripheral nervous systems; immunopharmacology in the immune system. Other divisions include cardiovascular, renal and endocrine pharmacology. Psychopharmacology, is the study of the effects of drugs on the psyche, mind and behavior, such as the behavioral effects of psychoactive drugs. It incorporates approaches and techniques from neuropharmacology, animal behavior and behavioral neuroscience, and is interested in the behavioral and neurobiological mechanisms of action of psychoactive drugs. The related field of neuropsychopharmacology focuses on the effects of drugs at the overlap between the nervous system and the psyche.

Pharmacometabolomics, also known as pharmacometabonomics, is a field which stems from metabolomics, the quantification and analysis of metabolites produced by the body. It refers to the direct measurement of metabolites in an individual's bodily fluids, in order to predict or evaluate the metabolism of pharmaceutical compounds, and to better understand the pharmacokinetic profile of a drug. Pharmacometabolomics can be applied to measure metabolite levels following the administration of a drug, in order to monitor the effects of the drug on metabolic pathways. Pharmacomicrobiomics studies the effect of microbiome variations on drug disposition, action, and toxicity. Pharmacomicrobiomics is concerned with the interaction between drugs and the gut microbiome. Pharmacogenomics is the application of genomic technologies to drug discovery and further characterization of drugs related to an organism's entire genome. For pharmacology regarding individual genes, pharmacogenetics studies how genetic variation gives rise to differing responses to drugs. Pharmacoepigenetics studies the underlying epigenetic marking patterns that lead to variation in an individual's response to medical treatment.

Clinical Practice and Drug Discovery

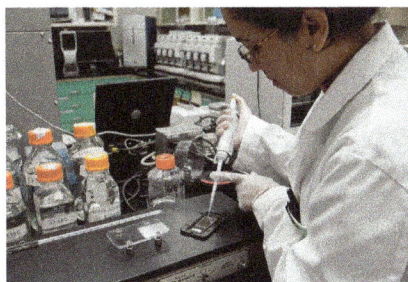

A toxicologist working in a lab.

Pharmacology can be applied within clinical sciences. Clinical pharmacology is the basic science of pharmacology focusing on the application of pharmacological principles and methods in the medical clinic and towards patient care and outcomes. An example of this is posology, which is the study of how medicines are dosed.

Pharmacology is closely related to toxicology. Both pharmacology and toxicology are scientific disciplines that focus on understanding the properties and actions of chemicals. However, pharmacology emphasizes the therapeutic effects of chemicals, usually drugs or compounds that could become drugs, whereas toxicology is the study of chemical's adverse effects and risk assessment.

Pharmacological knowledge is used to advise pharmacotherapy in medicine and pharmacy.

Drug Discovery

Drug discovery is the field of study concerned with creating new drugs. It encompasses the subfields of drug design and development. Drug discovery starts with drug design, which is the inventive process of finding new drugs. In the most basic sense, this involves the design of molecules that are complementary in shape and charge to a given biomolecular target. After a lead compound has been identified through drug discovery, drug development involves bringing the drug to the market. Drug discovery is related to pharmacoeconomics, which is the sub-discipline of health economics that considers the value of drugs Pharmacoeconomics evaluates the cost and benefits of drugs in order to guide optimal healthcare resource allocation. The techniques used for the discovery, formulation, manufacturing and quality control of drugs discovery is studied by pharmaceutical engineering, a branch of engineering. Safety pharmacology specialises in detecting and investigating potential undesirable effects of drugs.

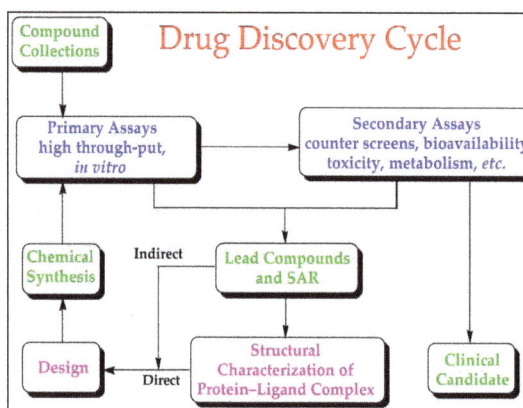

The drug discovery cycle.

Development of medication is a vital concern to medicine, but also has strong economical and political implications. To protect the consumer and prevent abuse, many governments regulate the manufacture, sale, and administration of medication. In the United States, the main body that regulates pharmaceuticals is the Food and Drug Administration and they enforce standards set by the United States Pharmacopoeia. In the European Union, the main body that regulates pharmaceuticals is the EMA and they enforce standards set by the European Pharmacopoeia.

The metabolic stability and the reactivity of a library of candidate drug compounds have to be assessed for drug metabolism and toxicological studies. Many methods have been proposed for quantitative predictions in drug metabolism; one example of a recent computational method is SPORCalc. If the chemical structure of a medicinal compound is altered slightly, this could slightly or dramatically alter the medicinal properties of the compound depending on the level of alteration as it relates to the structural composition of the substrate or receptor site on which it exerts its medicinal effect, a concept referred to as the structural activity relationship (SAR). This means that when a useful activity has been identified, chemists will make many similar compounds called analogues, in an attempt to maximize the desired medicinal effect(s) of the compound. This development phase can take anywhere from a few years to a decade or more and is very expensive.

These new analogues need to be developed. It needs to be determined how safe the medicine is for human consumption, its stability in the human body and the best form for delivery to the desired organ system, like tablet or aerosol. After extensive testing, which can take up to 6 years, the new medicine is ready for marketing and selling.

As a result of the long time required to develop analogues and test a new medicine and the fact that of every 5000 potential new medicines typically only one will ever reach the open market, this is an expensive way of doing things, often costing over 1 billion dollars. To recoup this outlay pharmaceutical companies may do a number of things:

- Carefully research the demand for their potential new product before spending an outlay of company funds.

- Obtain a patent on the new medicine preventing other companies from producing that medicine for a certain allocation of time.

The inverse benefit law describes the relationship between a drugs therapeutic benefits and its marketing.

When designing drugs, the placebo effect must be considered to assess the drug's true therapeutic value.

Drug development uses techniques from medicinal chemistry to chemically design drugs. This overlaps with the biological approach of finding targets and physiological effects.

Experimentation and Analysis

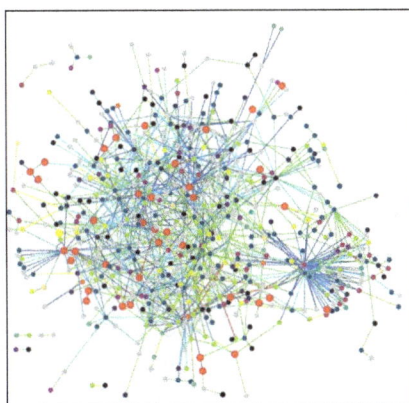

Interactions between proteins are frequently visualized and analyzed using networks. This network is made up of protein–protein interactions from Treponema pallidum, the causative agent of syphilis and other diseases.

Theoretical pharmacology is a field of research uses techniques from computational chemistry, and molecular mechanics. Theoretical pharmacology aims at rationalizing the relation between the observed activity of a particular drug to its structural features. It aims to find relations between structure and activity. Furthermore, on the basis of the structure theoretical pharmacology aims to predict the biological activity of new drugs based on their properties and to predict new classes of drugs. Theoretical pharmacology uses pharmacometrics, which are mathematical models of biology, pharmacology, disease, and physiology used to describe and quantify interactions between drugs with pharmacology, including beneficial effects and adverse effects. Pharmacometrics can be applied to quantify drug, disease and trial information to aid efficient drug development, regulatory decisions and rational drug treatment in patients.

Experimental pharmacology involves the study of pharmacology through bioassay, to test the efficacy and potency of a drug. Systems pharmacology or network pharmacology is the application of systems biology principles in the field of pharmacology. Pharmacoinformatics relates to the broader field of bioinformatics. Ethopharmacology relates to ethology and studies drugs in the context of animal behaviours.

Wider Contexts

Pharmacology can be studied in relation to wider contexts than the physiology of individuals. For example, pharmacoepidemiology is the study of the effects of drugs in large numbers of people and relates to the broader fields of epidemiology and public health. Pharmacoenvironmentology or environmental pharmacology is a field intimately linked with ecology and public health. Human health and ecology are intimately related so environmental pharmacology studies the environmental effect of drugs and pharmaceuticals and personal care products in the environment.

Drugs may also have ethnocultural importance, so ethnopharmacology studies the ethnic and cultural aspects of pharmacology.

Emerging Fields

Photopharmacology is an emerging approach in medicine in which drugs are activated and deactivated with light. The energy of light is used to change for shape and chemical properties of the drug, resulting in different biological activity. This is done to ultimately achieve control when and where drugs are active in a reversible manner, to prevent side effects and pollution of drugs into the environment.

Pharmacogenomics

Pharmacogenomics is the branch of pharmacology which deals with the influence of genetic variation on drug response in patients by correlating gene expression or single-nucleotide polymorphisms with a drug's efficacy or toxicity. It aims to develop rational means to optimize drug therapy, with respect to the patients genotype, to ensure maximum efficacy with minimal adverse effects. Such approaches promise the advent of personalized medicine, in which drugs and drug combinations are optimized for each individual's unique genetic makeup. Pharmacogenomics is the whole genome application of pharmacogenetics, which examines the single gene interactions with drugs.

Pharmacogenomics is the study of how an individual's genetic inheritance affects the body's response to drugs. The term comes from the words pharmacology and genomics and is thus the intersection of pharmaceuticals and genetics. Pharmacogenomics holds the promise that drugs might one day be tailor-made for individuals and adapted to each person's own genetic makeup. Environment, diet, age, lifestyle, and state of health all can influence a person's response to medicines, but understanding an individual's genetic makeup is thought to be the key to creating personalized drugs with greater efficacy and safety. The way a person responds to a drug (this includes both positive and negative reactions) is a complex trait that is influenced by many different genes. Without knowing all of the genes involved in drug response, scientists have found it difficult to develop genetic tests that could predict a person's response to a particular drug . Once scientists discovered that people's genes show small variations (or changes) in their nucleotide (DNA base) content, all of that changed: genetic testing for predicting drug response is now possible. Pharmacogenomics combines traditional pharmaceutical sciences such as biochemistry with annotated knowledge of genes, proteins, and single nucleotide polymorphisms.The most common variations in the human genome are called single nucleotide polymorphisms (SNPs). There is estimated to be approximately 11 million SNPs in the human population, with an average of one every 1,300 base pairs.

Genomics was established by Fred Sanger when he first sequenced the complete genomes of a virus and a mitochondrion. His group established techniques of sequencing, genome mapping, data storage, and bioinformatic analyses in the 1970-1980s. The actual term genomics is thought to have been coined by Dr. Tom Roderick, a geneticist at the Jackson Laboratory (Bar Harbor, ME) over beer at a meeting held in Maryland on the mapping of the human genome in 1986.

In 1972, Walter Fiers and his team at the Laboratory of Molecular Biology of the University of Ghent (Ghent, Belgium) were the first to determine the sequence of a gene: the gene for Bacteriophage MS2 coat protein. In 1976, the team determined the complete nucleotide-sequence of bacteriophage MS2-RNA. The first DNA-based genome to be sequenced in its entirety was that of bacteriophage Φ-X174 (5,368 bp), sequenced by Frederick Sanger in 1977.

The first free-living organism to be sequenced was that of Haemophilus influenzae in 1995, and since then genomes are being sequenced at a rapid pace. A rough draft of the human genome was completed by the Human Genome Project in early 2001, creating much fanfare.

As of September 2007, the complete sequence was known of about 1879 viruses, 577 bacterial species and roughly 23 eukaryote organisms, of which about half are fungi. Most of the bacteria whose genomes have been completely sequenced are problematic disease-causing agents, such as Haemophilus influenzae. Pharmacogenomics combines traditional pharmaceutical sciences such as biochemistry with annotated knowledge of genes, proteins, and single nucleotide polymorphisms.

Importance of Pharmacogenomics

Adverse Drug Reaction conveys little of the horror of a severe negative reaction to a prescribed drug. But such negative reactions can nonetheless occur. A 1998 study of hospitalized patients published in the Journal of the American Medical Association reported that in 1994, adverse drug reactions accounted for more than 2.2 million serious cases and over 100,000 deaths, making adverse drug reactions (ADRs) one of the leading causes of hospitalization and death in the United States . For instance, the daily doses required to treat patients vary by 20-fold for the warfarin, by 40-fold for the antihypertensive drug propranolol and by 60-fold for L-dopa for parkinsons disease. Other drugs have clinical utility in a subset of patients with given pathology, e.g., antipsychotics that are ineffective in 30% of schizophrenics, suggesting that such drugs are only effective in patients with specific disease etiologies . Many of the deaths could be avoided if the physician had prior knowledge of patients genetic profile, which determines the drug response. Currently, there is no simple way to determine whether people will respond well, badly, or not at all to a medication; therefore, pharmaceutical companies are limited to developing drugs using a one size fits all system . This system allows for the development of drugs to which the average patient will respond. But, as the statistics above show, one size does not fit all, sometimes with devastating results. What is needed is a way to solve the problem of ADRs before they happen. The solution is in sight though, and it is called pharmacogenomics.

Pharmacogenomics eventually can lead to an overall decrease in the cost of health care because of decreases in: (1) the number of adverse drug reactions; (2) the number of failed drug trials; (3) the time it takes to get a drug approved; (4) the length of time patients are on medication; (5) the number of medications patients must take to find an effective therapy; (6) the effects of a disease on the body (through early detection).

The cytochrome P450 (CYP) family of liver enzymes is responsible for breaking down more than 30 different classes of drugs. DNA variations in genes that code for these enzymes can influence their ability to metabolize certain drugs. Less active or inactive forms of CYP enzymes that are unable to break down and efficiently eliminate drugs from the body can cause drug overdose in patients. Today, clinical trials researchers use genetic tests for variations in cytochrome P450 genes to screen and monitor patients. In addition, many pharmaceutical companies screen their chemical compounds to see how well they are broken down by variant forms of CYP enzymes.

Another enzyme called TPMT (thiopurine methyltransferase) plays an important role in the chemotherapy treatment of a common childhood leukemia by breaking down thiopurines. A small percentage of Caucasians have genetic variants that prevent them from producing an active form of this protein. As a result, thiopurines elevate to toxic levels in the patient because the inactive form of TMPT is unable to break down the drug. Today, doctors can use a genetic test to screen patients for this deficiency, and the TMPT activity is monitored to determine appropriate thiopurine dosage levels.

New developments in this field will impact on drug design at three main levels: (1) the interaction of the drug with its receptor binding site; (2) the absorption and distribution of the drug; (3) the elimination of the drug from the body.

Benefits of Pharmacogenomics

Pharmacogenomics combines traditional pharmaceutical sciences such as biochemistry with annotated knowledge of genes, proteins, and single nucleotide polymorphisms. Following are the benefits.

More Powerful Medicines

Pharmaceutical companies will be able to create drugs based on the proteins, enzymes, and RNA molecules associated with genes and diseases. This will facilitate drug discovery and allow drug makers to produce a therapy more targeted to specific diseases. This accuracy will not only maximize therapeutic effects but also decrease damage to nearby healthy cells.

Better and Safer Drugs the First Time

Instead of the standard trial-and-error method of matching patients with the right drugs, doctors will be able to analyze a patient's genetic profile and prescribe the best available drug therapy from the beginning. Not only will this take the guesswork out of finding the right drug, it will speed recovery time and increase safety as the likelihood of adverse reactions is eliminated.

Methods of Determining Appropriate Drug Dosages

Current methods of basing dosages on weight and age will be replaced with dosages based on a person's genetics; how well the body processes the medicine and the time it takes to metabolize it. This will maximize the therapy's value and decrease the likelihood of overdose.

Advanced Screening for Disease

Knowing one's genetic code will allow a person to make adequate lifestyle and environmental changes at an early age so as to avoid or lessen the severity of a genetic disease. Likewise, advance knowledge of particular disease susceptibility will allow careful monitoring, and treatments can be introduced at the most appropriate stage to maximize their therapy.

Better Vaccines

Vaccines made of genetic material, either DNA or RNA, promise all the benefits of existing vaccines without all the risks. They will activate the immune system but will be unable to cause infections. They will be inexpensive, stable, easy to store, and capable of being engineered to carry several strains of a pathogen at once.

Improvements in the Drug Discovery and Approval Process

Pharmaceutical companies will be able to discover potential therapies more easily using genome targets. The drug approval process should be facilitated as trials are targeted for specific genetic population groups and providing greater degrees of success. The cost and risk of clinical trials will be reduced by targeting only those persons capable of responding to a drug.

Decrease in the Overall Cost of Health Care

Decreases in the number of adverse drug reactions, the number of failed drug trials, the time it takes to get a drug approved, the length of time patients are on medication, the number of medications patients must take to find an effective therapy, the effects of a disease on the body (through early detection), and an increase in the range of possible drug targets will promote a net decrease in the cost of health care.

Barriers to Pharmacogenomics Progress

Pharmacogenomics is a developing research field that is still in its infancy. Several of the following barriers will have to be overcome before many pharmacogenomics benefits can be realized.

Complexity of Finding Gene Variations that affect Drug Response

Single nucleotide polymorphisms (SNPs) are DNA sequence variations that occur when a single nucleotide (A, T, C, or G) in the genome sequence is altered. SNPs occur every 100 to 300 bases along the 3-billion-base human genome, therefore millions of SNPs must be identified and analyzed to determine their involvement (if any) in drug response. Further complicating of the process is our limited knowledge of which genes are involved with each drug response. Since many genes are likely to influence responses, obtaining the big picture on the impact of gene variations is highly time-consuming and complicated.

Limited Drug Alternatives

Only one or two approved drugs may be available for treatment of a particular condition. If patients have gene variations that prevent them using these drugs, they may be left without any alternatives for treatment.

Drug Companies to make Multiple Pharmacogenomic Products

Most pharmaceutical companies have been successful with their one size fits all approach to drug development. Since it costs hundreds of millions of dollars to bring a drug to market, will these companies be willing to develop alternative drugs that serve only a small portion of the population?

Impact on Pharmacy Profession

Presently doctors diagnose and prescribe a drug on the trial and error basis and pharmacist advices about side effects and drug-drug interaction. But a day will come when you will take a gene report instead of blood reports .Thus after the diagnosis, pharmacist would interpret the panels of genetic results and advice you which drug would be best for your particular gene so that you have fast recovery.

Pharmacognosy

Pharmacognosy is the study of plants or other natural sources as a possible source of drugs. The American Society of Pharmacognosy defines pharmacognosy as "the study of the physical, chemical, biochemical and biological properties of drugs, drug substances or potential drugs or drug substances of natural origin as well as the search for new drugs from natural sources".

The term "pharmacognosy" was used for the first time by the Austrian physician Schmidt in 1811 and 1815 by Crr. Anotheus Seydler in work titled *Analecta Pharmacognostica*.

Originally—during the 19th century and the beginning of the 20th century—"pharmacognosy" was used to define the branch of medicine or commodity sciences (*Warenkunde* in German) which deals with drugs in their crude, or unprepared, form. Crude drugs are the dried, unprepared material of plant, animal or mineral origin, used for medicine. The study of these materials under the name *pharmakognosie* was first developed in German-speaking areas of Europe, while other language areas often used the older term *materia medica* taken from the works of Galen and Dioscorides. In German the term *drogenkunde* ("science of crude drugs") is also used synonymously.

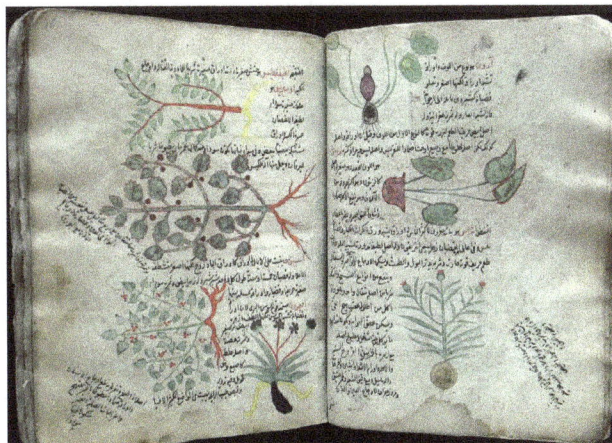

Dioscorides' Materia Medica, c. 1334 copy in Arabic, describes medicinal features of various plants.

As late as the beginning of the 20th century, the subject had developed mainly on the botanical side, being particularly concerned with the description and identification of drugs both in their whole state and in powder form. Such branches of pharmacognosy are still of fundamental importance, particularly for pharmacopoeial identification and quality control purposes, but rapid development in other areas has enormously expanded the subject. The advent of the 21st century brought a renaissance of pharmacognosy and its conventional botanical approach has been broadened up to molecular and metabolomic level.

In addition to the previously mentioned definition, the American Society of Pharmacognosy also defines pharmacognosy as "the study of natural product molecules (typically secondary metabolites) that are useful for their medicinal, ecological, gustatory, or other functional properties." Other definitions are more encompassing, drawing on a broad spectrum of biological subjects, including botany, ethnobotany, marine biology, microbiology, herbal medicine, chemistry, biotechnology, phytochemistry, pharmacology, pharmaceutics, clinical pharmacy and pharmacy practice.

- Medical ethnobotany: the study of the traditional use of plants for medicinal purposes.

- Ethnopharmacology: the study of the pharmacological qualities of traditional medicinal substances.

- The study of phytotherapy (the medicinal use of plant extracts).

- Phytochemistry, the study of chemicals derived from plants (including the identification of new drug candidates derived from plant sources).

- Zoopharmacognosy, the process by which animals self-medicate, by selecting and using plants, soils, and insects to treat and prevent disease.

- Marine pharmacognosy, the study of chemicals derived from marine organisms.

The carotenoids in primrose produce bright red, yellow and orange shades.

All plants produce chemical compounds as part of their normal metabolic activities. These phytochemicals are divided into (1) primary metabolites such as sugars and fats, which are found in all plants; and (2) secondary metabolites—compounds which are found in a smaller range of plants, serving a more specific function. For example, some secondary metabolites are toxins used to deter predation and others are pheromones used to attract insects for pollination. It is these secondary metabolites and pigments that can have therapeutic actions in humans and which can be refined to produce drugs—examples are inulin from the roots of dahlias, quinine from the cinchona, THC and CBD from the flowers of cannabis, morphine and codeine from the poppy, and digoxin from the foxglove.

Plants synthesize a variety of phytochemicals, but most are derivatives:

- Alkaloids are a class of chemical compounds containing a nitrogen ring. Alkaloids are produced by a large variety of organisms, including bacteria, fungi, plants, and animals, and are part of the group of natural products (also called secondary metabolites). Many alkaloids can be purified from crude extracts by acid-base extraction. Many alkaloids are toxic to other organisms.

- Polyphenols (also known as phenolics) are compounds that contain phenol rings. The anthocyanins that give grapes their purple color, the isoflavones, the phytoestrogens from soy and the tannins that give tea its astringency are phenolics.

- Glycosides are molecules in which a sugar is bound to a non-carbohydrate moiety, usually a small organic molecule. Glycosides play numerous important roles in living organisms. Many plants store chemicals in the form of inactive glycosides. These can be activated by enzyme hydrolysis, which causes the sugar part to be broken off, making the chemical available for use.

- Terpenes are a large and diverse class of organic compounds, produced by a variety of plants, particularly conifers, which are often strong smelling and thus may have had a protective function. They are the major components of resin, and of turpentine produced from resin. When terpenes are modified chemically, such as by oxidation or rearrangement of the carbon skeleton, the resulting compounds are generally referred to as *terpenoids*. Terpenes and terpenoids are the primary constituents of the essential oils of many types of plants and flowers. Essential oils are used widely as natural flavor additives for food, as fragrances in perfumery, and in traditional and alternative medicines such as aromatherapy. Synthetic variations and derivatives of natural terpenes and terpenoids also greatly expand the variety of aromas used in perfumery and flavors used in food additives. The fragrance of rose and lavender is due to monoterpenes. The carotenoids produce the reds, yellows and oranges of pumpkin, corn and tomatoes.

Natural Products Chemistry

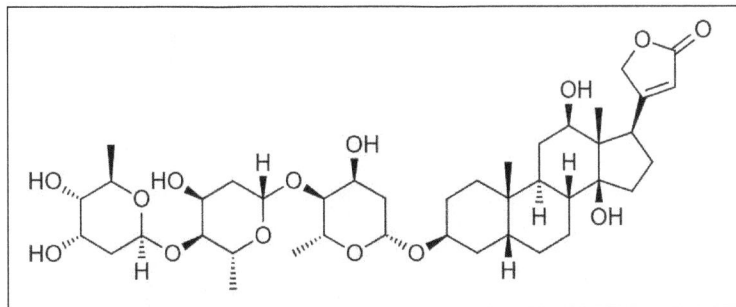

Digoxin is a purified cardiac glycoside that is extracted from the foxglove plant, *Digitalis lanata*. Digoxin is widely used in the treatment of various heart conditions.

A typical protocol to isolate a pure chemical agent from natural origin is bioassay-guided fractionation, meaning step-by-step separation of extracted components based on differences in their physicochemical properties, and assessing the biological activity, followed by next round of separation and assaying. Typically, such work is initiated after a given crude drug formulation (typically prepared by solvent extraction of the natural material) is deemed "active" in a particular *in vitro* assay. If the end-goal of the work at hand is to identify which one(s) of the scores or hundreds of compounds are responsible for the observed *in vitro* activity, the path to that end is fairly straightforward:

- Fractionate the crude extract, e.g. by solvent partitioning or chromatography.

- Test the fractions thereby generated with *in vitro* assay.

- Repeat steps 1) and 2) until pure, active compounds are obtained.

- Determine structure(s) of active compound(s), typically by using spectroscopic methods.

In vitro activity does not necessarily translate to activity in humans or other living systems.

Herbal

In some countries in Asia and Africa, 80% of the population relies on traditional medicine (including herbal medicine) for primary health care. Native American cultures have also relied on traditional medicine such as ceremonial smoking of tobacco, potlatch ceremonies, and herbalism, to name a few, prior to European colonization. Knowledge of traditional medicinal practices is disappearing, particularly in the Amazon.

Pharmacognosy involves the identification, physicochemical characterization, cultivation, extraction, preparation, quality control, and biological assessment of drugs. A plant leaf, flower, root, animal or plant extract may be used to isolate the bioactive chemical.

Any plant preparation used for health purposes rather than simply for nutritional supplementation or to add flavor to food is called a medicinal preparation. Some examples of such compounds include caffeine, salicylic acid, and some chemotherapeutic, inotropic, and anti-gout agents.

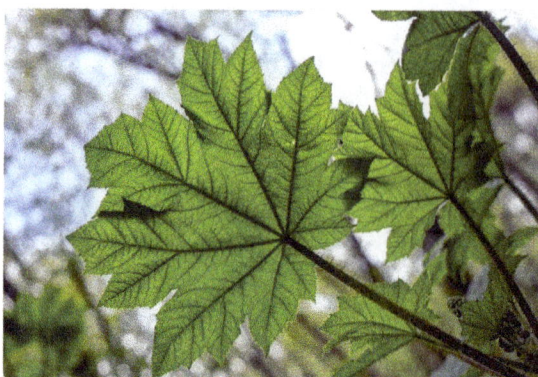

Even today, about a quarter of all prescription drugs in the US have one or more bioactive compounds derived from plants.

Pharmacognosy in Drug Development

Pharmacognosy is used by pharmaceutical companies to screen, characterize and produce new drugs for the treatment of human disease. Often, naturally occurring drugs cannot be mass produced, so they must be studied in order to develop synthetic biosimilars.

Producing these compounds synthetically allows modifications to be made such as increases in bioavailability, altered pharmacokinetics and increased efficacy. These modifications can transform a crude inactive plant extract into a powerful drug, as observed in some anticancer drugs. Thus, natural compounds could provide excellent models to produce novel drugs.

Pharmacognosy includes botanical knowledge to classify and name the plant; understand its genetic pattern and its cultivation; chemical knowledge to isolate, identify, and quantitatively assess the bioactive compounds in the plant sources; and pharmacology to detect and evaluate their biological properties and effects on living systems.

It also needs a working knowledge of quality control to ensure correct identification and purity of the drug as well as accurate testing of its efficacy and safety.

Importance of Pharmacognosy

Traditionally, pharmacognosy was recognized as a vital part of drug development processes and pharmacy education, but began to be neglected with the advent of new miracle drugs that can be synthesized in the laboratory.

However, many scientists are now recognizing that indigenous knowledge about the medicinal virtue of many plants should never be lost as it offers great insight into the development of new drugs. For example, artemisinin from the Artemisia annua or ginghaosu tree, which is recognized as an ancient Chinese drug for malaria.

The respect for ancient wisdom is reflected in the form of phytotherapy and phytopharmaceuticals. The use of plant products to treat illness is well known in South American nations, China, and India where billions of dollars are spent on pharmacognosy research to identify and market natural medicinal drugs.

The importance of medicinal plants should also be studied in other countries in order to fight currently untreatable, life-threatening diseases such as Alzheimer's, HIV, chronic pain, and malaria. Several natural drugs are under investigation in clinical trials, at present.

Pharmacometrics

Pharmacometrics is mathematical models of biology, pharmacology, disease, and physiology used to describe and quantify interactions between xenobiotics and patients (human and non-human), including beneficial effects and adverse effects. It is normally applied to quantify drug, disease and trial information to aid efficient drug development, regulatory decisions and rational drug treatment in patients.

Pharmacometrics uses models based on pharmacology, physiology and disease for quantitative analysis of interactions between drugs and patients. This involves Systems pharmacology, pharmacokinetics, pharmacodynamics and disease progression with a focus on populations and variability.

Mould and Upton provide an overview of basic concepts in population modeling, simulation, and model-based drug development.

A major focus of pharmacometrics is to understand variability in drug response. Variability may be predictable (e.g. due to differences in body weight or kidney function) or apparently unpredictable (a reflection of current lack of knowledge).

Types of Models

- Pharmacokinetics (PK): Models of pharmacokinetic processes.

- Pharmacodynamics (PD): Models of pharmacodynamic processes.

- Physiologically Based Pharmacokinetics: Physiologically based pharmacokinetic models

- Exposure-response: Exposure-response models describe the relationship between exposure (or pharmacokinetics), response (or pharmacodynamics) for both desired and undesired effects.

- Disease Progression: Disease progression models describe the time course of disease and placebo effects. Disease and exposure-response models are used to understand the relationship between treatment, biomarker changes and clinical outcomes.

- Trial: Trial models describe variations from the nominal trial protocol due to things such as patient dropout and lack of adherence to the dosing regimen.

Pharmacometrics uses models based on pharmacology, physiology and disease for quantitative analysis of interactions between drugs and patients. This involves pharmacokinetics, pharmacodynamics and disease progression with a focus on populations and variability, Pharmacometrics is defined as the science that quantifies drug, disease and trial information to aid efficient drug development, regulatory decisions and rational drug treatment in patients. Drug models describe the relationship between exposure, response for both desired and undesired effects. Disease models describe the time course of disease and placebo effects. Disease and drug models are used to understand the relationship between treatment, biomarker changes and clinical outcomes. Trial models describe variations from the nominal trial protocol due to things such as patient dropout and lack of adherence to the dosing regimen. A major focus of pharmacometrics is to understand variability in drug response. Variability may be predictable or apparently unpredictable.

Pharmacometric Modelling

An understanding of pharmacometric modelling and simulation, and how it can give insights into the dose–concentration–effect relationship, will be useful to all clinical pharmacists and pharmacologists.

Understanding the dose–concentration–effect relationship is a fundamental component of clinical pharmacology. Interpreting data arising from observations of this relationship requires the use of mathematical models; i.e. pharmacokinetic (PK) models to describe the relationship between dose and concentration and pharmacodynamic (PD) models describing the relationship between concentration and effect. Drug development requires several iterations of pharmacometric model-informed learning and confirming. This includes modelling to understand the dose–response in preclinical studies, deriving a safe dose for first-in-man, and the overall analysis of Phase I/II data to optimise the dose for safety and efficacy in Phase III pivotal trials. However, drug development is not the boundary at which PKPD understanding and application stops. PKPD concepts will be useful to anyone involved in the prescribing and administration of medicines for purposes such as determining off-label dosing in special populations, individualising dosing based on a measured biomarker (personalised medicine) and in determining whether lack of efficacy or unexpected toxicity maybe solved by adjusting the dose rather than the drug. In clinical investigator-led study design, PKPD can be used to ensure the optimal dose is used, and crucially to define the expected effect size, thereby ensuring power calculations are based on sound prior information. In the clinical setting the most likely people to hold sufficient expertise to advise on PKPD matters will be the pharmacists and clinical pharmacologists.

When a medicine is prescribed, the purpose is to derive an effect that usually evolves with time. Whilst the definition of a medicine now encompasses small molecules, biologics and gene therapy, there remains a fundamental requirement to understand the dose–response relationship in order to determine how much and how frequently to administer a treatment. Paracelsus, widely regarded as the founder of modern toxicology, wrote: "Poison is in everything the dosage makes it either a poison or a remedy". This should be considered regardless of the treatment in question: for example, marathon runners often poison themselves by drinking too much water 1. It is important to consider dosing in both clinical practice and research, which requires an understanding of pharmacokinetics (PK) and pharmacodynamics (PD).

The mathematical model is defined as an equation used to relate known covariates (dose given, time of dose, time of observations) with observed measurements. In the case of the PK 1 compartment intravenous bolus model, the concentration measured at time t is given by: $\hat{c}(t) = D/Ve^{-CL/Vt}$, where D is the known dose, V and CL are the model parameters volume of distribution and clearance, and ĉ(t) is the model prediction of concentration at some time t. Using this assumed mathematical model, the values of the parameters V and CL are sought that minimise the difference between the model prediction and observed concentrations; this is the statistical model, which in the simplest case of single subject data, is given by: $c(t) = \hat{c}(t) + \varepsilon$, where $c(t)$ is an observed concentration at time t, and ε denotes the deviation of the model prediction from the observation. Statistical modelling seeks to minimise the value of ε by searching for the optimal values of the model parameters (V and CL). All models are gross simplifications of the system under study, and so the goal of PKPD modelling is often to test a range of models to determine which fits best.

In clinical practice and research, the study of PK only is usually confined to a limited set of circumstances where the PD can be readily inferred from a measured concentration. An example of this is antimicrobial chemotherapy, where the relationship between the minimal inhibitory concentration (determined *in vitro*) is linked with maximum concentration (C_{max}), area under the (concentration–time) curve (AUC) or fraction of a dose interval is spent with concentrations above the minimal inhibitory concentration 2. In many situations one wishes to also model the PD in order to understand the full dose–concentration–effect relationship, or occasionally one may not have easy access to PK measures and seek to model the dose–response, otherwise known as K-PD models. PD can encompass a wide variety of measurement types, all of which can be described in mathematical terms with parameter values estimated using statistical modelling. In recent years, the term pharmacometrics has gained popularity. Pharmacometrics encompasses the analysis of PK and PD data, and then uses resulting models to make inferences (often using simulation) on optimum dosing for clinical trials or practice.

Mathematical and Statistical Models Required to Understand pharmacometric Data

Biological systems are inherently nonlinear, and defining a target exposure or concentration through simple observations of raw data can be difficult. For example, in a plot of the PK model-predicted remifentanil concentrations *vs.* observed mean arterial blood pressure (MAP) measurements have been made using data collected on a study in infants prior to craniofacial surgery 3. The anaesthetists in this study used remifentanil to control MAP in order to reduce bleeding in the operative field. The aim of this study was to therefore combine measurement of remifentanil PK with measures of MAP (PD) to estimate the parameters of a PKPD model that would be used to define a target concentration (along with appropriate dose to reach that concentration) to yield a 30% drop in MAP. Through simple observation of these data, defining an appropriate target concentration is challenging for two main reasons:

Firstly, hysteresis is clearly present in that the same effect (MAP) can be seen at different observed concentrations within a patient. This comes about due to the fact that circulating concentrations are in flux coupled to the delay in the drug reaching the site of action, binding to its target and eliciting its effect. Nonlinear mathematical PK and PD models coupled with an effect compartment model were used to describe this phenomenon, define the target effect site concentration, and then to suggest a dose yielding this concentration in a typical patient. Here the word *nonlinear* refers to the fact that the PK (a two-compartment model) and the PD (sigmoidal E_{max} model) were not expressed as linear $y = mx + c$ type models. The term *effect compartment* refers to an additional compartment with first order equilibration rate constant between it and the central compartment, which was used in the PD model to account for hysteresis.

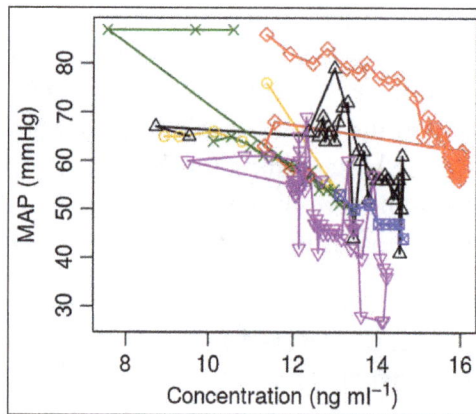

Model predicted remifenatanil concentration vs. mean arterial pressure (MAP) in infants prior to craniofacial surgery 3. Different symbols and colours represent data points from each patient.

The concept of a typical patient, or average expected response in the population of interest, brings us to the second challenge for interpreting these data: namely that there is a clear interindividual variability between patients. Ignoring the correlation between each individual's data points when fitting the PKPD model (the so-called naïve pooled approach) may bias parameter estimates and will inflate the amount of unexplained variability in the model. For this reason, mixed effects analysis, or the so-called *population approach*, must be used for parameter estimation during statistical model fitting.

Pharmacometric Modellers use to Inform Model Choices

Beware the mathematician or statistician who, upon seeing PK or PD data, questions the proposed pharmacological model and suggests an empirical alternative. At its extreme, statisticians are now suggesting multimodel approaches whereby several models are simultaneously fitted, the weight given to each model adjusted according to how well it fits the data 9. Whilst such approaches are undoubtedly useful for fitting and describing observed data, large sample sizes and exposure ranges will be required to characterise the population response and extrapolation outside the studied population will not be straight-forward without biologically interpretable parameters. By ignoring the extensive biological prior information that we, as pharmacologists, have on the system that generated the data, empirical modelling approaches are rarely useful for application in clinical settings where small datasets are available, and the goal is often to extrapolate findings in one population to another, to use findings of one study to plan another (the learning and confirming paradigm 10), or to apply findings to dose adjustment in direct patient care.

In the case of a physiologically-based PK (PBPK) model, with tissue volumes, blood flows and partition coefficients added to the model *a priori* rather than fitted to observed PK data, it is clear from where the biological priors come. However, even the simple 1-compartment PK model 11 parametrised with clearance (CL) and volume (V) carries biological interpretation.

The fact that CL is a parameter with units of volume per time, which match blood flows and glomerular filtration rates (GFRs) for example, and is related to the AUC through CL = dose/AUC allows one to leverage prior information. For example, the CL of tobramycin, which is eliminated primarily by glomerular filtration, in a typical 70 kg individual is around 140 ml min^{-1} 12, or slightly higher than a normal GFR. Say tobramycin was a new drug, and from its physicochemical properties (large polar molecule) and preclinical data (excreted unchanged in the urine) one knew it was likely to be excreted by glomerular filtration, first-in-man dosing could be rationally planned to attain target concentrations (recall that average concentration is given by $AUC_{(0-t)}/t$) in the desired nontoxic ranges, and it would come as no surprise to the pharmacologist to find CL to be similar to GFR in these studies. This biological prior knowledge would then allow dosing to be planned to attain target concentrations in subsequent studies in populations with different GFRs (e.g. elderly, hyperfiltrating ICU patients, children).

In the case of V, the apparent volume of distribution, whilst it does not represent the volume of an actual physiological compartment, biological prior information can still be utilised. For example, diclofenac is highly bound to plasma proteins, so it should come as no surprise that its estimated central V for a typical 70 kg individual is around 3.68 l 8, which is similar to normal plasma volume 13. For a highly protein bound drug such as diclofenac, one would expect V to have a linear relationship with body weight since blood volume is proportional to weight 13. For drugs with larger distribution volumes, particularly where partition to body fat maybe important in obese patients, models for predicting lean body weight or fat-free mass are now available for adults 14, 15 and children 16. Using biological prior information such as this can help to predict maximal concentrations and elimination half-lives in populations of interest.

With regard to PD models, there are two main considerations. The first is on the observed response, its time course and its type (usually a measured biomarker or clinical outcome such as disease score). The observed response will be heterogeneous and disease specific and whether biological prior information can be used to inform modelling is variable. For example, drug-induced neutropaenia has been successfully described using a mechanistic model of the simplified life-span of a neutrophil, with most cytotoxic chemotherapy agents acting on the proliferating precursor cells 17. On the other hand, sometimes PD endpoints are measured by a score (for example the Paediatric Crohn's Disease Activity Index 18) whereby the introduction of biological prior information on probabilistic PD models is less straightforward. The second consideration with PD models is the concentration–response effect at the site of drug action, which is then often used to drive the observed PD time course, often through an effect compartment, or using indirect response models 19. Here, the well-established Hill (or Emax) model is used, which can be derived from the law of mass action, and provides a mechanistic basis for the concentration–effect relationship.

Pharmacometric Models Scalling

In paediatrics, it is well established that smaller children need smaller doses, but this is often lost in the one-dose-fits all world of adult medicine. Adult clinical studies in high-profile journals often do not recognise that body size is an important determinant of drug exposure and consequently ought to be corrected for. This is particularly important for drugs requiring optimised exposure for effect (e.g. anti-infective agents) or those with a narrow therapeutic index. For example, Nijland et al 21 state that rifampicin exposure is *strongly reduced* in patients with type II diabetes whereas the majority of the difference in exposure between nondiabetics and Type II diabetics is explained by the Type II diabetics being heavier. Takahashi et al 22 meanwhile emphasised genetic differences as the major causative factor behind an observation that a cohort of African–American, Caucasian and Japanese patients needed different doses of warfarin. Body weights in these cohorts were not matched, and the African–American patients were heavier than the Caucasian patients, who in turn were heavier than the Japanese patients. Dividing the dose by the weight shows all ethnic groups in this study were on 0.06 mg kg^{-1}, and from the reported regression coefficients being heterozygous for any CYP2C9 polymorphism or VKORC1 1173 C > T has the same effect as a 55 kg or 42 kg difference in body weight, respectively. This poses the question as to why a flat 10 mg induction regimen is recommended in all adults whether they weigh 40 kg or 120 kg, whereas prescribers are warned about potential genotypic effects in the summary of product characteristics.

Accepting that PK scales with size, it is then important to consider how important PK parameters scale. In 1947, in his treatise on scaling of basal metabolic rate with size and it implications, Kleiber 23 stated:

> "For the dosage of drugs one should know whether or not the action depends on reaching a certain concentration in the blood stream without regard to its further maintenance. In this case the dosage should be proportional to body weight, since the amount of blood is proportional to body weight. If, however, the action of the biotic depends on the maintenance of a given concentration over a period of time, and if the rate of destruction or excretion of the biotic is proportional to the metabolic rate, then the dosage should be based on the metabolic body size."

In other words, volumes scale with linear body weight, and hence drugs for which a threshold concentration is required (e.g. aminoglycoside C_{max} targets) should be dosed by body weight, whereas, in the case of most drugs, where PD is driven by exposure (recall $AUC = dose/CL$) metabolic weight, meaning weight raised to a power of 3/4, should be used. This metabolic weight is quite similar to body surface area (weight raised to a power of 2/3) and paediatricians have long since known to dose narrow therapeutic index drugs by surface area 24. Scaling of clearance by metabolic weight does not only apply to small molecules, but also biologics 25. Here it must be noted that these principles apply to drugs with both linear and nonlinear pharmacokinetics, but with Michaelis–Menten elimination it is Vm that should scale allometrically, with Km constant across size and ages.

Returning to the linear PK case, this difference in the way that CL and V scale with size means that smaller people have shorter half-lives due to their proportionally higher CL and therefore elimination rate constant. gives an illustration of how CL, V and half-life are expected to vary with size and age according to the principles described above. Unfortunately, this subtlety was lost in a *British Medical Journal* study finding shorter caffeine half-lives (the paper incorrectly asserts half-life to be a proxy for CL) in pregnant women were associated with lower birth weights ($P = 0.06$), caffeine with its metabolites being somehow responsible for fetal growth restriction 26. There are three fundamental problems with the analysis of these data that would be spotted by a competent PK expert. Firstly, one cannot estimate half-life from oral PK data without also estimating an absorption rate constant (which might reasonably be fixed to a sensible value if no data in the absorption phase were gathered), V (to transform the dose input into a concentration) and CL (from which and V, the elimination rate constant can be derived along with half-life should one wish). The authors do not mention V or absorption rate constant, so immediately the reader will be concerned about how exactly half-life was estimated. The second problem is that empirical linear covariate analysis was done on half-life, including correlated items such as age and weight, without prior consideration of the biological system that derived the data. Caffeine is largely eliminated by CYP1A2-mediated hepatic metabolism 27 so one would expect larger individuals with larger livers to have a greater capacity for caffeine metabolism. Given the weight range reported, the caffeine half-life for the smallest woman would be approximately 20% shorter than that of the largest woman based on allometric principles, and this relationship would be nonlinear. Given that we therefore expect smaller women to have shorter half-lives, and given that birth weight and maternal weight are correlated so we expect smaller women to have smaller babies, ideally one would correct for size *a priori* to delineate this effect from other covariates of interest. Finally, half-life is a continuous variable yet the authors arbitrarily dichotomised the group **into** *fast* **and** *slow* finding a weak ($P = 0.06$) association between *fast* half-life and low birth weight. It would have been interesting to see whether this relationship would have held had CL been estimated and the test conducted on this continuous variable.

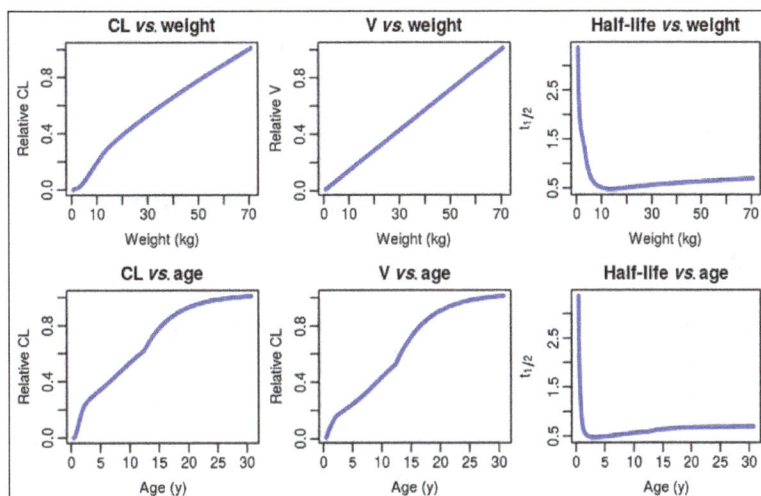

Illustration of the relative expected changes in clearance (CL) volume of distribution (V) and elimination half-life with weight (based on allometric principles) and age for the one-compartment intravenous bolus model. The standard value for weight here is set to 70 kg, so CL and V take the value 1.

Size scaling, when done properly as described above, tends to work well in children older than 2 years but, in younger patients, maturation of drug metabolising enzyme expression and glomerular filtration means that age needs to be taken into account. Various methods for size and age scaling are available, the most sensible of which was recently set out and proposed as a standard scaling method 28. Whilst size and age scaling are now well established for PK models, and it has been proposed in many cases that with proper PK scaling PD can be predicted in children 29, there are some PD endpoints (e.g. drug effects on the developing adaptive immune system 30) where size and age may need to be considered in PD modelling.

Population PKPD

The population approach when applied in pharmacometrics is used to refer to the statistical aspect of model fitting called mixed effects or multilevel modelling. By fitting models, the goal is to estimate the most likely values of parameters (e.g. CL and V) from a set of observed data (e.g. concentrations) along with known covariates (e.g. dose, time, body weight). Whilst the standard goal of model fitting by regression is to minimise a residual departure of model predictions from observed data points, since PKPD data include multiple data points from several individuals, it is necessary to account for the correlations of data points within individuals so as not to bias parameter estimates and inflate unexplained variability. For this reason, in addition to a data point level of variability, mixed effects modelling has a parameter level of variability, allowing parameters to vary between individuals. Population analysis can be used for rich or sparse data. The rule-of-thumb definition for rich data is at least as many samples per subject as model parameters, with fewer samples per subject than model parameters being called sparse data. This definition may, however, be too simplistic because the timing of samples can be more important than the total number. For example, multiple samples towards the end of an oral administration PK curve will give little information on volume and absorption parameters. It is now possible to use optimal design, a technique using a previous or assumed model, to define optimally informative sampling times so that data collected will give precise estimates of model parameters. The end result of a population pharmacometric model fitting exercise is a set of typical population model parameters, their variance, and the variance of the residual unexplained variability. This can then be used to generate new hypotheses (e.g. what will be the expected concentrations under different dosing conditions) or as a Bayesian prior for personalised medicine. There are several excellent reviews explaining the population approach to PKPD analysis.

Examples of Pharmacometric Models used in the Clinic

Dosing in Special Populations

Prescribing medicines outside the terms of their product license (off-label) is common in hospital-based settings, particularly in paediatrics. Often when this is the case it may be appropriate to adjust dosing and here the clinical pharmacist or pharmacologist with a sound understanding of PKPD principles will be able to help. An example of this arose in around 2009 when the infectious diseases team at Great Ormond Street Hospital wanted to use posaconazole, which was unlicensed in children. At the time, there were published PK data on only two children (aged 8 and 10 years) so to predict dosing in younger patients required extrapolation. It was known that posaconazole is hepatically metabolised (so CL should follow allometric 3/4 scaling) and that the major metabolic pathway was glucuronidation. The maturation of glucuronidation was known through studies on paracetamol and morphine. Assuming that the target exposure should be achieved by a dose achieving a similar AUC to the licensed adult dose (200 or 400 mg), simply multiplying this dose by a scaled typical weight for age and additionally the published maturation function (which takes values between 0 and 1, increasing with age) gave the following target doses to give a similar exposure to 200 mg in adults: neonates 1.5 mg kg^{-1}; infants aged 1 month-1 year 3 mg kg^{-1}; infants and children aged 1 year or over 4 mg kg^{-1} (maximum 200 mg). These doses were then put forward to be used in the hospital prescribing guidelines.

Personalised Medicine

The term personalised medicine, which in recent years has been hijacked by reductionist (pharmaco-)geneticists, can have two meanings. Firstly, there is stratified medicine, whereby treatment is personalised before a dose is given. Sometimes this might be a genetic or other clinical/biomarker that determines treatment choice, sometimes this might be a clinical/biomarker that determines treatment dose. Paediatricians practice this second type of stratified medicine every time a drug is prescribed, the dosing being based on weight, age or surface area. Population PKPD models can be used to identify important covariates that determine response, and this may include genetic or metabolomic markers alongside other factors, ideally informed by biological prior information.

The second interpretation of personalised medicine arises where a treatment is adjusted according to response (this may also be called individualised medicine). Typically, this is done with therapeutic drug monitoring, where the biomarker is drug concentration, although the biomarker can just as easily be a PD endpoint (e.g. International Normalized Ratio in response to warfarin). In this context, rather than empirically adjusting the dose until a target is reached, there is increasing interest in using population PKPD models as Bayesian priors, with the observed patient biomarker and covariate information being used to construct a posterior set of most likely individual model parameters to be used to predict/adjust future treatment. A wide range of software applications are now available for this, and applications beyond traditional therapeutic drug monitoring such as prediction of drug-induced neutropaenia and International Normalized Ratio under warfarin therapy.

Managing Overdose

PK principles are crucial in some overdose situations, most notably with paracetamol where a PK-derived nomogram is available to guide acetylcysteine therapy based on measured paracetamol concentration. The PKPD-literate clinical pharmacist or pharmacologist does not, however, need to limit advice giving solely to agents that have readily available nomograms. One example was a query received regarding persistent hypotension in a child following an accidental intravenous clonidine overdose. Using a published PKPD model linking clonidine and mean arterial pressure (MAP), the trajectory of the expected hypotensive time course given the dose received was easily plotted to show that resolution of the effect would be expected to take several more hours.

Examples of Pharmacometric Models in Clinical Pharmacology Research

Developing dosing Guidelines for a Clinical Trial

Pivotal clinical trials are often costly and time consuming so getting the dose right, particularly for narrow therapeutic index agents, is of critical importance. Whilst many pharmaceutical companies integrate PKPD information throughout early-phase development to get the dose right for Phase III, it is also important that investigator-led clinical studies are supported by clinical pharmacist or pharmacologist colleagues in study design. An example of this was during the design of a study to use insulin-like growth factor (IGF-1) in children with Crohn's disease. It was proposed that IGF-1 supplementation could be used to promote growth in adolescents with Crohn's disease and IGF-1 deficiency, but since high IGF-1 levels may be carcinogenic, it was important to ensure that the dosing would only correct levels up to the normal range and not too far beyond. A small PK study was performed in the target population, and covariate analysis showed that in addition to the biological priors of size and age (normal IGF-1 levels increase during adolescent growth), disease severity measured by the PCDAI was required to tailor dosing to endogenous IGF-1 production.

Defining the effect Size for a Clinical Trial

The number of patients recruited to a clinical trial is governed by the expected effect size of the tested treatment. In many cases, investigators make over-optimistic predictions on the expected effect size leading to trail failure due to inadequate sample size. This is an area where PKPD model predicted outcomes are underutilised. In the planning of a randomised double blind noninferiority trial of clonidine *vs.* midazolam for sedation in neonatal and paediatric intensive care, the clinician's estimate of successful sedation with midazolam (the control arm) was 85%, which led to a sample size of 90 (45 patients per group). The midazolam effect size was also evaluated through simulation of expected concentrations using the planned dose scheme, a published PK model, and a target PD concentration. This gave an expected sedation success rate of 75%, which meant the necessary sample size increased more than three-fold to 300 patients (150 per group), and indeed this more conservative effect size will be used in the proposed study.

Pharmacometric Model Parameters as Trial Endpoints

In the drive to make clinical trials more efficient, an interesting idea has recently been proposed whereby the drug effect parameter in a PKPD model could be used as a trial endpoint. Often trial endpoints are tested as being a biomarker or clinical observation at a specific, somewhat arbitrary time, whereas if a drug effect parameter were used, data from the whole response time course within a patient could be used. Using the example of a viral kinetic model in hepatitis C infection, Laouenan et al. showed that the power to detect a difference in drug effect between two competing therapies could in some circumstances increase study power by 10-fold as compared with using the single time-point outcome of change in viral load at Day 14 of treatment. For diseases where there are sufficient data to build a prior population PKPD model, this approach could be a paradigm for small investigator-led clinical trial design.

References

- Bitstream: inflibnet.ac.in, Retrieved 1 February, 2019

- Nordberg M, Duffus J, Templeton DM (1 January 2004). "Glossary of terms used in toxicokinetics (IUPAC Recommendations 2003)". Pure and Applied Chemistry. 76 (5): 1033–1082. Doi:10.1351/pac200476051033

- Importance-pharmacokinetics-testing-beginning-clinical-trials: pharmamodels.net, Retrieved 29 March, 2019

- Ashauer R. "Toxicokinetic-Toxicodynamic Models – Ecotoxicology and Models". Swiss Federal Institute of Aquatic Science and Technology. Archived from the originalon 2012-04-05. Retrieved 2011-12-03

- Luch A, ed. (2009). Molecular, clinical and environmental toxicology. Springer. P. 20. ISBN 978-3-7643-8335-0

- Importance-of-Pharmacognosy.aspx, health: news-medical.net, Retrieved 30 April, 2019

- Dhami, N. (2013). "Trends in Pharmacognosy: A modern science of natural medicines". Journal of Herbal Medicine. 3(4): 123–131. Doi:10.1016/j.hermed.2013.06.001

- Pharmacometrics, definition: definitions.net, Retrieved 31 May, 2019

- "Native American/Alaska Native Traditional Healing | aidsinfonet.org | The AIDS infonet". Www.aidsinfonet.org. Retrieved 2016-02-24

Compounds used in Medicinal Chemistry

3

- **Inorganic Compounds**
- **Organic Carbamates**

Some of the major compounds used in medicinal chemistry are inorganic compounds and organic carbamates. The chemical compounds that lack carbon-hydrogen bonds are known as inorganic compounds. Organic carbamates are the organic compounds which are derived from carbamic acid. The diverse uses of these compounds in medicinal chemistry have been thoroughly discussed in this chapter.

Inorganic Compounds

Neurological Agents

Lithium like alcohol can influence mood. Lithium drugs such as lithium carbonate $Li_2 Co_3$, are used for the treatment of manic-depressive disorders, most likely through an effect on the transmission of neuronal signals. Li(I) interferes with the biochemistry of Mg (II) which is of similar size. Lithium (I) acts as an uncompetitive inhibitor of inositol monophosphatase that hydrolyses inositol. phosphate into inositol and phosphate. According to the 'inositol depletion' theory of bipolar disorder treatment, the therapeutic effect of lithium is to block inositol recycling via inositol monophosphatase inhibition, and thus reduce inositol levels in the cell. Li+ blocks the release of the aquation product phosphate from the active site by binding to Mg-Inosine monophosphate and thereby forming MgLi -Inosine monophosphate, which is inactive. Glycogen synthase kinase-3 (GSK-3) is a critical, negative regulator of diverse signaling pathways. Growing evidence also suggests a link between GSK3, bipolar disorder, and the therapeutic effects of Li+. Li+ acts as a specific inhibitor of the GSK-3 family of protein kinases in vitro and in intact cells. For example, lithium is known to increase the inhibitory N-terminal phosphorylation of GSK-3, but the target of lithium responsible for this indirect regulation has not been identified.

Anticancer Agents

Metal compounds can bind tightly to biomolecules such as DNA to kill cancer cells. Cisplatin [cis-diamminedichloro platinum (II)], one of the leading metal-based drugs, is widely used in the treatment of testicular cancer. It is a neutral square planar complex of platinum (II). The mode of action of cisplatin is due to release of chloride ions on crossing cell membrane. Then a charged species is formed on hydrolysis, which is attracted to anionic DNA. For the drug to work according to the proposed mechanism, it must hydrolyze in the right place; if it hydrolyzes in the blood before it gets to the chromosomes within the cell, it will be more likely to react with the nontarget species. Fortunately for the stability of the complex, the blood has approximately O.lM in chloride ions, forcing the hydrolysis equilibrium back to the chloro complex. Once the drug crosses the cell membrane into the cytoplasm it finds a chloride ion concentration of only 4mM. The cytotoxicity of cisplatin originates from its binding to DNA through N_7 site of guanine and the formation of covalent cross-links involving 1,2-intrastrand d(GpG). Binding of cisplatin to DNA causes distortion of helical structure and results in inhibition of DNA replication and transcription. Platinum complexes that are currently in clinical use or approved for clinical use or in clinical trials are shown in figure.

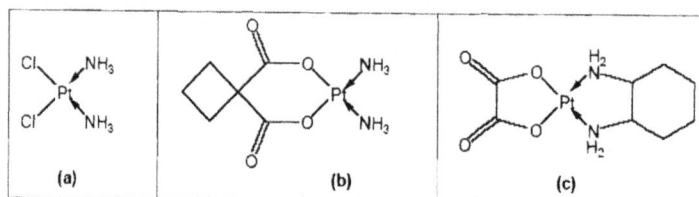

(a)　　　　(b)　　　　(c)

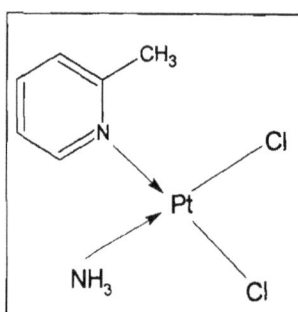

Cis-amminedichloro(2-methylpyridine) platinum(II) called ZD0473 is a new platinum based therapeutic compound to overcome resistance to standard platinum drugs mentioned above. The second class of multinuclear platinum complexes that bind to DNA in a manner different from that of cisplatin contain two, three or four platinum centers with both cis and/or trans configuration. A representative trinuclear complex BBR 3464 exhibits activity against pancreatic, lung and melanoma cancers. BBR 3464 is a highly charged (4+) species and binds to DNA. The interstrand cross-links appear to account for antitumour activity.

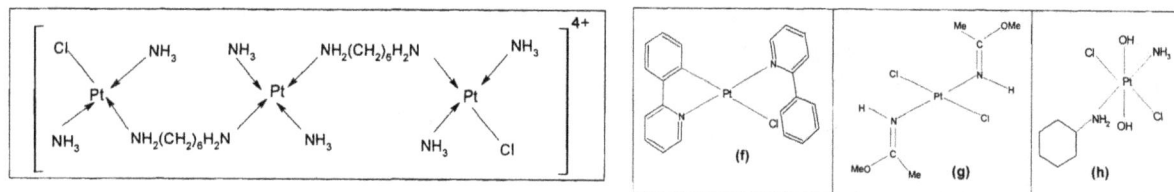

(f)　　　　(g)　　　　(h)

Monofunctional platinum(II) complexes with one normal and one cyc1ometalated 2-phenylpyridine ligand show high antitumour activity against cisplatin resistant cell lines. The trans analog of cisplatin (II) is inactive but substitution of one or both ammine ligands in trans-diamminedichloro platinum (II) with more bulky ligands such as planar aromatic amines, alkyl amines, imino ethers, piperidine, piperazine or 4- pi coline has displayed significantly cytotoxicity against cisplatin resistant cancer cells. Representative examples of trans complexes are shown in Figures Ig-h and these have different DNA binding modes from that of cisplatin.

During the recent years many ruthenium compounds were found to have very promising anti-cancer activity. Ruthenium complexes with oxidation state 2+ or 3+ display anti tumour activity. Due to the octahedral structure of Ru(lI) and Ru(III) complexes as opposed to the square-planar geometry of Pt(II), ruthenium anti tumour complexes probably function in a manner different-ly than cisplatin. The ruthenium (III) complexes namely Na trans-[Ru(Im)(Me$_2$ SO)CI$_4$], (ImH) trans- [Ru(Im) (Me$_2$SO)CI$_4$ and [Ru(II) (η^6- arene) (en)X]$^+$ display antitumour activity especially against metastatic cancers Ru(III) complexes tend to be more biologically inert than related Ru(II) complexes.

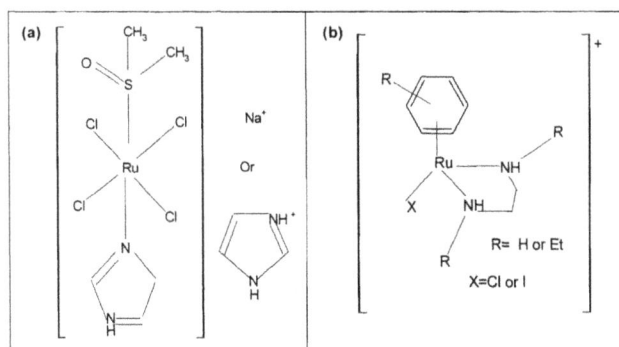

Interestingly, it has been demonstrated that Ru(II) complexes are far more reactive towards DNA than Ru(III) and it is therefore possible that the anticancer activity of Ru(III) involves initial reduction to Ru(II) at the tumour site, promoted by the altered physicochemical envi-ronment in tumour cells (vide supra). If this hypothesis is correct then Ru(III) complexes are essentially prodrugs1 In addition to DNA binding, ruthenium compounds interact with proteins including serum transferrin and albumin, and it is likely that both activities contribute to the anticancer properties of the compounds. Since tumors rapidly utilize oxygen and other nutri-ents and the development of new blood vessels (known as neovascularization or angiogenesis) often fails to keep pace with tumor growth, there is usually a lower o2 content (hypoxia) in tu-mor. Consequently, cancer cells depend more on glycolysis for energy and generate an excess of lactic acid, which lowers the pH in tumor cells. Due to these metabolic differences, the relative electrochemical potential inside tumors is generally lower than in the surrounding normal tis-sue, particularly at the center of the tumor. These differences in tumor relative to normal cell me-tabolism should favor the production of Ru(II) relative to Ru(III) in tumors, compared with normal tissue.

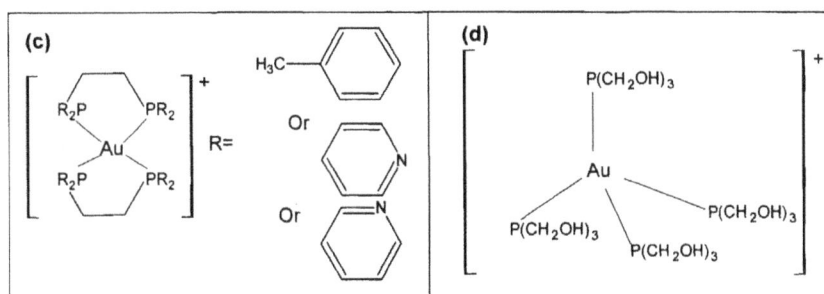

Tetrahedral gold (I) complexes with 1,2-bis-(diphenylphosphino) ethane; 1,2,-bis-(dipyridylphosphino)ethane; tetrakis-" tris (hydroxymethyl)-phosphine) gold (I) complex and chlorotriphenylphosphine-1,3-bis-(diphenyiphosphino) propane gold (I) complex display anti tumour activity. Their cytotoxicity is mediated by their ability to modify mitochondrial function and inhibit protein synthesis. Other examples include titanocene dichloride and bis (p-diketonato) Ti (IV) complex called budotitane.

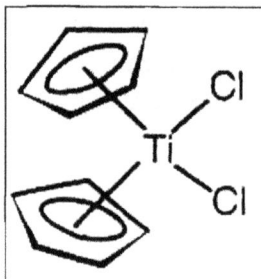

Antimicrobial Agents

EIrich in 1910 introduced 'Salvarsan' for the treatment of syphilis. A few other arsenic compounds namely tryparsamide (sodium Ncarbamoylmethylarsanilite), melarsen [N - (4,6- diamino-s-triazin-2-yl)arsanilic acid], diphetarsone (disodium N -N -ethylenediarsanilate) and puriodobenzenearsonic acid are being currently used for the treatment of trypanosome and amoeba mediated diseases. The therapeutic effectiveness of Salvarsan is due to its oxidized arsenoso compound, which is the active form. This form binds to sulphydryl (-SH) compounds present in and essential for microbial cells through covalent bond, and thus causes their toxic effect.

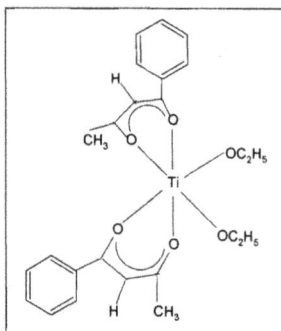

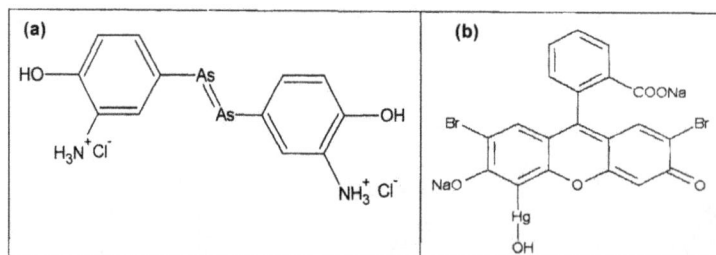

Mercurochrome, an organic mercury compound, in 2% aqueous solution is used as a topical antiseptic. The application of silver-containing solution to the burned skin is an effective protection against the cha~ge of second-degree burn (redness and blistering) into third degree burn (complete destruction of all layers of skin). Silver sulphadiazine, an insoluble polymeric compound releases Ag (I) ions slowly and is used clinically in the form of cream as an antimicrobial and antifungal agent to prevent bacterial infections in case of severe burns. This compound in colloidal silver form disables oxygen metabolism enzymes of virus, fungi, bacterium or any other single celled pathogen. Unlike pharmaceutical agents (for example sulfonamides) which destroy beneficial enzymes, colloidal silver leaves these tissue-cell enzymes intact. Antimony (V) drugs namely sodium stibogluconate and N-methylglucamine antimonate (Glucantime) are used clinically for the treatment of leishmaniasis, a disease caused by intracellular parasites.

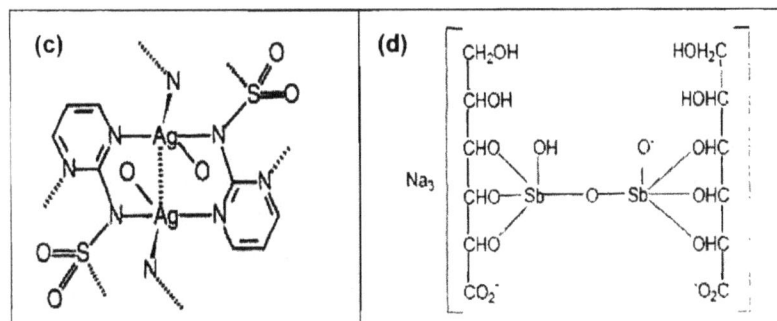

Nmethylglucamine antimonate has the same structure to that of sodium stibogluconate but with the CO_2^- groups being replaced by deprotonated $CH_2 N(H)CH_3$.

Antiviral Agents

Polyoxometallates, for example, $[NaW_{21}Sb_9O_{86}] [NH_4]_{17}$ and $K_{12}H_2[P_2W_{12}O_{48}]$. $24H_2O$ exhibit antiviral activity. These are nanoscale assemblies of early transition metals (for example, vanadium, tungsten, molybdenum) with oxygen to form a variety of cage-like structures. Being negatively charged, these compounds bind to positive patches of HIV gp120 blocking binding to lymphocyte CXCR4 receptor.

Anti-inflammatory Agents

Gold-based drugs prescribed for the treatment of rheumatoid arthritis are disease-modifying anti-rheumatoid drugs and are known to inhibit the progression of the disease and, in some cases, cause remission. Gold (I) is the most stable state in vivo and this fact has been used in the design of drugs of most of the gold compounds that have been approved for clinical use. There are two classes of gold (I) complexes used in chrysotherapy: (i) the gold (I) thiolates, and (ii) phosphine gold (I) thiolate. The representative examples of class 1 drugs are (a) Myocrisin, sodium aurothiomalate, (b) Solganol, aurothioglucose, (c) Allochrysine Limiere, sodium aurothiopropanol sulphonate, and (d) Sanocrysin, sodium aurothiosulphate.

The examples of class I drugs are generally polymeric complex (gold: ligand ratio of 1: 1) with linear Au (I) thiolate-S bridging. The second class comprises only one example namely, auranofin, triethylphosphino gold (I) tetraacetylatethioglucose. This drug is monomeric and gold atom exists as linear geometry. Aauranofin, in the presence of calcium ions, is a highly efficient inducer of mitochondrial membrane permeability transition, potentially referable to its inhibition of mitochondrial thioredoxin reductase.

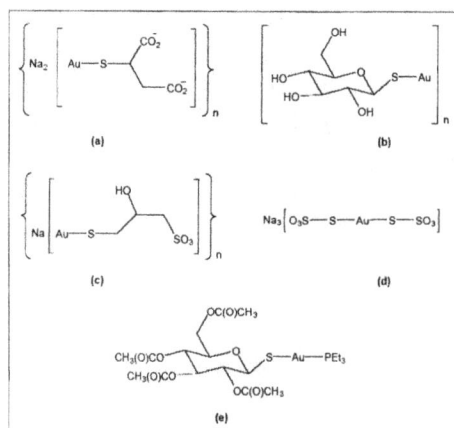

Basically gold drugs should be prodrugs, in that upon administration to patients, metabolism occurs with bond cleavage within the drug, which releases Au that is bonded to biologically relevant thiol and/or selenol groups. Selenols are able to bind some heavy metals more efficiently than thiols and, therefore, the selenocysteine of thioredoxin reductase appears as the target of organic gold inhibitors. Gold (I) compounds exhibit also a marked and specific reactivity with selenoenzymes such as glutathione peroxidase (GPx), iodothyronine deiodinase type I, and thioredoxin reductase; an enzyme recently shown to possess selenium at its catalytic site. Considering glutathione peroxidase, gold (I) derivatives such as aurothiomalate, aurothioglu- Figure. cose and auranofin have been shown to exert their inhibitory action by forming a glutathionate-gold (I)-selenocysteine glutathione peroxidase ternary complex (GPxSe-Au-SG). Gold drugs are almost certainly transformed inside the body into more active species. It was found that most of the gold in circulation had become protein bound. The small amount of gold left in plasma that could be identified was the dicyangold (I) anion [Au (CN) $_2^-$].

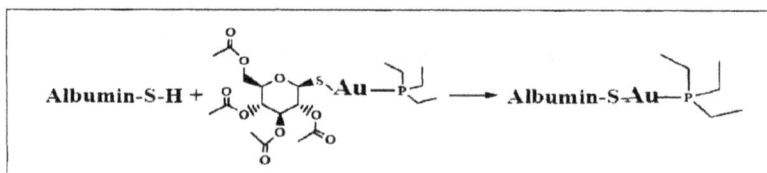

One target site is the abundant blood protein albumin, to which gold binds very specifically at a single amino acid residue, the sulfur atom at amino acid residue number 34. Gold bound to albumin circulates in blood and is delivered to cells and tissues where it can inhibit enzymes which break down joint tissue.

There are two possible mechanisms for interaction between dicyanogold (I) and serum albumin that retain a two-coordinate gold (I): covalent or electrostatic. A covalent binding mechanism similar to that observed for gold drugs would involve the loss of a cyanide ligand in order to bind to the sulfur of cysteine34. In an electrostatic binding mechanism, the dicyanogold (I) anion would bind intact to some positively charged region of the protein.

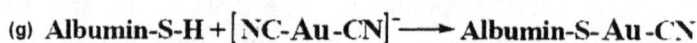

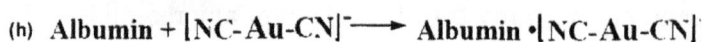

(g) Albumin-S-H + [NC-Au-CN]⁻ ⟶ Albumin-S-Au-CN

(h) Albumin + [NC-Au-CN]⁻ ⟶ Albumin •[NC-Au-CN]⁻

The other explanation relates to conversion of gold (I) administered in various drug formulations to aurocyanide and oxidized to gold (III) by the immune system.

Selenium is an essential micronutrient in all known forms of life; it is a component of the unusual amino acid selenocysteine. Selenium, long known to be an important dietary 'antioxidant', is now recognized as an essential component of the active sites of a number of enzymes, and several additional mammalian selenoproteins. Mammalian thioredoxin reductase (TrxR) enzymes are important selenoproteins that, together with Trx and additional Trx-dependent enzymes, carry out several antioxidant and redox regulatory roles in cells. These roles include synthesis of deoxyribonucleotides with ribonucleotide reductase, reduction of peroxides or oxidized methionine residues with peroxiredoxins or methionine sulfoxide reductases, respectively, regulation of several transcription factor or protein kinase activities, as well as regeneration of many low molecular weight antioxidant compounds.

Se deficiency is associated with two human diseases (Keshena disease and Kashimbeck disease). Keshena disease is cardiomyopathy where multifocal necrosis and fibrosis of the myocardium occurs, presenting with muscle weakness and myalgia. Kashimbeck disease is an endemic osteoarthropathy and is characterized by chronic osteoarthrosis affecting fingers, toes and long bones and is found in children aged between 5 and 12 years. It is a progressive disorder that results in deformity and growth retardation. These conditions are improved by administration of sodium selenite or selenomethionine.

Other synthetic selenium-containing compounds have been reported to be undergoing evaluation as potential pharmacological agents. Ebselen [2-phenyl-l,2-benzisoselenazol-3(2H)-one (PZ 511 DR3305)], a seleno-organic compound, which was designed to mimic the enzymatic activity of glutathione peroxidase, also reacts with peroxynitrite and can inhibit enzymes such as lipoxygenases, NO synthases, NADPH oxidase protein kinase C and H^+/K^+-ATPase.

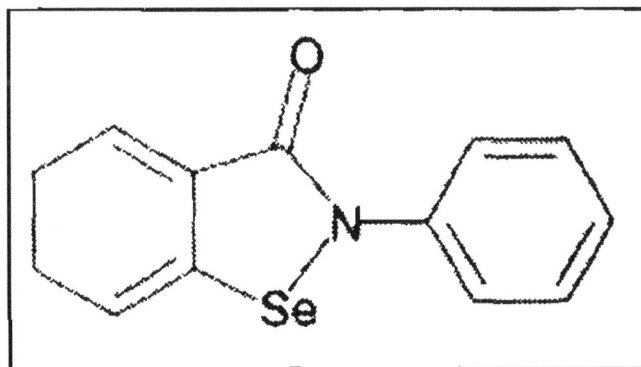

Ebselen is one of the promising synthetic antioxidants and a potential chemopreventive agent in inflammation-associated carcinogenesis and is currently undergoing clinical testing for the inhibition of stroke. Unlike many inorganic and aliphatic selenium compounds, Ebselen has low toxicity as metabolism of the compound does not liberate the selenium moiety, which remains within the ring structure. Both selenazofurin (2-P-Dri bofuranosylselenazole-4-carboxamide, selenazole), as an antineoplastic and antiviral agent, and selenotifen, as an anti-allergic agent, are examples of pharmacologically active figure organoselenium compounds that offer significant advantages over their corresponding sulfur analogs.

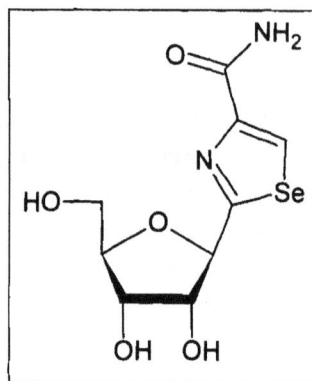

Cardiovascular Agents - Metal-based no Donors and Scavengers

NO is produced in the body and the physiological processes mediated by NO include neurotransmission, blood pressure regulation and immunological response. The low spin ferrous complex, sodium nitroprusside $Na_2[Fe(CN)_sNO]$ $2H_2O$ is often employed for the treatment of hypertension to lower blood pressure in human subjects. The therapeutic effect of this compound depends on release of nitric oxide (NO), which relaxes muscles. It is activated by reduction in vivo to [Fe(CN)sNOPin which an antibonding orbital becomes populated to facilitate the loss of NO. Ruthenium complexes exhibit both nitric oxide release and scavenging functions that can affect vasodilation. Structure of the ruthenium NO-releasing complex, trans- $[(NO)(P(OCH_2CH_3)(NH_3)_4Ru(II)]$ is shown in figure.

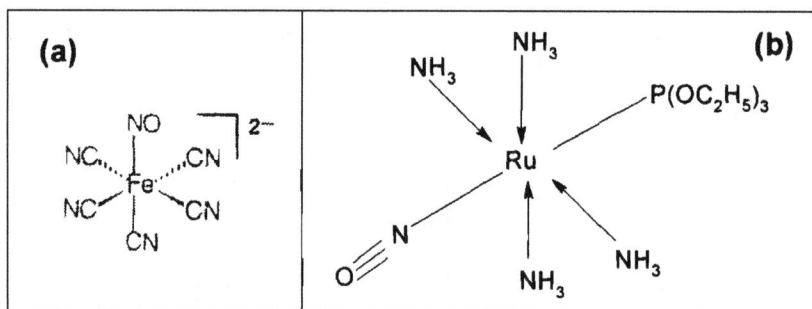

On the other hand, overproduction of NO contributes to diseases such as sepsis, arthritis, diabetes and epilepsy. Effective scavengers of NO, such as K[CI(EDT A)Ru(III)], may be useful in treating toxic shock syndrome by lowering the dangerously high level of NO in the bloodstream.

Insulin Mimetics

Vanadium supplementation has a potential role in maintaining blood glucose levels in diabetics. Bis (maltolato)-oxo-vanadium (IV) has been marketed as a dietary supplement and is chelated form of vanadyl ion. In the solid-state complex, it has five coordinate square pyramid geometry with the oxo-ligand in the axial position and trans maltolato ligands. It is neutral, water-soluble and 2-3 times more potent than vandadyl sulphate $VOSO_4$ .H_2O. Other vanadium compounds of promise are bis-(glycinato) oxovanadium (BGOV) and bis-(methylpicolinato) oxovanadium (IV). These compounds exert their action by regulating the cellular levels of tyrosine phosphorylation. In general, the vanadium insulin like behaviour seems to improve glucose management in insulindependent diabetes (Type I) while vanadium improves glucose tolerance and lower glucose levels in Type II diabetes.

Low-molecular weight chromium binding substance, a naturally occurring oligopeptide consisting of chromium (III), aspartic acid, glutamic acid, glycine and cysteine in 4:2:4:2:2 ratios activate insulin-dependent tyrosine protein kinase activity of insulin receptor.

Future Perspectives

There is enormous scope for the development of novel square planar gold (III) complexes for their anti tumour activity as gold (III) is isoelectronic with platinum (II) and forms square planar complexes similar to that of cisplatin. Moreover, gold (III) also offers more synthetic variability. The understanding of the physiological processing of metal complexes, chemical mechanisms underlying cleavage of RNA and DNA targets and the application of combinatorial chemistry may be helpful for the development of inorganic drugs. The coming years should be an exciting time for inorganic drugs.

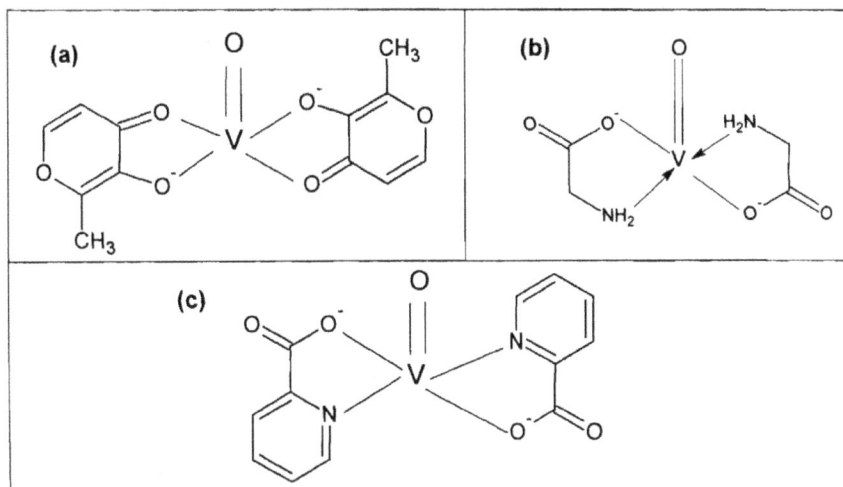

Organic Carbamates

Organic carbamates (or urethanes) are structural elements of many approved therapeutic agents. Structurally, the carbamate functionality is related to amide-ester hybrid features and, in general, displays very good chemical and proteolytic stabilities. Carbamates are widely utilized as a peptide bond surrogate in medicinal chemistry. This is mainly due to their chemical stability and capability to permeate cell membranes. Another unique feature of carbamates is their ability to modulate inter- and intramolecular interactions with the target enzymes or receptors. The carbamate functionality imposes a degree of conformational restriction due to the delocalization of nonbonded electrons on nitrogen into the carboxyl moiety. In addition, the carbamate functionality participates in hydrogen bonding through the carboxyl group and the backbone NH. Therefore, substitution on the O- and N-termini of a carbamate offers opportunities for modulation of biological properties and improvement in stability and pharmacokinetic properties.

Carbamates have been manipulated for use in the design of prodrugs as a means of achieving first-pass and systemic hydrolytic stability. Carbamate derivatives are widely represented in agricultural chemicals, such as pesticides, fungicides, and herbicides. They play a major role in the chemical and paint industry as starting materials, intermediates, and solvents. Furthermore, organic carbamates serve a very important role as optimum protecting groups for amines and amino acids in organic synthesis and peptide chemistry.

Peptide-based molecules are an important starting point for drug discovery, especially in the design of enzyme inhibitors. Because of their high affinity and specificity toward biological functions, peptide-based molecules also serve as valuable research tools. However, the poor *in vivo* stability, inadequate pharmacokinetic properties, and low bioavailability have generally limited their broader utility. Hence, a variety of peptide mimics are being developed to improve drug-like character along with increased potency, target specificity, and longer duration of action. To this end, several classes of peptidomimetics are tailored by replacing the native amide bond with unnatural linkages such as retro-amide, urea, carbamate, and heterocycles as peptide bond surrogates. These functionalities confer metabolic stability toward aminopeptidases, the enzymes involved in the metabolism of peptide-like drugs. The carbamate's emerging role in medicinal chemistry is also due to its chemical stability and to its capability to increase permeability across cellular membranes. These attributes of organic carbamates have been exploited in drug design. As a result, the carbamate motif is becoming the choice for peptide bond surrogates.

Other uses of carbamates are well-known. Particularly, the employment of carbamates in various industries as agrochemicals, in the polymer industry, and also in peptide syntheses. In addition, among the various amine-protecting groups, carbamates are commonly used to enhance their chemical stability toward acids, bases, and hydrogenation.

One important feature of organic carbamates is represented by the amide resonance. The amide resonance in carbamates has been studied in detail employing both experimental and theoretical methods by estimating the C–N bond rotational barriers. The amide resonance in carbamates has been shown to be about 3–4 kcal mol^{-1} lower than those of amides, owing to the steric and electronic perturbations due to the additional oxygen. Three possible resonance structures (A, B, and C, figure) contribute to the stabilization of the carbamate moiety.

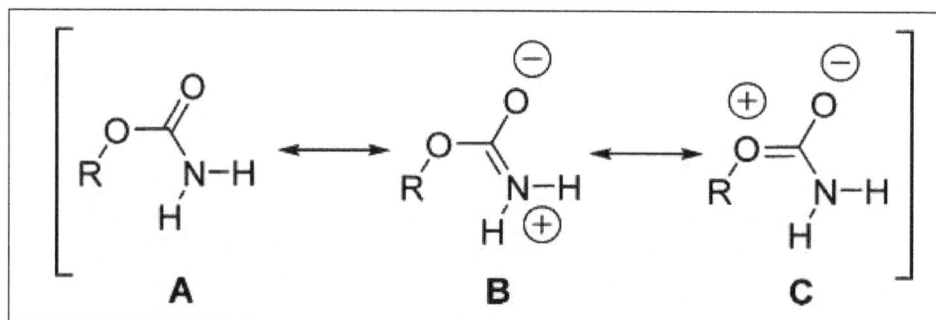

Possible resonance structures for the carbamate moiety.

Carbamate motifs are characterized by a pseudo double bond. This implies the potential deconjugation of the heteroatom-(σ-bond)-carbon-(π-bond)-heteroatom system that restricts the free rotation about the formal single σ-bond. Therefore, two isomers, *syn* and *anti*, may coexist in carbamates.

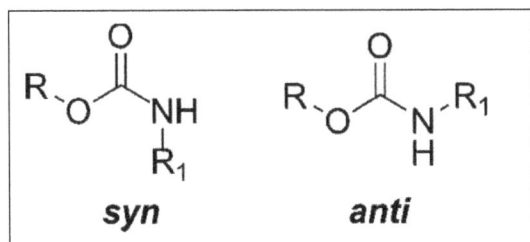

Syn and *anti* conformations of carbamates.

Although carbamates display close similarity to amides, they show preference for the *anti*-isomer conformation. The *anti* rotamer is usually favored by 1.0–1.5 kcal mol^{-1} for steric and electrostatic reasons with respect to the *syn* counterpart. In many cases, the energy difference may be close to zero. As a result, those carbamates are found as an approximately 50:50 mixture of *syn* and *anti* isomers, as in the case of a number of Boc-protected amino acid derivatives. This issue is of key importance since this balanced rotamer equilibria and the low activation energies render carbamates as optimal conformational switches in molecular devices.

The influence of the R and R$_1$ substituents on the free-energy difference between the two conformations has been investigated. Beyond steric effects, electronegativity of R$_1$ must be considered since it may affect the conformation in many ways, including changes in the dipole moment and bond angles. Only the *anti* conformation would be expected in five-, six-, and seven-membered cyclic carbamates. Calculations of the dipole moment for the carbamate group support this expectation. Solvent, concentration, salts, and pH strongly influence the free energy difference of the *syn* and *anti* isomers of carbamates as well. Intra- and intermolecular hydrogen bonding may also perturb the *syn–anti* isomer equilibrium of carbamates.

A representative example of hydrogen bonding and concentration dependence was provided by Gottlieb, Nudelman, and collaborators. The authors took into consideration *N*-Boc-amino acids and their corresponding methyl esters. An unusual abundance of *syn*-rotamer for *N*-Boc-amino acids was detected. *N*-Boc-amino acid esters give the expected spectra, consistent with previous reports of only a single species being observed at room temperature. Concentration-dependent ^{1}H NMR spectra indicate that the proportion of the *syn*-rotamers increases with concentration, supporting the existence of an aggregation process.

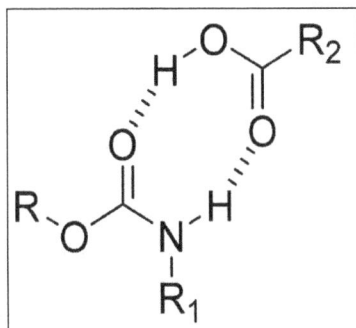

Possible dimer between a *syn*-carbamate and an acid group.

Since decreasing temperature is another method for stabilizing oligomerization, NMR experiments were also performed at different temperatures. As expected, when the temperature increases, the favored rotamer switches from *syn* to *anti*. Overall, the collected data strongly supports the concept that the *syn* rotamers of *N*-carbamoylated amino acids form intermolecularly H-bonded species and the OH of the carboxylic acid must be involved in this process, as the corresponding esters do not behave similarly. To explain this phenomenon, the formation of a dimer was suggested.

Support of this hypothesis was provided by adding increasing amounts of acetic acid to a solution of a carbamoylated amino acid ester. As expected, the *syn*rotamer appeared, and its concentration increased as a function of the amount of acid added. In contrast, addition of acetic acid to a solution of the corresponding carbamoylated amino acid did not affect the *anti/syn* ratio. In this context, Moraczewski and co-workers designed a more effective hydrogen-bonding system that selectively perturbs the *syn/anti* rotamer equilibrium of a target carbamate group. The authors examined the abilities of acetic acid and 2,6-bis(octylamido)pyridine (3) to perturb the *syn/anti* ratio of carbamates 1 and 2.

In a CDCl$_3$ solution, acetic acid moderately stabilizes double hydrogen bonding of the *syn* rotamer of phenyl carbamate 1 , with no relevant effect on the syn/anti ratio for 2-pyridyl carbamate 2. In the second case, the carboxylic acid favors donation of a hydrogen bond to the more basic pyridyl nitrogen and forms the complex shown in Figure. On the contrary, in the case of the donor–acceptor–donor triad 3, it strongly stabilizes the syn rotamer of 2 over the *anti* rotamer. There is no effect on the *syn/anti* ratio for 1, presumably because of a steric deterrent to the formation of a hydrogen-bonded complex.

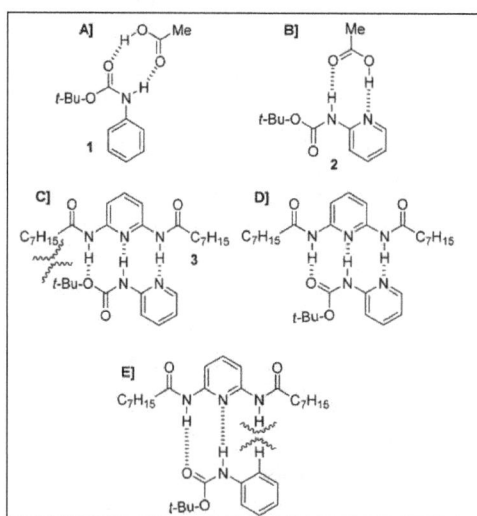

(A) *Syn*-carbamate of 1 is stabilized by hydrogen bonding with acetic acid; (B) acetic acid is associated with the *anti* rotamer of 2; (C) association of 3with anti-rotamer of 2; (D) association of 3 with the syn-rotamer (preferred); (E) association of 3 with the syn rotamer of 1 is disfavored.

The carbamate moiety plays a noteworthy role in medicinal chemistry, not only because it is found in drugs but also for its presence in a number of prodrugs. The rate and level of their hydrolysis is a key issue for the duration and intensity of their pharmacological activity. Fast hydrolysis of carbamate-bearing drugs may result in weak or shortened activity. On the contrary, carbamate-based prodrugs must undergo extensive hydrolysis at a suitable rate for releasing an active drug and obtaining the expected activity profile.

Vacondio et al. recently proposed an interesting study in which they compiled a large number of reliable literature data on the metabolic hydrolysis of therapeutic carbamates. The authors were able to exploit the collected data to gain a qualitative relationship between molecular structure and lability to metabolic hydrolysis. A trend was extrapolated, according to which the metabolic lability of carbamates decreased in the following series: aryl-OCO-NHalkyl ≫ alkyl-OCO-NHalkyl ~ alkyl-OCO-N(alkyl)$_2$ ≥ alkyl-OCO-N(endocyclic) ≥ aryl-OCO-N(alkyl)$_2$ ~ aryl-OCO-N(endocyclic) ≥ alkyl-OCO-NHAryl ~ alkyl-OCO-NHacyl ≫ alkyl-OCO-NH$_2$ > cyclic carbamates. Therefore, carbamates derived from ammonia or aliphatic amines are sufficiently long-lived. An example is represented by cefoxitin (4), a second-generation cephalosporin antibiotic. Cyclic five- or six-membered carbamates are quite stable and do not usually undergo metabolic ring opening. The antibacterial agent linezolid (5) is a representative example of this class. For these drugs, carbamate hydrolysis is not necessarily the half-life-determining metabolic reaction. On the contrary, fatty acid amide hydrolase (FAAH) inhibitor 6 (URB524) showed significant hydrolysis in buffer at physiological pH after 24 h.

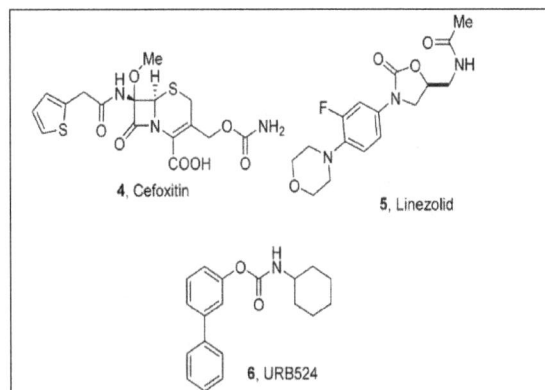

Example of carbamate drugs displaying different metabolic stability.

Methods for the Synthesis of Carbamates

Organic carbamates play an important role in organic synthesis, especially as subunits of biologically active compounds. Accordingly, simple and efficient methods for the synthesis of carbamates are of great interest. A number of methods have been developed for the synthesis of carbamates.

Carbamate Synthesis via Traditional Methods

Over the years, a variety of carabamates have been prepared by utilizing the Hofmann rearrangement of amides, the Curtius rearrangement of acyl azides, the reductive carbonylation of nitroaromatics, the carbonylation of amines, the reaction of alcohols with isocyanates, and carbon dioxide alkylation.

The Hofmann rearrangement is well-recognized as a useful method to convert primary carboxamides to amines or carbamates, characterized by the reduction of one carbon in the structure. Much effort has been devoted to the development of modified reagents to optimize the Hofmann rearrangement since the classical method for this transformation, involving the use of an alkaline solution of bromine, is unsatisfactory and unreliable. A variety of oxidants and bases have been proposed as modified agents, e.g., iodine(III) reagents such as PhI(OAc)$_2$, MeOBr, NBS-CH$_3$ONa, NBS-KOH, lead tetraacetate, and benzyltrimethylammonium tribromide. These modified methods, however, require more than 1 equiv or an excess amount of the oxidizing reagent, which is not very convenient.

The Curtius rearrangement is the thermal decomposition of acyl azides into the isocyanate intermediate. This method is widely employed in the transformation of carboxylic acids into carbamates and ureas. Acyl azides are usually prepared from carboxylic acid derivatives such as acyl chlorides, mixed anhydrides, and hydrazides. Subsequent isocyanate intermediates can be trapped by a variety of nucleophiles to provide the carbamate derivatives. The acid chloride method is not suitable for acid-sensitive functionalities. One-pot transformations of carboxylic acids into carbamates avoids the isolation of unstable acyl azides. However, protocols involving the use of diphenylphosphoryl azide (DPPA) for the one-pot Curtius reaction are also characterized by issues related to toxicity and the high boiling point of DPPA, which creates difficulties during workup and purification. Other general methods for carbamate preparation involve the use of the highly toxic phosgene, phosgene derivatives, or isocyanates.

Significant efforts have been made to find an alternative to the phosgene process. A very attractive substitute for phosgene is carbon dioxide because it is a classic renewable resource. In addition, its use is also very attractive due to its environmentally benign nature (nontoxic, noncorrosive, and nonflammable). Carbon dioxide is well-known to react rapidly with amines to form carbamic acid ammonium salts. The majority of the approaches in this context rely on the creation of the carbamate anion via the reaction of carbon dioxide and amines, followed by the reaction with electrophiles. Nevertheless, since the nucleophilicity of the carbamate anion is lower than that of the amine formed in the equilibrium of the salt formation, the subsequent reaction of the carbamate salts with alkyl halides does not selectively provide urethanes.

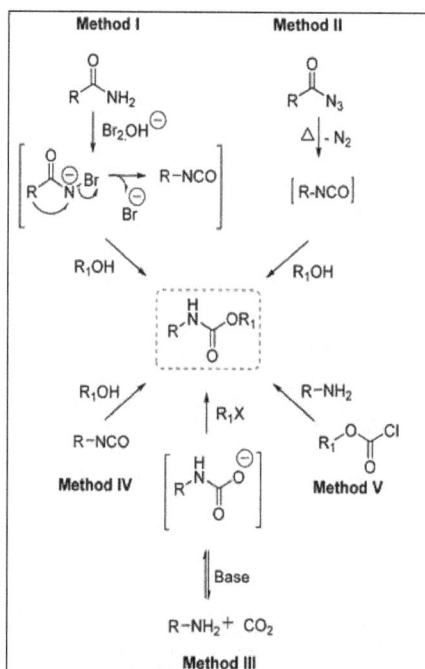

Traditional Synthetic Methodologies Adopted for the Synthesis of Carbamates.

The formation of carbamates from isocyanates is fundamentally important to polyurethane industries. Synthetic limitations and toxicity issues, however, are associated with the use of phosgene, the most common route to obtain isocyanates. The readily available alkyl chloroformates are the most frequently used reagents for the preparation of carbamates. However, these reagents display major drawbacks, as a large excess of base and a long reaction time are required in order to gain acceptable reaction efficiency. Moreover, excess reagents are not suitable for the synthesis of molecules bearing multiple functionalities in which the chemoselectivity is critical.

Carbamate Synthesis via Activated Mixed Carbonates

A number of organic carbonates have been developed as low-cost and benign alternatives to the phosgene-based routes for the synthesis of organic carbamates. In this context, several new alkoxy-carbonylating agents (7–11) based on mixed carbonates have been developed. These methods are often used for the synthesis of carbamates in drug design.

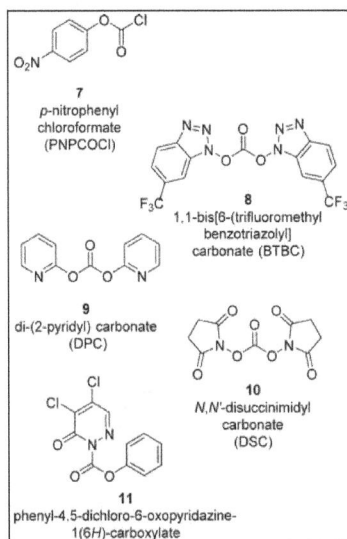

Most commonly employed carbonate reagents for carbamate synthesis.

Mixed carbonates with a *p*-nitrophenyl moiety are frequently used for the preparation of a large range of carbamates. For this, *p*-nitrophenyl chloroformate (7, PNPCOCl), when treated with the suitable alcohol in the presence of base, furnishes the corresponding activated carbonates, which have been shown to be useful and effective alkoxycarbonylating reagents for suitable amines. Examples of carbamate derivatives are shown in table.

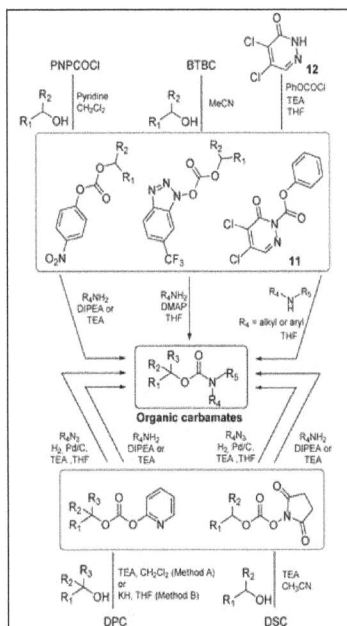

Carbamate Synthesis via Activated Mixed Carbonates (Highlighted in the Red Box).

Table: Examples of Carbamate Formation from **p**-Nitrophenyl-Based Mixed Carbonates.

Several alkoxycarbonylating reagents for amino groups having heterocyclic groups, such as *N*-hydroxyimide, have been reported. Moreover, the utility and versatility of carbonates and oxalates containing an electron-withdrawing group, such as *N*-hydroxyimide and benzotriazole derivatives as reagents for various tranformations, have been described.

Takeda et al. reported that 1-alkoxy[6-(trifluoromethyl)benzotriazolyl]carbonates easily derived from 1,1-bis[6-(trifluoromethyl)benzotriazolyl]carbonate (**8**, BTBC) showed high acylating reactivity toward alcohols as well as amino groups. BTBC was prepared from 6-trifluoromethyl-1-hydroxybenzotriazole and trichloromethyl chloroformate and purified by washing with dry ether. Moreover, it can be stored for several months in a freezer. BTBC was allowed to react with primary alcohols in acetonitrile at room temperature to give stable activated carbonates. The carbonates were treated with amines in the presence of 4-dimethylaminopyridine (DMAP), providing the corresponding carbamates.

Table. Examples of Carbamate Formation from 1,1-Bis[6-(trifluoromethyl)benzotriazolyl] Mixed Carbonates

In connection with our research work aimed at synthesizing biologically active polyfunctional molecules for probing enzyme active sites, we required a more general and synthetically reliable method for the synthesis of various carbamate derivatives. In 1991, we described the utility of di(2-pyridyl) carbonate (9, DPC) as an efficient, high-yielding, and convenient alkoxycarbonylation reagent for amines overcoming many of the limitations of existing methodologies. DPC was readily prepared from commercially available 2-hydroxypyridine and triphosgene in the presence of triethylamine and subsequently reacted with the suitable primary or secondary alcohol (e.g., (+)-menthol) to provide a mixed carbonate. Alkoxycarbonylation of primary and secondary amines with the mixed carbonates was carried out in the presence of triethylamine and furnished the corresponding carbamates in good yields. Potassium hydride was used in the place of triethylamine in the preparation of the mixed carbonates containing tertiary alcohols.

Table: Examples of Carbamate Formation from 2-Pyridyl-Based Mixed Carbonates.

Entry	Alcohol	Amine	Carbamate	Method	Yield (%)
1	35	36	37	A	81
2	35	38	39	A	70
3	40	38	41	B	68

Subsequently, we investigated the scope of *N,N'*-disuccinimidyl carbonate (10, DSC) promoted alkoxycarbonylation of amines with a host of alcohols under mild conditions. Rich and co-workers highlighted the convenience of succinimidyl-based mixed carbonates for the high-yielding introduction of a 2-(trimethylsilyl)ethoxycarbonyl (Teoc) protecting group to amino acids, without oligopeptide byproduct formation. DSC was found to be a highly effective alkoxycarbonylating reagent for a variety of primary and sterically hindered secondary alcohols. DSC is commercially available, or it can be conveniently prepared from *N*-hydroxysuccinimide following a procedure tracing out the synthesis of DPC. The ready availability of DSC, the stability of the mixed carbonates, and the mildness of the reaction procedure render this method a reliable route to organic carbamates.

Since azides were extensively employed as incipient amines in the context of amino sugar and amino acid syntheses, their conversion into the corresponding carbamate derivatives could provide a novel, effective route for medicinal chemistry applications. In this context, a facile synthetic protocol to transform various azides into the corresponding functionalized urethanes in high yields has been developed. In general, mixed carbonates of variously protected alcohols were prepared by reaction of excess DSC or DPC. Exposure of mixed carbonates to catalytic hydrogenation conditions with azides in the presence of 10% palladium on charcoal in tetrahydrofuran furnished the corresponding carbamates. Interestingly, the use of triethylamine as a promoter has a notable effect on the yield and the rate of the alkoxycarbonylation process.

Table: Examples of Carbamate Formation from N,N′-Disuccinimidyl-Based Mixed Carbonates.

Table: Examples of Carbamate Formation from Mixed Carbonates and Azides.

More recently, Yoon and co-workers exploited 2-substituted-pyridazin-3(2H)-ones as electrophilic transfer reagents. the carbonylation potency of phenyl 4,5-dichloro-6-oxopyridazine-1(6H)-carboxylate (11) to amines for the preparation of phenylcarbamates. Compound 11 is stable in air and in organic solvents at high temperature and is prepared easily from cheap and commercially available 4,5-dichloropyridazin-3(2H)-one (12) in the presence of phenylchloroformate and triethylamine.

Table: Examples of Carbamate Formation from Phenyl 4,5-Dichloro-6-oxopyridazine-1(6H)-carboxylate

Entry	Amine	Carbamate	Yield (%)
1	60	61	95
2	62	63	93
3	64	65	98
4	66	67	94

Recent Methodologies for Carbamate Synthesis

The application of carbon dioxide in organic synthesis has recently attracted much interest. Most of the approaches rely on the generation of the carbamate anion via the reaction of carbon dioxide and amines, followed by the reaction with electrophiles, usually alkyl halides.

In this context, a mild and efficient preparation of alkyl carbamates on solid supports was described by Jung et al. Amines and anilines were coupled with Merrifield's resin through a CO_2 linker in the presence of cesium carbonate and tetrabutylammonium iodide (TBAI). Carbon dioxide was supplied by bubbling it into the reaction suspension, where N,N-dimethylformamide (DMF) was the solvent of choice.

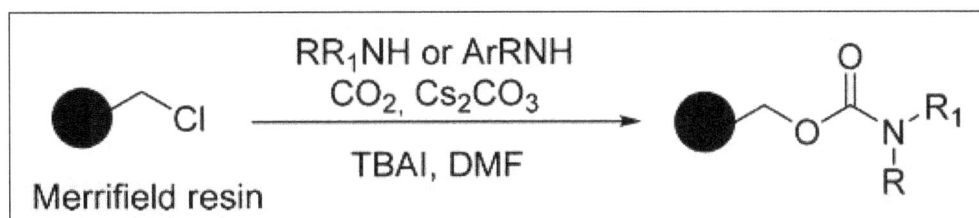

Scheme. Solid-Phase Synthesis of Carbamates Using Aromatic Amines and Merrifield Resin

The reaction conditions are convenient for purification, and the reactions undergo complete conversions. The method is convenient for the generation of large combinatorial libraries for rapid screening of bioactive molecules. Chiral substrates susceptible to racemization have survived the conditions.

Table: Solid-Phase Synthesis of Carbamates Using Merrifield Resin with Primary and Secondary Amines and Anilines.

Entry	Amine	Carbamate	Yield (%)
1	**68**		90
2	**69**		73
3	**70**		95
4	**71**		97

One-pot synthesis of *N*-alkyl carbamates starting from primary amines. Carbamates were generated via a three-component coupling of primary amines, CO_2, and an alkyl halide in the presence of cesium carbonate and TBAI in anhydrous DMF.

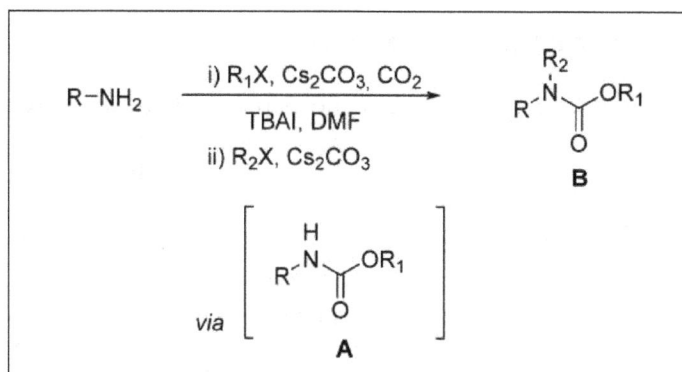

Synthesis of *N*-Alkyl Carbamates by a Three-Component Coupling of Primary Amines, CO_2, and an Alkyl Halide in the Presence of Cesium Carbonate and TBAI.

Direct *N*-alkylation of the intermediate carbamate A in the presence of additional cesium carbonate by using a different alkyl halide gave rise to the desired *N*-alkyl carbamate B. Isolation of the intermediate A proved to be unnecessary, offering shortened synthetic sequences. It is interesting to note that TBAI helps to minimize the overalkylation of the produced carbamate, presumably by enhancing the rate of CO_2 incorporation and/or stabilizing the incipient carbamate anion through conjugation with the tetrabutylammonium cation.

Sakakura and co-workers reported urethane synthesis by the reaction of dense carbon dioxide with amines and alcohols by a procedure that is not only phosgene-free but also completely halogen-free Dialkyl carbonate synthesis from an alcohol and CO_2 is catalyzed by metal complexes such as dialkyl(oxo)tin and dialkyl(dichloro)tin. However, the alcohol conversion is very poor.

Similarly, the direct reaction of an amine, an alcohol, and carbon dioxide in the presence of dialkyltin compounds produced urethane only in a poor yield.

Table: One-Pot Synthesis of **N**-Alkyl Carbamates Starting from Primary Amines.

Entry	Amine	R$_1$X	R$_2$X	Carbamate	Yield (%)
1	**72**	MeI, **73**	**74**	**75**	87
2	rac-**69**	**76**	**74**	**77**	75
3	**64**	**76**	**74**	**78**	72
4	**79**	**76**	**80**	**81**	62

The low conversion observed was attributed to thermodynamic limitations and catalyst deactivation by coproduced water. In order to overcome this issue, a new reaction system utilizing acetals as a chemical dehydrating agent, with subsequent alcohol regeneration, was developed.

In order to obtain urethane in good yields, dense-phase CO$_2$ under high pressure was necessary to lower the major side reactions, namely imine formation from acetone and alkylation of amines by alcohols.

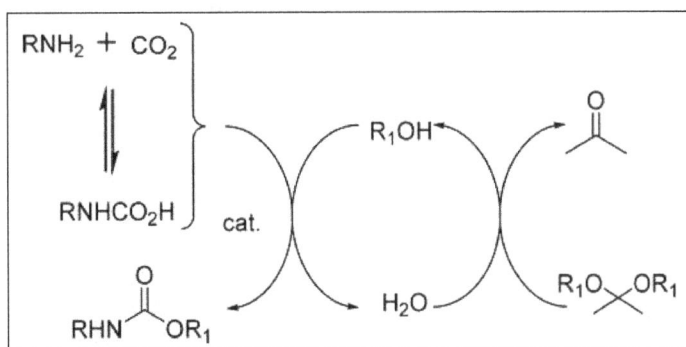

Halogen-Free Carbamate Synthesis Employing Dense Carbon Dioxide in the Presence of Amines and Alcohols.

However, developing less toxic and more active catalysts based on metals other than tin was required. Interestingly, adding nitrogen-based bidentate ligands efficiently improved the catalytic activity of Ni(OAc)$_2$-based catalysts. Bipyridines and phenanthrolines with strong coordinating abilities (low steric hindrance and high electron densities) were the better choice for obtaining urethanes in high yields. It is important to note that the Ni-phenanthroline system is more active and less toxic than dialkyl(oxo)tin under the same reaction conditions. It is also noteworthy that the catalytic activity of the Ni(OAc)$_2$-(4,4′-dimethylbipyridine) system is highly dependent on the ligand/metal ratio.

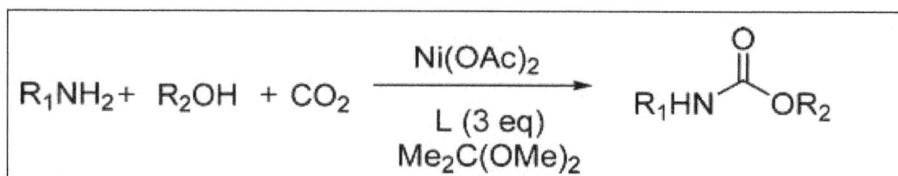

Ni-Based Catalytic Systems for Dehydrative Urethane Formation from Carbon Dioxide, Amine, and Alcohol.

Table: Nickel-Catalyzed Urethane Synthesis from CO$_2$.

Entry	Amine	Alcohol	Ligand (L)	Carbamate	Conv.[a] (%)	Select.[b] (%)
1	CyNH$_2$ 82	MeOH	84	85, CyNHCOOMe	83	81
2	t-BuNH$_2$ 83	MeOH	86	87, t-BuNHCOOMe	44	94
3	83	MeOH	88	87	18	34[c]
4	83	MeOH	88	87	41	100[d]

Peterson and co-workers proposed a method for rapid SAR development of compounds bearing urea or carbamate functionalities For carbamate formation, an amine, in principle, could proceed through the carbamic acid–isocyanate reaction, and subsequent reaction with an alcohol may provide a carbamate product.

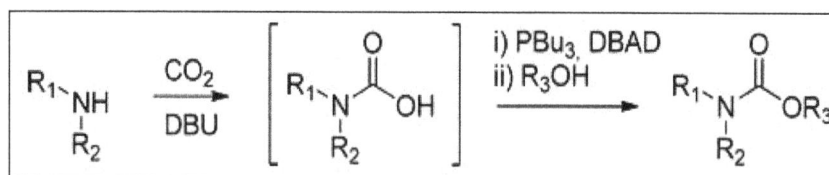

DBU-Catalyzed Carbamate Formation in the Presence of Gaseous Carbon Dioxide.

While this is precedented by an intramolecular reaction variant to produce cyclic carbamates, the desired intermolecular coupling was not fruitful under the proposed reaction conditions. Carbamic acids produced from secondary amines, however, did react with alcohols under Mitsunobu conditions (dibenzyl azodicarboxylate, DBAD, and tributylphosphine) in a DBU-catalyzed reaction with gaseous carbon dioxide, providing the corresponding carbamates. This reaction did not proceed through the isocyanate intermediate but rather through an S$_N$2 displacement of the activated alcohol. This hypothesis is supported by the observed inversion of stereochemistry upon conversion of a chiral secondary alcohol to the corresponding carbamate.

Table: Carbamates from Secondary Carbamic Acids.

Entry	Amine	Alcohol	Carbamate	Yield (%)
1	89	29	90	96
2	89	91	92	46
3	93	94	95	50
4	89	96	97	80

Very recently, Jiao and co-workers reported a practical, PdCl$_2$-catalyzed efficient assembly of organic azides, carbon monoxide, and alcohols for the direct synthesis of carbamates via isocyanate formation and application *in situ*.

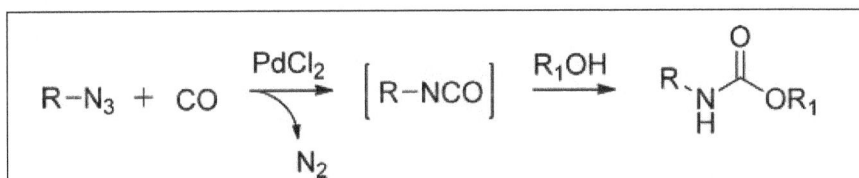

Carbamate Formation by a PdCl$_2$-Catalyzed Efficient Assembly of Organic Azides, Carbon Monoxide, and Alcohols.

Mild and neutral reaction conditions and generation of harmless N$_2$ as the byproduct render this protocol very useful, particularly for the synthesis of bioactive compounds. Moreover, the employment of CO at atmospheric pressure and the use of a small amount of PdCl$_2$ catalyst (2 mol %) in the absence of any ligand represent a real alternative to customary carbamate synthetic methods.

The synthesis of carbamates through the generation of carbamoyl chlorides is not convenient because of the requirement of the toxic phosgene. Also, such carbamoyl chlorides are highly reactive, prone to hydrolysis, unstable, and not suitable for long-term storage. For these problems, Batey and co-workers identified the use of carbamoylimidazolium salts as convenient *N,N'*-disubstituted carbamoyl transfer reagents, showing increased reactivity over carbamoylimidazoles as a result of the imidazolium effect.

Table: Carbamates from Organoazides, CO (1 atm) and Alcohols.

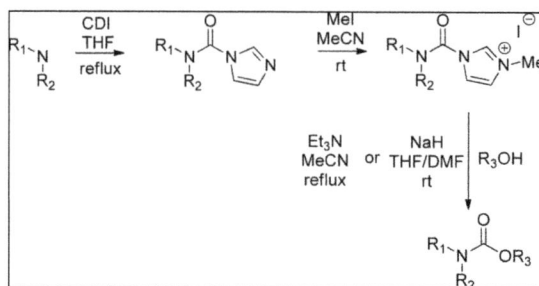

Carbamate Synthesis by the Use of Carbamoylimidazolium Salts.

These salts are readily prepared by the sequential treatment of secondary amines with N,N′-carbonyldiimidazole (CDI) and iodomethane. In the case of phenols, tertiary amines are appropriate bases for the in situ generation of the reactive phenoxides. The lower acidity of aliphatic alcohols presumably prevents the formation of the alkoxide anion, which would serve as the reactive nucleophile. Less acidic alcohols react with carbamoylimidazolium after their conversion into more nucleophilic sodium alkoxides.

Table: Carbamates from Carbamoylimidazolium Salts and Phenols or Alcohols.

The use of solid-supported reagents has become ubiquitous due to enhanced reactivity and selectivity, milder reaction conditions, convenient work-ups, and decreased solvent waste. The modified Hofmann rearrangement, proposed by Gogoi et al., is operationally simple, inexpensive and applicable to a variety of aliphatic and aromatic amides for the synthesis of methyl carbamates.

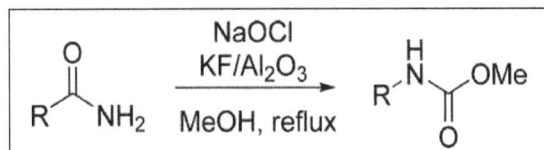

Synthesis of Methyl Carbamates by a Modified Hofmann Rearrangement.

KF/Al_2O_3 represents a useful and interesting solid-supported strong base, which replaces organic bases in a variety of reactions. Sodium hypochlorite is an inexpensive, convenient, and safe alternative to the currently employed oxidants. KF/Al_2O_3 basicity stems from the formation of KOH in the initial preparation of the solid-supported material by the reaction of KF with alumina supports. Under these highly basic reaction conditions, hypochlorite ion is the predominant form of chlorine, reacting with the amide to form an *N*-chloroamide, which later undergoes rearrangement to the isocyanate. In the presence of methanol, the isocyanate is rapidly converted into the corresponding methyl carbamate.

Table: Carbamates from Modified Hofmann Rearrangement.

Entry	Amine	Carbamate	Yield (%)
1	117	118	94
2	60	119	84
3	120	121	91
4	122	123	83

Modifications of the Curtius rearrangement have also been explored. Lebel and co-workers have reported a useful protocol for the preparation of *tert*-butyl carbamates from the corresponding carboxylic acids. Their reaction with di-*tert*-butyl dicarbonate and sodium azide led to the formation of the corresponding acyl azides, which then undergo a Curtius rearrangement, in the presence of tetrabutylammonium bromide and zinc(II) triflate, providing carbamates through trapping of the isocyanate intermediate.

In particular, the reaction of a chloroformate or di-*tert*-butyl dicarbonate and sodium azide with an aromatic carboxylic acid produced the corresponding acyl azide, presumably through the formation of an azidoformate. In contrast to what was observed with aliphatic carboxylic acids, using similar reaction conditions, aromatic carboxylic acids led mainly to the formation of the corresponding *tert*-butyl ester, likely via the displacement of an azide leaving group with *tert*-butoxide. This may be ascribed to the higher stability of aromatic acyl azides with respect to their aliphatic counterparts. Therefore, for these substrates, the Curtius rearrangement can be promoted only at higher temperatures (40 vs 75 °C).

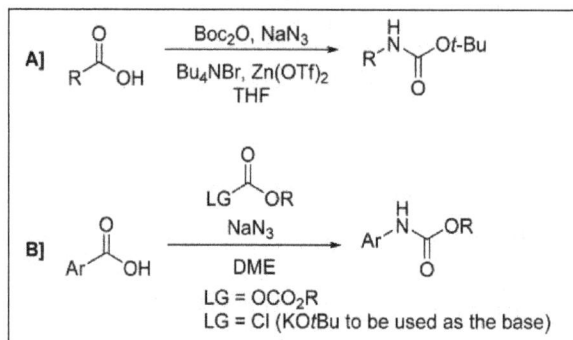

Synthesis of Carbamates by Modified Curtius Rearrangement.

Table: Carbamates from Modified Curtius Rearrangement.

As mentioned, alkyl chloroformates are the most frequently used reagents for the preparation of carbamates, although the need of an excess amount limits their usefulness. A promising method for preparing carbamates involves the use of a catalytic promoter. Lately, indium-mediated reactions have gained significant consideration due to the high reactivity and unique properties of indium reagents, among them nontoxicity and inertness toward air and water. Moreover, pretreatment is not required for activating indium metal. In this context, Jang and co-workers developed a simple, efficient, and selective method for synthesizing carbamates from amines, employing a catalytic amount of indium and only an equimolar amount of alkyl chloroformate.

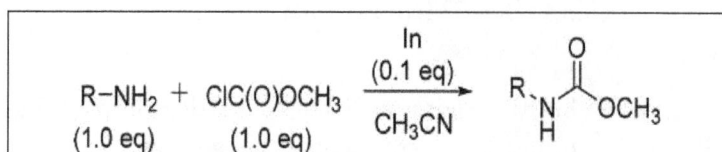

Indium-Catalyzed Carbamate Formation.

The method shows the generality for a wide variety of sterically diverse amines and alcohols and can also be applicable for the selective protection of amino groups under mild conditions.

Table. Carbamates from Indium-Catalyzed Reaction of Amines and Chloroformates

Entry	Amine	Chloroformate	Carbamate	Yield (%)
1	25	131	133	90
2	108	134	135	84
3	117	134	136	84
4	137	134	138	86

Arndtsen et al. proposed another application of indium-based reagents for the generation of N-protected amines in a single step.

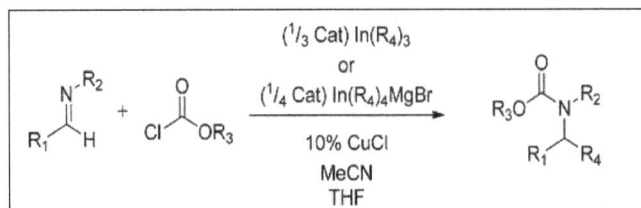

Coupling of Organoindium Reagents with Imines via Copper Catalysis.

Since organoindium reagents readily transfer their organic groups to an imine carbon, only one-third of an equivalent is required, and the only byproduct is represented by indium trichloride. Tetraorganoindium reagents can also be employed in a similar fashion for transferring all four organic groups. Therefore, one-fourth of an equivalent of indium is necessary for their reaction with imines. Copper(I) chloride (10%) was found to be the most efficient catalyst.

Table: Carbamates from Imines and Organoindium Reagents.

Entry	Imine	Chloroformate	R₄	Carbamate	Yield (%)
1	139	131	Et	140	92[a] (94)[b]
2	141	131		142	89[a] (91)[b]
3	143	144		145	77[a] (75)[b]

Sodeoka and colleagues reported the use of 1-alkoxycarbonyl-3-nitro-1,2,4-triazole reagents as useful intermediates for the preparation of carbamates To achieve a rapid and clean reaction, the features of the leaving group have a key role. An ideal leaving group should have a highly electron-withdrawing element in order to increase the electrophilicity of the carbonyl carbon, and the nucleophilicity should be low to avoid side reactions. It should also be easily separated from the reaction product. 3-Nitro-1,2,4-triazole (NT), although showing nucleophilicity, could be easily removed from the reaction due to its insolubility in dichloromethane or chloroform.

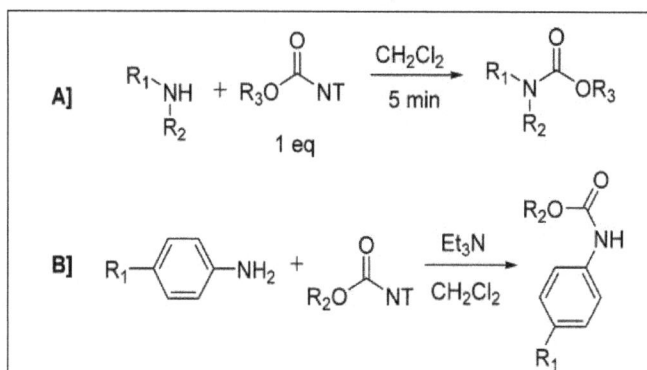

Carbamate Synthesis Employing 1-Alkoxycarbonyl-3-nitro-1,2,4-triazole Reagents.

NT-based reagents have a series of benefits such as high stability, since they can be stored for long periods without decomposition. Reactions of these NT reagents with primary and secondary amines proceeded quickly to give the corresponding carbamates in >95% yield. In contrast to aliphatic amines, aromatic amines were less reactive. However, the addition of triethylamine was found to be effective in promoting the reactions.

Table: Carbamates from NT-Based Reagents and Amines or Anilines.

Entry	Amine	NT reagent	Carbamate	Yield (%)
1	146	147	148	89
2	149	150	151	94
3	152	153	154	quant.
4	64	153	155	94

The reductive carbonylation of aromatic nitro compounds to the corresponding carbamates has remained a subject of great interest both from mechanistic and application standpoints.

$$ArNO_2 + 3CO + ROH \longrightarrow ArNHCOOR + 2CO_2$$

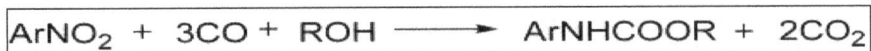

Carbamate Preparation by Reductive Carbonylation of Aromatic Nitro Compounds.

Cheng and collaborators report the use of $Ru(CO)_4^-$ and $Ru_3(CO)_{12}$ complexes for the catalysis of this reaction and highlighted the key effect of alcohol on the selectivity of carbamates The results clearly indicate that low selectivity of carbamate is closely related to the ability of the alcohol to reduce nitroarenes to amino derivatives. Therefore, the employment of an alcohol that cannot reduce nitroarene greatly increases the selectivity of carbamate. Later, the binuclear rhodium complex $[(Ph_3P)_4Rh_2(\mu\text{-}OH)_2]\cdot2C_6H_6$ was employed as an effective catalyst for the reductive carbonylation of nitrobenzenes to carbamate esters Palladium-based catalysts have also been explored.

Table: Carbamates from Reductive Carbonylation of Nitro Compounds.

Entry	ArNO$_2$	ROH	Catalyst	Carbamate	Conv. (%)	Selectivity ArNH$_2$ vs ArNHCOOR	Yield (%)
1	156 (NO$_2$)^a	t-BuOH	Rh(CO)$_4^-$	157 (OtBu)	100	8/96	-[124]
2	156 (NO$_2$)^a	t-BuOH	Ru$_3$(CO)$_{12}$	157 (OtBu)	100	3/97	-[124]
3	156 (NO$_2$)^b	MeOH	[(Ph$_3$P)$_4$Rh$_2$(μ-OH)$_2$]	158 (OMe)	-	-	94[125]
4	156 (NO$_2$)^c	EtOH	PdCl$_2$(PPh$_3$)$_2$	159 (OEt)	-	-	80[127]
5	156 (NO$_2$)^d	EtOH	PdCl$_2$(4-MePy)$_2$	159 (OEt)	-	-	27[128]

Carbamate synthesis via transfunctionalization of substituted ureas and carbonates in the presence of di-*n*-butyltin oxide (DBTO) as the catalyst was reported by Chaudhari and colleagues.

The carbonate reactivity pattern seems to be driven by the leaving group ability of the alkoxides and phenoxide to form the carbamate observed in aminolysis of carbonates. It has been shown that basicity of reacting urea plays a vital role in the catalytic activity of this reaction. Indeed, aliphatic ureas show higher reactivity compared to aromatic ureas due to their higher basicity. The basic DBTO is supposed to work as a nucleophile by attacking the carbonyl carbon of the carbonate, thus generating the catalytically active species dibutyl alkoxy carbonato tin [a]. As shown, species [a] interacts with substituted urea to eliminate one molecule of carbamate, forming dibutyl alkoxy carbamato tin [b]. A further reaction of species [b] with a carbonate results in the formation of one more molecule of carbamate with regeneration of the active species [a].

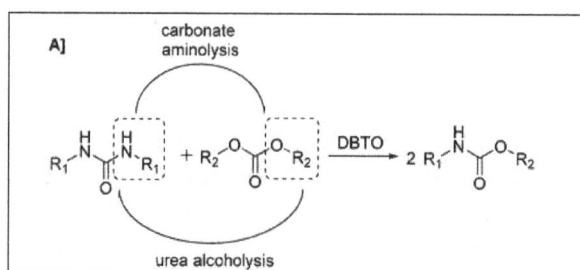

Carbamate Synthesis via Transfunctionalization of Substituted
Ureas and Carbonates in the Presence of DBTO.

Table: Carbamates Formed via Transfunctionalization of Substituted Ureas and Carbonates Using DBTO Catalyst.

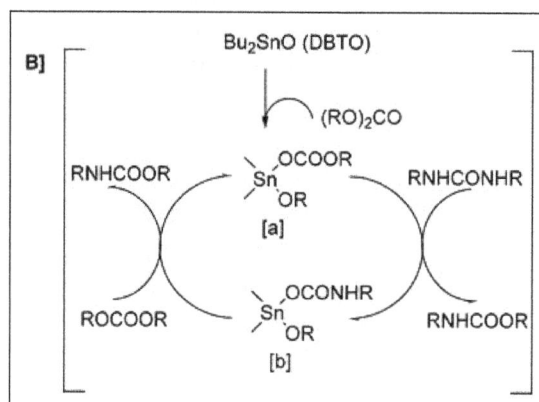

Entry	Urea	Carbonate	Carbamate	Yield (%)
1	160	161	162	89
2	163	161	164	90
3	165	166	167	50
4	168	169	170	91

Use of dialkyl carbonates as environmentally friendly and nontoxic phosgene substitutes in alkoxy-carbonylation reactions has also been exploited by Porco et al.

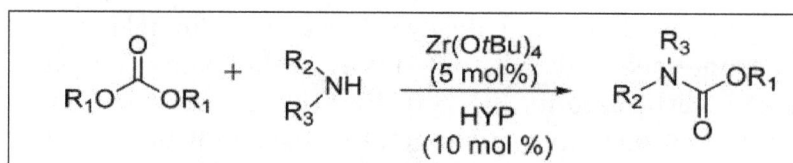

Zr(IV)-Catalyzed Carbonate–Carbamate Exchange.

Table: Carbamates Formed via Zr(IV)-Catalyzed Exchange Process.

Entry	Amine	Carbonate	Carbamate	Yield (%)
1	25	169	171	88
2	172	169	173	97
3	174	175	176	98
4	38	177	178	95

Recently, Padiya and co-workers reported a useful method for preparing carbamates in an aqueous media.

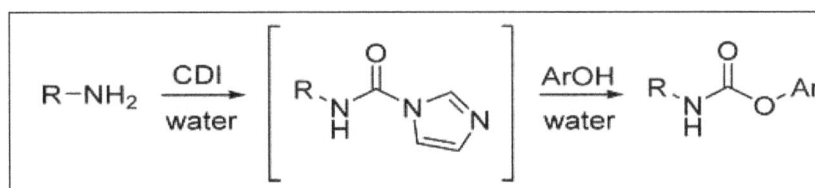

Carbamates Synthesis in Aqueous Media by the Use of CDI.

Interestingly, they found that 1,1'-carbonyldiimidazole (CDI), although unstable in water, rapidly reacts in aqueous media with amine to give good yields of the corresponding N-substituted carbonylimidazolide. Carbonylimidazolide derived from the primary amine reacts *in situ* with a nucleophile such as phenol, providing the corresponding carbamate. The product precipitates out from the reaction mixture and can be obtained in high purity by filtration, making the method simple and scalable.

Table: Carbamates from in Situ Generation of Carbonylimidazole in Water.

Entry	Amine	Phenol	Carbamate	Yield (%)
1	179	180	181	75
2	182	112	183	78
3	184	112	185	98
4	184	180	186	73

CDI was also found to mediate the Lossen rearrangement, which occurs in the transformation of an activated hydroxamic acid into the corresponding isocyanate.

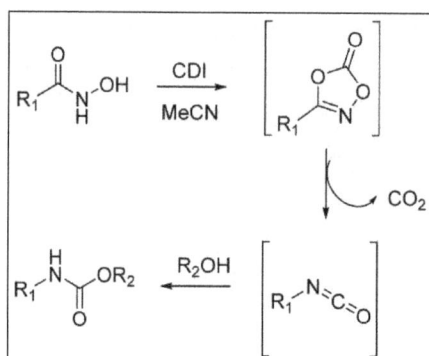

CDI-Mediated Lossen Rearrangement for Carbamate Synthesis.

The proposed methodology is experimentally efficient and mild, being characterized by imidazole and CO_2 as the only stoichiometric byproducts. This method is a green and unconventional alternative to the Curtius and Hofmann rearrangements. Another method based on the Lossen rearrangement was recently proposed. The methodology envisaged the reaction of a hydroxamic acid with an alcohol, promoted by 2,4,6-trichloro-1,3,5-triazine (cyanuric chloride; TCT) in the presence of an excess of N-methyl morpholine (NMM).

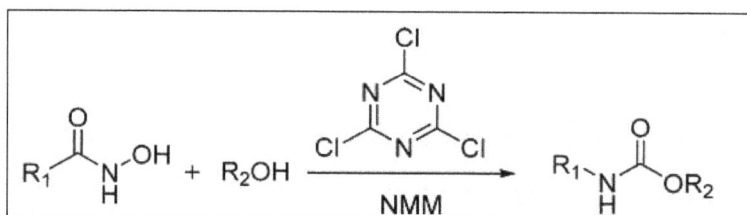

TCT-Mediated Lossen Rearrangement for Carbamate Synthesis.

Table: Carbamates from CDI- and TCT-Mediated Lossen Rearrangement.

Entry	Hydroxamic acid	Alcohol	Promoter	Carbamate	Yield (%)
1	187	29	CDI	188	93
2	189	29	CDI	190	99
3	187	191	TCT	192	84
4	187	35	TCT	193	77

Carbamates with Clinical Potential

Carbamates are inherent to many FDA approved drugs. This structural motif is also a key functionality in numerous medicinal agents with clinical potential.

Miscellaneous Carbamates with Clinical Relevance

Rivastigmine

Rivastigmine tartrate (Exelon, Novartis Pharma) is a carbamate derivative that reversibly inhibits the metabolism of acetylcholinesterase (AChE) and butyrylcholinesterase (BuChE) preferentially in the central nervous system (CNS). It is used for the treatment of mild-to-moderate Alzheimer's disease (AD) dementia and dementia due to Parkinson's disease. The drug can be administered orally or via a transdermal patch. The transdermal patch reduces side effects such as nausea and vomiting. Rivastigmine undergoes extensive metabolism by ChE-mediated hydrolysis to the de-carbamylated metabolite, without involvement of the major cytochrome P450 (CYP450) isozymes. The metabolite may undergo *N*-demethylation as well as conjugation. The pharmacokinetic half-life of rivastigmine in AD patients is around 1.5 h. When given orally, rivastigmine is well-absorbed, with a bioavailability of about 40% administered as a 3 mg dose.

Muraglitazar

Muraglitazar (195) contains a carbamate functionality. It is a potent, novel nonthiazolidindione peroxisome proliferator-activated receptor dual agonist (PPARα/γ) that demonstrated highly efficacious glucose and lipid lowering activities *in vivo*, along with an excellent ADME profile. In a double-blind randomized clinical trial, muraglitazar resulted in a statistically significant improvement in plasma triglyceride, HDL cholesterol, apoB, and non-HDL cholesterol concentrations at week 12. Muraglitazar reduced triglyceride concentrations to a larger extent than did pioglitazone, regardless of baseline triglyceride levels. Muraglitazar and pioglitazone treatment was associated with slight (3–4%) increases in LDL cholesterol. However, muraglitazar development was discontinued due to major adverse cardiovascular side effects.

Roxifiban

Roxifiban (196) is a carbamate derivative with a methyl ester prodrug. It is a potent, nonpeptide antagonist of the glycoprotein IIb/IIIa receptor. The free acid resulting from roxifiban hydrolysis blocks the binding of fibrinogen to the receptor, thereby inhibiting platelet aggregation and providing a mechanism for antithrombotic therapy. However, clinical development of roxifiban was discontinued in October 2001.

Entinostat

Entinostat (197, MS-275) contains a pyridylmethyl carbamate functionality. It is undergoing clinical trials for the treatment of various cancers. Entinostat preferentially inhibits HDAC1 (IC_{50} = 300 nM) over HDAC3 (IC_{50} = 8 μM) and is reported to have no inhibitory activity toward HDAC8 (IC_{50} > 100 μM). This drug induces cyclin-dependent kinase inhibitor 1A (p21/CIP1/WAF1), thereby slowing cell growth, differentiation, and tumor development *in vivo*. Recent studies suggest that 197 may be particularly useful as an antineoplastic agent when combined with other drugs like adriamycin.

Albendazole and Mebendazole

Albendazole (198, Albenza, Teva Pharmaceuticals) is a broad-spectrum anthelmintic carbamate drug. It undergoes rapid hepatic oxidation by liver microsomal enzymes, producing the active metabolite albendazole sulfoxide, which is then oxidized to the inactive metabolites albendazole sulfone and albendazole-2-amino sulfone.

Mebendazole (199) is a methyl carbamate derivative showing broad-spectrum anthelmintic properties. It demonstrated efficacy in the oral treatment of ascariasis, uncinariasis, oxyuriasis, and trichuriasis. Like other benzimidazole anthelmintics, mebendazole's primary mechanism of action is consistent with tubulin binding. Mebendazole was discontinued in 2011.

Flupirtine and Retigabine

Flupirtine (200) and retigabine (201) are ethyl carbamate derivatives. Flupirtine is a centrally acting nonopioid analgesic that was identified within an antiepileptic drug discovery program by the U.S. National Institutes of Health. The doses used in a small clinical trial exceeded those established for analgesic activity. On the basis of this data, subsequent structural optimization resulted in retigabine. Retigabine has anticonvulsant properties that appear to be mediated by opening or activating neuronal voltage-gated potassium channels. Flupirtine showed N-methyl-d-aspartate (NMDA) receptor antagonist properties.

Felbamate

Felbamate (202, Felbatol, Meda Pharmaceuticals) is an alkyl carbamate derivative. It is an antiepileptic drug. The mechanism of action of felbamate involves a dual mechanism involving inhibition of N-methyl-d-aspartate (NMDA) receptor response and positive modulation of γ-amino butyric acid subtype A (GABA$_A$) receptor, thus decreasing neuronal excitation. Felbamate is rapidly absorbed (t_{max} = 2–6 h) with an oral bioavailability > 90%. Felbamate undergoes moderate metabolism via CYP3A4 and CYP2E1 isoenzymes, which are amenable to inhibition and induction effects. The clinical use of felbamate has declined in recent years due to its serious adverse side effects.

Efavirenz

Efavirenz (203, Sustiva or Stocrin, Bristol-Myers Squibb) is a cyclic carbamate derivative. It is a non-nucleoside reverse transcriptase inhibitor (NNRTI). The drug is used as part of highly active antiretroviral therapy (HAART). However, its use is associated with variable treatment response and adverse effects, in most part because of the large differences in pharmacokinetics. CYP2B6 is the main enzyme catalyzing the major clearance mechanism of efavirenz (8-hydroxylation to 8-hydroxyefavirenz) *in vivo*.

Zafirlukast

Zafirlukast (204, Accolate, AstraZeneca) is a cyclopentyl N-aryl carbamate derivative. It is a selective and competitive receptor antagonist of the cysteinyl leukotrienes D-4 and E-4, which is indicated for the prophylaxis and treatment of mild-to-moderate persistent and chronic asthma. Both O → CH$_2$ and O → NH bioisosteric analogues of Zafirlukast were found to be potent. The carbamate moiety present in zafirlukast provided an excellent *in vitro* and *in vivo* profile and high oral bioavailability. Zafirlukast undergoes hepatic metabolism, where hydroxylation by cytochrome CYP2C9 is the major biotransformation pathway. The metabolites of zafirlukast do not significantly contribute to its overall activity.

Mitomycin C

Mitomycin C (205, MMC, Mutamycin) is a complex carbamate derivative. It is an antitumor antibiotic that was identified in the 1950s in fermentation cultures of the Gram-negative bacteria *Streptomyces caespitosus*. MMC is a site-specific, nondistorting DNA cross-linking agent. However, recent reports suggest that DNA may not be the primary target of the drug. In particular, interaction of MMC with rRNA and subsequent inhibition of protein translation has been proposed. MMC is customarily used as a chemotherapeutic agent in the treatment of several types of cancer, such as bladder, colon, and breast cancers.

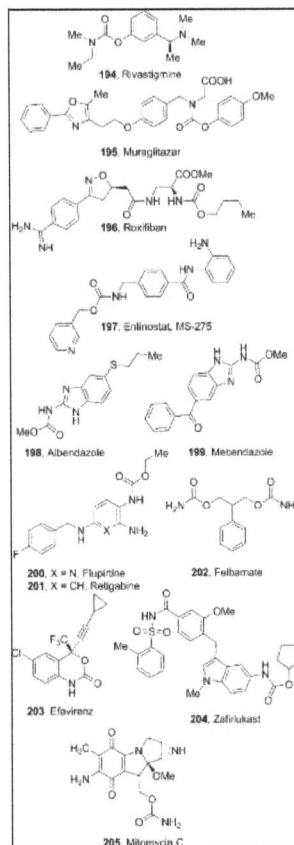

Carbamates with clinical potential.

Therapeutic Carbamates as HIV Protease Inhibitors

HIV protease is an aspartic acid protease responsible for the cleavage of the Gag–pol polyprotein into functional proteins essential for the production of infections progeny virus. Inactivation of HIV-1 protease either by site-directed mutagenesis or by chemical inhibition results in the formation of immature, noninfections virus particles. As a consequence, HIV-1 protease is an attractive target in antiviral therapy. HIV protease is a C_2-symmetric, 198-amino acid homodimeric aspartyl protease in which each protein subunit contributes one Asp-Thr-Gly motif to the single active site. The X-ray crystallographic analysis of the native protein and subsequent protein–ligand complexes and extensive research programs on other aspartyl proteases, including human renin, provided a path toward accelerated drug discovery programs targeting HIV protease. A number of FDA-approved HIV protease inhibitor drugs contain an important carbamate functionality.

Ritonavir

Ritonavir (206, Norvir, ABT-538, A-84538, AbbVie, Inc.) structure possesses a thiazolyl methyl carbamate functionality. It is a peptidomimetic inhibitor of both the HIV-1 and HIV-2 proteases and was approved by the FDA in March 1996. This first-generation protease inhibitor was developed at Abbott Laboratories. The discovery of ritonavir was based on studies with C_2-symmetric diamine subunits. Ritonavir showed EC_{50} of 0.025 μM, bioavailability of 78%, and a plasma half-life of 1.2 h. Ritonavir has a high molecular weight; however, it showed excellent pharmacokinetic properties. This is possibly due to the increased stability of the thiazole groups to oxidative metabolism and also due to its effect on cytochrome P450 oxidative enzymes. Ritonavir is a type II heme ligand that fits into the CYP3A4 active site cavity and irreversibly binds to the heme iron via the thiazole nitrogen. Inhibiting CYP3A4, ritonavir increases plasma concentrations of other anti-HIV drugs oxidized by CYP3A4, thereby improving their clinical efficacy.

Amprenavir

Amprenavir (46, Agenerase, VX-478, GlaxoSmithKline, Vertex) is a tetrahydrofuranyl carbamate derivative. It was approved by the FDA in April 1999. Amprenavir was identified as a potent, orally bioavailable HIV-1 protease inhibitor with a low molecular weight and a mean IC_{50} of 12 nM. It is marketed with a twice-a-day dosing format. Amprenavir structure bears a stereochemically defined tetrahydrofuranylcarbamate engaging in a weak backbone interaction with the protease. *In vitro* and *in vivo* studies have shown that amprenavir is primarily metabolized by CYP3A4, and the two major metabolites result from oxidation of the tetrahydrofuran and aniline moieties.

Atazanavir

Atazanavir (207, ATV, Reyataz (ATV sulfate), BMS-232632, Bristol-Myers Squibb) is a methyl carbamate derivative. It is a hydroxyethylene hydrazide-based second-generation HIV-protease inhibitor developed in the late 1990s and approved by the FDA in June 2003. ATV contains two methylcarbamate functionalities. It showed potent enzyme inhibitory activity (K_i = 2.66 nM), and its antiviral IC_{50} in HIV_{MN}-infected MT-2 cells was 26 nM. ATV displayed excellent bioavailability. The favorable pharmacological profile for ATV raised the possibility of once-daily dosing.

Darunavir

Darunavir (48, DRV TMC-114) possesses a structure-based designed bis-tetrahydrofuranyl (bis-THF) carbamate functionality. It is a new generation HIV-1 protease inhibitor with improved bioavailability, potency, and drug properties. DRV also maintains high potency against multidrug-resistant HIV-1 strains. The design of DRV originated from the backbone binding concept envisaging that an effective protease inhibitor maximizes rich networks of hydrogen-bonding interactions with the backbone atoms throughout the active site of the protease. The bis-THF moiety present in DRV was designed based on the X-ray structure of inhibitor-HIV-1 protease complexes. The bis-THF carbamate moiety of DRV was found to be essential for enzyme affinity. DRV demonstrated exceptional potency against both wild-type HIV isolates and a wide range of resistant variants. DRV received FDA approval in 2006 for the treatment of HIV/AIDS patients harboring multidrug-resistant HIV-1 variants. In 2008, DRV received full approval for the treatment of therapy-naive adults and children. DRV is metabolized by the isoenzyme CYP3A4. However, in the presence of a low dose of ritonavir, DRV exhibits very good pharmacokinetic properties in patients.

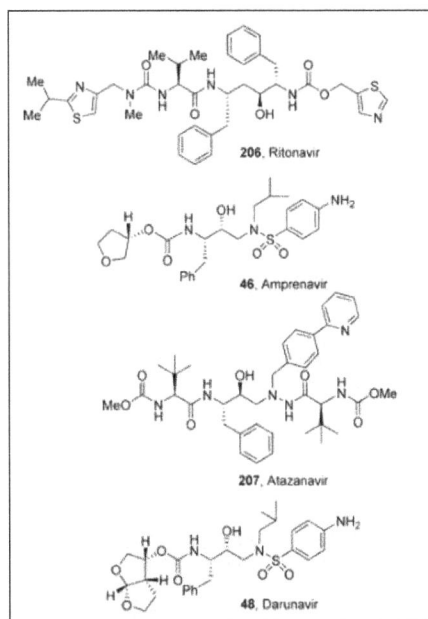

Representative carbamate-containing therapeutic HIV protease inhibitors.

Carbamate Prodrugs and their Metabolism

Prodrugs are chemically modified forms of the actual pharmacologically active drug that undergo *in vivo* transformation to release the active drug molecule. This is a well-established strategy to improve drug disposition properties (physicochemical, biopharmaceutical, or pharmacokinetic properties) of pharmacologically relevant compounds and thereby increase their drug-like profile. A prodrug strategy helps to overcome a variety of hurdles in drug formulation and delivery such as (i) poor oral absorption and aqueous solubility, (ii) poor lipid solubility, (iii) chemical instability, (iv) rapid presystemic metabolism, (v) toxicity and local irritation, and (vi) lack of site-selective delivery.

A functional group on the parent drug may be used to form a chemical bond with the promoiety. Generally, the linker should be self-removing or cleavable so that the parent drug can be released spontaneously or under a certain triggering condition, such as the presence of an enzyme or a change in pH. The promoiety coupled to the parent drug provides the ability to improve the drug-like properties or overcome the barriers in delivering the drug to its target cells.

Carbamates are the esters of carbamic acid, preferentially used in the design of prodrugs as a means of achieving first-pass and systemic hydrolytic stability. Carbamates are typically enzymatically more stable than the corresponding esters. They are, in general, more susceptible to hydrolysis than amides. Thus, bioconversion of carbamate prodrugs requires esterases for the release of the parent drug. Upon hydrolysis, carbamate esters release the parent phenol or alcohol drug and carbamic acid, which, due to its chemical instability, breaks down to the corresponding amine and carbon dioxide. Carbamates of primary amines can also fragment into isocyanates and alcohols on treatment with bases, a further potential pathway for metabolic degradation. The OH-catalyzed hydrolysis of these carbamate esters (R′-NHCO-OR) is strongly dependent on both the pK_a of the proton on the leaving group (ROH) and the degree of substitution on the nitrogen of the carbamate ester. Since phenols have a lower pK_a with respect to alcohols, carbamate esters of phenols are generally more chemically labile than those of alcohols. In the case of alcohols, both the N-monosubstituted and N,N-disubstituted carbamates are chemically stable toward hydrolysis. In phenols, N,N-disubstituted carbamates are chemically stable, whereas N-monosubstituted carbamates are the most labile toward chemical hydrolysis. Short-lived carbamates have also been used as prodrugs of heteroaromatic amines (e.g., capecitabine, 217) and amidines (lefradafiban (221), dabigatran).

Alcohol and Phenol Carbamate Prodrugs

Most of the therapeutically relevant carbamate prodrugs have been designed as substrates of specific enzymes. Antibody-directed enzyme prodrug therapy (ADEPT) and gene-directed enzyme prodrug therapy (GDEPT) are new strategies for targeting tumors. Carboxypeptidase G2 (CPG2), an enzyme of bacterial origin, has been shown to catalyze the cleavage of an amide, carbamate, or urea linkage between glutamic acid and an aromatic group. On the basis of this specificity, a large number of prodrugs have been designed and synthesized for CPG2. As shown in Figure, the prodrug 208 (ZD2767P) is activated by hydrolysis at the carbamate bond by CPG2 to the corresponding potent di-iodophenol mustard (209). 208 was found to possess the best profile in terms of enzymatic kinetics, cytotoxicity, and *in vivo* efficacy. It was selected for clinical development. The half-life ($t_{1/2}$) of the drug is approximately 2 min, which is enough for diffusion into the tumor cell from the local release site and to minimize peripheral toxicity.

Irinotecan was designed to deliver camptothecin as a predominant topoisomerase I inhibitor for anticancer therapy. Irinotecan hydrochloride salt 210 (CPT-11, Camptosar; Pfizer) is a parenteral aqueous soluble carbamate prodrug of antineoplastic topoisomerase I inhibitor 211 (SN-38, 7-ethyl-10-hydroxy-camptothecin). The potent antitumor activity of irinotecan is due to rapid formation of active metabolite 211*in vivo*. In this molecule, a dipiperidino ionizable promoiety is linked to the phenol functionality by a carbamate bond, thus improving the overall aqueous solubility. The bioconversion back to 211 occurs primarily by human liver microsomal carboxylesterases, CES 1A1 and CES2, which release the ionizable piperidinopiperidine promoiety and 211, the active form of the drug.

Beyond minimizing the rate of enzymatic hydrolysis of its prodrug, sustained drug action can also be provided by decreasing the rate of drug metabolism. This is the case of bambuterol (212, Bambec, AstraZeneca), a bis-dimethyl carbamate prodrug of the β2-agonist terbutaline (213), which is used as a bronchodilator in the treatment of asthma. The phenolic moiety of terbutaline is subjected to rapid presystemic metabolism. In bambuterol, protection of this functionality also avoids first-pass intestinal and hepatic metabolism. This prodrug is inactive, however, after oral administration; it is slowly converted to terbutaline, mainly outside the lungs, by a series of hydrolysis and oxidation reactions (maily catalyzed by plasma cholinesterase, pChE, and by CYP450, Figure). This allows a once-daily bambuterol treatment with respect to the three daily terbutaline administrations.

An N,N'-dimethyl ethylenediamine spacer, used for the evaluation of cyclization-elimination-based prodrugs of phenols and alcohols, has been used for the development of prodrugs as a part of the ADEPT activation strategy. When activated by a specific enzyme, the terminal amino group on the spacer activates and initiates an intramolecular cyclization reaction to eliminate a phenol or alcohol parent drug with parallel release of the cyclized spacer. In one such application, Scherren et al. explored paclitaxel-2'-carbamates. This is particularly interesting because a free 2'-hydroxyl group is important for biological activity. In general, carbamate linkages are more stable *in vivo* than esters and carbonates. Since the proteolytic active form of plasmin is located in the tumor, linking a cytotoxic drug to a plasmin substrate may result in tumor-selective delivery. On the basis of this rationale, following plasmin hydrolysis, the spacer is expected to undergo spontaneous cyclization to yield a cyclic urea derivative (imidazolidinone), thereby releasing paclitaxel (214), as illustrated in Scheme.

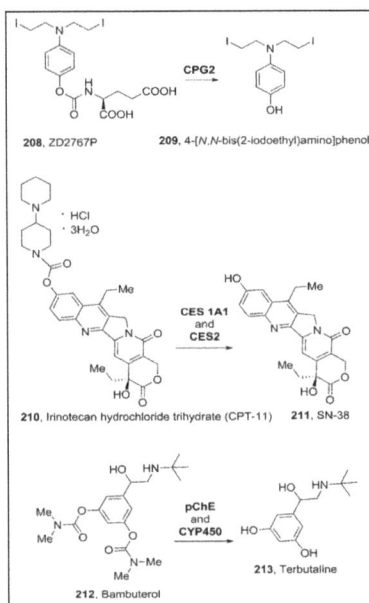

Examples of phenol carbamate prodrugs and their metabolic activation.

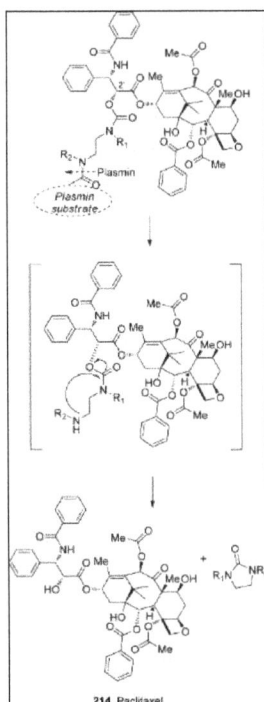

Plasmin Hydrolysis and Subsequent Spontaneous Cyclization of
the *N,N'*-Dimethyl Ethylenediamine Spacer and Release of Paclitaxel.

Amine and Amidine Carbamate Prodrugs

The amine group is one of the most common functional groups in many approved drugs. Amines in drugs can cause physicochemical hurdles that have the potential to limit their safety and effective delivery to desired sites of action. Therefore, a variety of prodrugs of amines have been designed to overcome formulation and delivery barriers. The carbamate functionality has been utilized in many prodrug strategies designed for amines. Short-lived carbamates are also used as prodrugs of heteroaromatic amines and amidines.

Gabapentin is a structural analogue of γ-aminobutyric acid (GABA). It is marketed as an anticonvulsant and an analgesic agent. Gabapentin shows a number of limitations, including saturable absorption, high interpatient variability, lack of dose proportionality, and a short half-life. Gabapentin enacarbil (215, Horizant, previously known as XP13512) is a carbamate prodrug of gabapentin. The prodrug is benefited by a monocarboxylate transporter type 1 (MCT1). MCT1 is expressed in all segments of the colon and upper gastrointestinal tract. The prodrug also helps the sodium-dependent multivitamin transporter (SMV T), responsible for absorption of multiple essential nutrients. Following absorption via these pathways, the prodrug is rapidly converted to gabapentin by nonspecific esterases, mainly in enterocytes and to a lesser extent in the liver. During conversion to gabapentin, each molecule of 215 also generates carbon dioxide, acetaldehyde, and isobutyrate. The oral bioavailability of 215 was improved from 25 to 84% in monkeys. It showed dose-proportional gabapentin exposure in humans. In 2011, Xenoport received FDA approval (Horizant) for the treatment of moderate-to-severe restless legs syndrome. In 2012, Horizant was also approved for the management of postherpetic neuralgia (PHN) in adults.

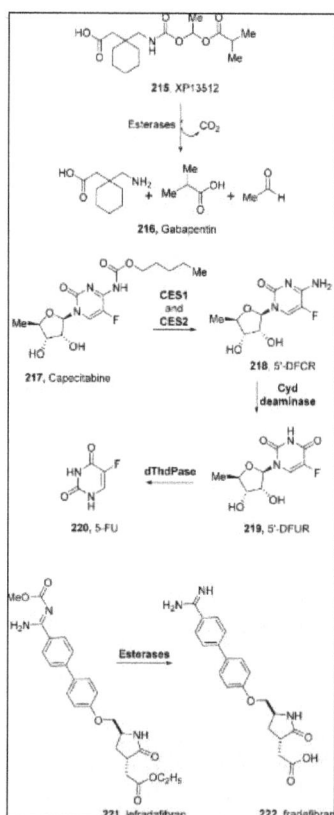

Examples of amine and amidine prodrugs and their metabolic activation.

Capecitabine (217, Xeloda, Roche) was designed to achieve greater selectivity than its active form, 5-fluorouracil (220, 5-FU). It is an orally administered carbamate prodrug of 5-FU, belonging to the fluoropyrimidine carbamate class. It requires a cascade of three enzymes for the bioconversion to the active drug. As shown in Figure, the enzymatic bioconversion starts in the liver, where human carboxylesterases 1 and 2 (CES1 and CES2) cleave the carbamate ester bond. Intact capecitabine is absorbed in the intestine, and its bioconversion in the liver releases the parent drug. To some extent, its bioconversion proceeds in tumors, thus avoiding any systemic toxicity. In particular, the remaining transformations to 5-FU are catalyzed by cytidine deaminase and thymidine phosphorylase. The latter enzyme is highly enriched in tumors, thus providing selective release of 5-FU in cancer cells. The absorption of capecitabine is evident since 95% of an orally administered dose is recovered in urine and the T_{max} of 5-FU is reached in approximately 1.5–2 h. Capecitabine is currently approved as a first line of therapy for colorectal and breast cancers and is also approved for use in combination with other anticancer drugs.

Alkoxycarbonyl derivatives can serve as useful prodrugs for benzamidines. For example, the methoxycarbonyl methyl ester lefradafiban (221, BIBU104, Boehringer Ingelheim, Germany) is effectively converted to the active platelet aggregation inhibitor fradafiban (222, BIBU 52) after oral administration. This was revealed by monitoring the plasma concentrations of 222 and by ex vivo platelet aggregation studies. Lefradafiban is the orally active prodrug of fradafiban, a glycoprotein IIb/IIIa receptor antagonist. Esterases, but not CYP450-dependent enzymes, are involved in the conversion of lefradafiban to fradafiban *in vivo*.

Cyclic Ether-derived Carbamates as HIV-1 Protease Inhibitors

Over the years, we have developed a series of novel HIV-1 protease inhibitors incorporating cyclic ether-derived carbamates designed based on the X-ray structures of inhibitor-HIV-1 protease complexes. In this endeavor, we have specifically developed stereochemically defined cyclic ether templates, where the cyclic ether oxygen could effectively replace a peptide carbonyl oxygen. The advantage of such replacement is to reduce peptidic features and improve metabolic stability of compounds. These cyclic ligands have been incorporated as carbamate derivatives. The evolution of the carbamate structural template is shown in Figure. On the basis of the X-ray crystal structure of saquinavir (223)-bound HIV-1 protease, we first investigated 3-(R)-tetrahydrofuranylglycine so that the 3-(R)-THF ring oxygen would interact with the Asp30 NH, similar to the asparagine side chain carbonyl oxygen of saquinavir (compound 224). In an effort to reduce molecular weight, the P3 quinoline was removed, and the amide bond was replaced with a carbamate to provide inhibitor 225 with significant reduction of molecular weight (515 Da from 670 Da). The X-ray crystal structure of 225-bound HIV-1 protease revealed that the ring oxygen of the 3-(S)-tetrahydrofuran (3-(S)-THF) is within proximity to form a hydrogen bond with the Asp29 NH bond in the S2 subsite. The importance of the carbamate moiety is evident. The carbamate NH forms a hydrogen bond with the backbone carbonyl of Gly27, and the carbamate carbonyl functionality makes a tightly bound water-mediated hydrogen bond with the backbone NH's of the flap Ile50 and Ile50' in the active site.

Our further investigation of the 3-(S)-THF in inhibitors containing a hydroxyethylene isostere led to a series of exceptionally potent inhibitors. As shown in table, -(S)-THF-containing carbamate drivatives (compounds 226–231) provided very potent inhibitors in antiviral assays. The potency enhancing effect of 3-(S)-THF carbamate was subsequently demonstrated in inhibitors containing the (R)-(hydroxyethyl)sulfonamide isostere. Clinical development of inhibitor 46 (VX476) led to FDA approval of amprenavir for the treatment of HIV/AIDS patients.

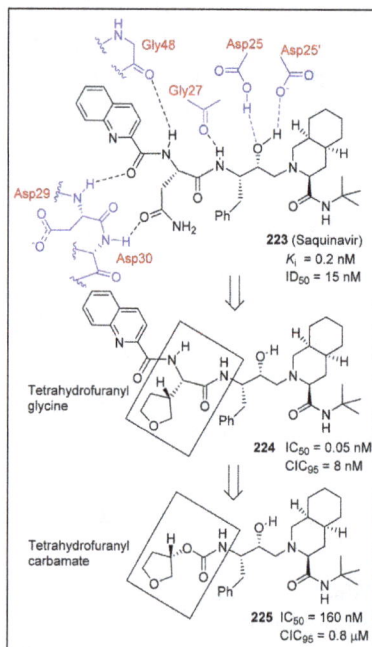

Evolution of 3-tetrahydrofuranyl carbamate as an HIV-1 protease inhibitor.

Table: Exploration of 3-Tetrahydrofuranyl Urethanes.

	Hydroxyethylene isostere			Hydroxyethylamine isostere		
	Compound	IC_{50}	CIC_{95}	Compound	IC_{50}	CIC_{95}
R =	226	0.3	400	229	>300 0	800
R =	227	<0.03	3	230	160	-
R =	228	0.03	100	231	694	-

Further development of carbamate-derived novel HIV-1 protease inhibitors is shown in Figure. We have designed a variety of inhibitors incorporating cyclic sulfones and bicyclic ligands. These ligands were conceived in order to maximize hydrogen-bonding interactions with the protease backbone as well as to fill in the hydrophobic pocket in the S2 subsite. On the basis of the X-ray structure of saquinavir-bound HIV-1 protease, we then designed a fused bicyclic tetrahydrofuran (bis-THF) ligand to form hydrogen bonds with backbone aspartates in the S2 subsite as well as to fill in the hydrophobic site adjacent to the P3-quinoline ring of saquinavir . An X-ray structural analysis of 236-bound HIV-1 protease revealed that the bis-THF carbamate mimics the majority of P2–P3-amide bonds of saquinavir. A detailed structure–activity study also established that the stereochemistry of the bis-THF ring, and the position of the ring oxygens is critical to potency.

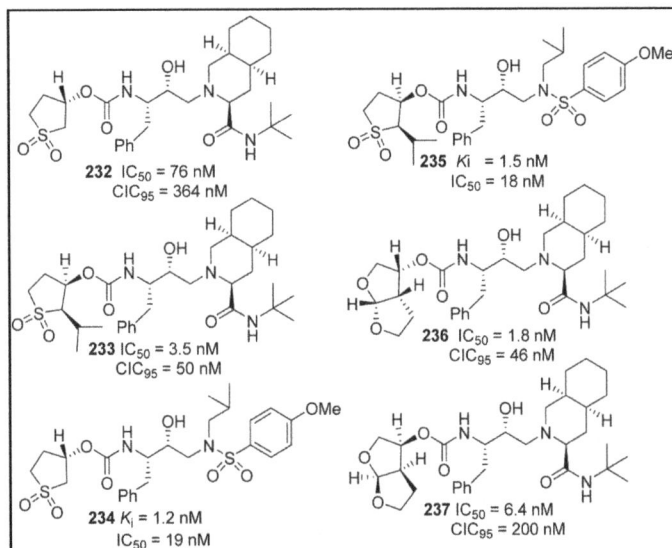

Cyclic sulfolane and bicyclic ligand-derived carbamates as HIV-1 protease inhibitors.

With the development of a bis-THF carbamate that could form a network of hydrogen bonds in the S2 subsite of HIV-1 protease, we investigated transition state isosteres that can be functionalized to form hydrogen bonds in the S2′ subsite. Our basic hypothesis was to design inhibitors that form a network of hydrogen bonds with the protease backbone atoms throughout the active site of HIV-1 protease, from S2 to S2′ subsites. This backbone binding strategy to combat drug resistance led to the development of a series of very potent carbamate-derived protease inhibitors. As shown in Figure, we incorporated the bis-THF ligand in the (R)-hydroxyethylsulfonamide isostere bearing p-methoxysulfonamide as the P2′ ligand so that the methoxy oxygen can interact with aspartate backbone atoms in the S2′ subsite. The resulting inhibitors exhibited notable potency. Inhibitor 239 with a (3R,3aS,6aR)-bis-THF as the P2 ligand is significantly more potent in an antiviral assay than corresponding inhibitor 238 with an enantiomeric bis-THF ligand. An X-ray structure of 239-bound HIV-1 protease revealed that the carbamate NH formed a hydrogen bond with the backbone Gly27 carbonyl group and that carbamate carbonyl of 239 is involved in an interesting tetra-coordinated hydrogen-bonding interaction with the structural water molecule, inhibitor sulfonamide oxygen, and the flap Ile 50 NH residues. Also, the structure revealed interactions with the backbone atoms in both the S2 and S2′ subsites.

Further replacement of the p-methoxy group at the S2′ to a p-amino group led to inhibitor 48. This inhibitor showed marked enzyme inhibitory activity as well as antiviral activity. An in-depth antiviral study revealed that 48 maintained excellent antiviral activity against multidrug-resistant HIV-1 variants. The X-ray structural studies of darunavir-bound HIV-1 protease showed extensive active site interactions. Particularly, it formed a network of hydrogen bonds with the protein backbone throughout the active site. Darunavir also exhibited favorable pharmacokinetic properties. Subsequently, clinical development led to its FDA approval as darunavir for the treatment of HIV/AIDS patients.

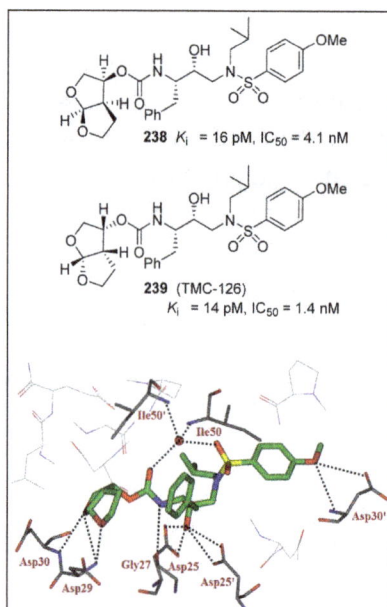

Design of bicyclic carbamate and inhibitor 239-bound HIV-1 protease X-ray structure.

The carbamate functionality of darunavir (48) was assembled as shown in Scheme. (3R,3aS,6aR)-3-Hydroxyhexahydrofuro[2,3-b]furan (bis-THF) 47 was treated with disuccinimidyl carbonate to provide activated mixed carbonate 240. Reaction of this activated carbonate with hydroxyethylsulfonamide isostere 45provided darunavir.

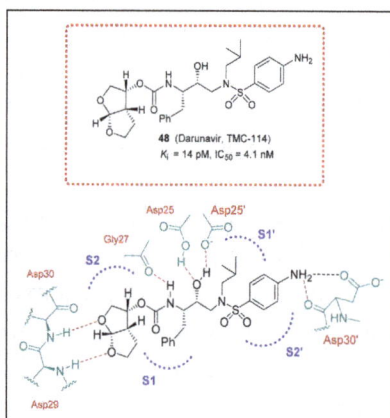

Darunavir and highlight of the X-ray structure of darunavir-bound HIV-1 protease showing the main interactions.

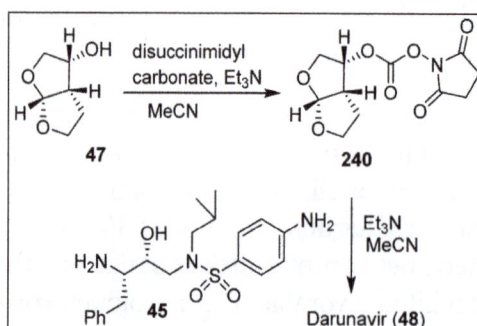

Assembly of Carbamate Functionality of Darunavir.

The backbone binding inhibitor design strategies to combat drug resistance have been further utilized by us and others to advance a number of other preclinical and clinical inhibitors with carbamates. Figure shows selected bis-THF-derived carbamates (241–244) with marked enzyme and antiviral activities. Like darunavir, inhibitor-bound X-ray structures of these inhibitors showed a network of hydrogen bonds in both S2 and S2′ subsites of HIV-1 protease. The inhibitor side chains as well as the bis-THF bicyclic framework also effectively filled the hydrophobic pockets in the active site.

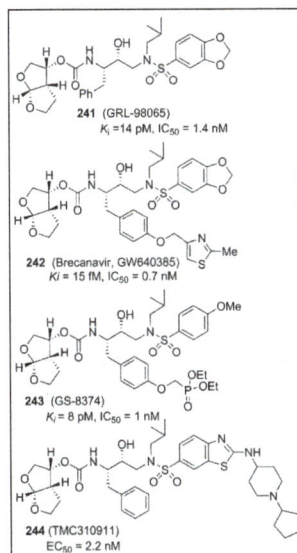

Bis-THF-derived protease inhibitors for preclinical and clinical development.

We have outlined a selected number of cyclic ether-derived carbamates that have been developed based on the backbone binding concept in Figure. Particularly, incorporation of these stereochemically defined oxacyclic ligands such as Cp-THF, Tp-THF, Tris-THF, and fluoro-bis-THF provided exceptionally potent inhibitors (51 and 245–249) with clinical potential. The importance of the carbamate functionality in these inhibitors is particularly worthy of note. X-ray crystal structures of these inhibitors in complex with HIV-1 protease provided the ligand-binding site interactions responsible for their respective antiviral potency against wild-type and multidrug-resistant viruses. In general, inhibitors are involved in hydrogen-bonding interactions with Asp29, Asp30, Gly27, Asp25, Asp25′, and Asp30′ in the HIV-1 protease active site. Furthermore, the ring cycles adequately fill the hydrophobic pockets in the active site.

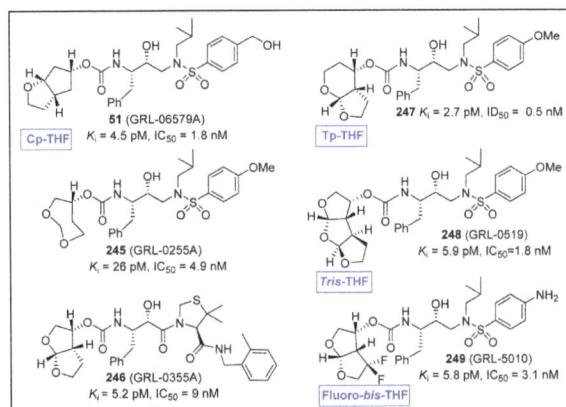

Cyclic ether carbamate-derived novel protease inhibitors.

Carbamates as β- and γ-secretase inhibitors

The search for an effective treatment for Alzheimer's disease (AD) remains a major challenge in medicine. One of the pathological hallmarks of AD is the formation of β-amyloid (Aβ) peptides in the cortex of AD patients. Aβ-peptides are generated from β-amyloid precursor protein (APP) by sequential cleavage by β-secretase (also known as BACE1 or memapsin 2) and γ-secretase. Due to this central role of Aβ-production, both β-secretase and γ-secretase have been implicated as important therapeutic targets for AD intervention. As a result, design and synthesis of selective β-secretase and γ-secretase inhibitors have become an intense area of research over the years.

Development of β-secretase Inhibitors

Following the discovery of β-secretase, the first-generation β-secretase inhibitors were designed and synthesized by Ghosh, Tang, and co-workers. As shown in Figure, utilizing a carbamate derivative of the Leu–Ala isostere 250, potent pseudopeptide inhibitors 251 and 252 were identified. The X-ray crystal structure of 252-bound β-secretase was determined to provide molecular insight into the ligand binding site interactions. The in-depth structural analysis thus provided critical drug design templates and led to the beginning of structure-based design approaches to peptido-mimetic/nonpeptide β-secretase inhibitors.

The X-ray structure of 252-bound β-secretase revealed that the P2 asparagine side chain carboxamide nitrogen formed an intermolecular hydrogen bond with the P4 glutamic acid carbonyl group.

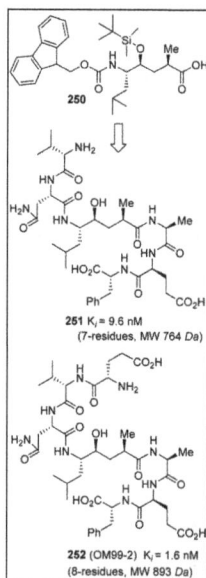

Design of pseudopeptide BACE1 inhibitors.

On the basis of this molecular insight, a number of 14–16-membered cycloamide-carbamate-based macrocyclic inhibitors were designed and synthesized. As shown in Figure, acyclic carbamate derivatives (253 and 254) were less potent than their corresponding cyclic inhibitors. Inhibitor 255, with a 16-membered macrocycle containing a *trans*-olefin, amide and carbamate functionalities within the macrocycle, showed good β-secretase inhibitory activity. Saturated inhibitor 256 is less potent against BACE1, but it showed enhanced potency for BACE2. X-ray structural studies of inhibitor 256-bound secretase revealed that the carbamate carbonyl forms a hydrogen bond with the Gln73 side chain carboxamide residue. Interestingly, unsaturated inhibitor 255 showed slight selectivity against memapsin 1 (K_i = 31 nM). The design of a selective inhibitor is important for reducing toxicity through off-target effects. Particularly, selectivity over other aspartic proteases, such as BACE2, pepsin, renin, cathepsin D (Cat-D), and cathepsin E, may be important for the reduction of side effects and drug efficiency.

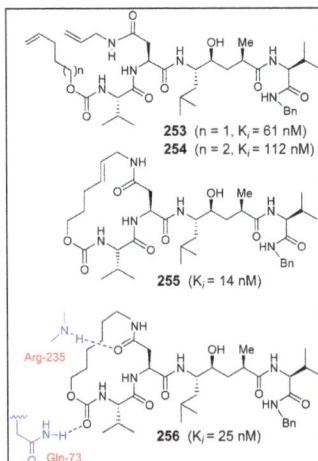

Carbamate-based macrocyclic BACE1 inhibitors.

On the basis of our detailed structure–activity studies and X-ray structural analysis, we have designed a variety of highly selective and potent BACE1 inhibitors. In this Perspective, we will highlight only the development of BACE1 inhibitors bearing carbamate functionalities. As shown in Figure, inhibitor 257 is a potent BACE1 inhibitor. However, it did not show selectivity against BACE2 or Cat-D. Subsequent structure-based design led to the development of selective inhibitors 258 and 259, which contain a pyrazolylmethyl and oxazolymethyl carbamate at the P3 position, respectively. Inhibitor 258 showed excellent BACE1 potency and selectivity over BACE2 and cathepsin D. The X-ray crystal structure of 258-bound β-secretase revealed that the carbamate carbonyl formed a hydrogen bond with the Thr-232 backbone NH. Also, the pyrazole nitrogen formed a strong hydrogen bond with the Thr-232 side chain hydroxyl group. The P2-sulfonyl functionality formed a number of hydrogen bonds in the S2 subsite as well. On the basis of this molecular insight, oxazole-derived 259 was designed to provide a more stable and selective inhibitor.

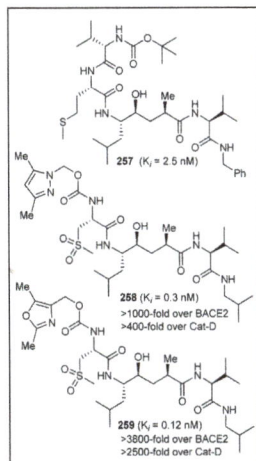

Carbamate-derived selective BACE1 inhibitors.

The synthesis of inhibitors 258 and 259 is outlined in Scheme. Urethanes 263 and 264 were prepared by treatment of 2,5-dimethylpyrazolylmethanol (260) or 2,5-dimethyl-4-oxazolemethanol (261) with triphosgene in the presence of triethylamine, followed by l-methionine methyl ester hydrochloride (262).

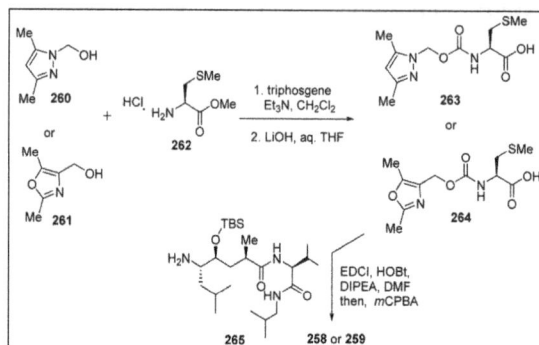

Synthesis of BACE1 Inhibitors 258 and 259.

Saponification of the resulting methyl esters provided the corresponding acids. Coupling of amine 265 with acids 263 and 264, as described previously, and subsequent oxidation of the sulfides with *m*-chloroperbenzoic acid furnished inhibitors 258 and 259.

Freskos and co-workers have reported a series of β-secretase inhibitors that incorporated polar carbamate derivatives as the P2 ligand. This strategy led to improve the Cat-D selectivity. It was hypothesized that the S2 subsite of Cat-D is more lipophilic and less tolerant of polar groups. As can be seen in Figure, benzyl carbamate derivative 266 displayed 6-fold selectivity over Cat-D. However, polar 3-pyridylmethyl derivative 267 improved selectivity nearly 90-fold. The corresponding 4-pyridyl methyl compound 268 provided a reduction in selectivity (~50-fold). 3-(S)-Tetrahydrofuranyl carbamate 269 showed a nearly 30-fold selectivity over Cat-D. These inhibitors have also shown good to excellent IC_{50} values in HEK cells.

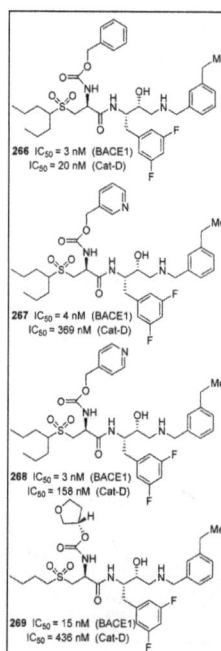

Butyl sulfone carbamate-derived selective BACE1 inhibitors.

Development of γ-secretase Inhibitors

Over the years, many structural classes of potent and selective γ-secretase inhibitors have been reported. A number of inhibitors displayed drug-like properties and also inhibited Aβ production in animal models. On the basis of γ-secretase inhibitor 270 (LY-411575), Peters and co-workers designed a series of carbamate derivatives of dibenzazepinone as potent and metabolically stable γ-secretase inhibitors. As shown in Figure, carbamate derivative 271 was prepared based on 270. Subsequently, carbamate 272 emerged as a potent γ-secretase inhibitor.

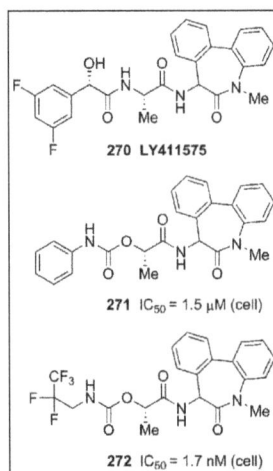

Carbamate-derived potent γ-secretase inhibitors.

Researchers at Pharmacopeia and Schering-Plough Research Institute developed a series of potent γ-secretase inhibitors containing tetrahydroquinoline sulfonamide and piperidine sulfonamide carbamates. As shown in Figure, a number of representative carbamate derivatives showed IC_{50} values in the low nanomolar range. Racemic carbamate 273 first showed a good IC_{50} value. Enantiomers were then separated by HPLC. One of the enantiomers showed an IC_{50} value of 39 nM, whereas the other enantiomer displayed an IC_{50} > 1000 nM. Absolute stereochemistry of the active enantiomer was not determined. Piperidine carbamate 274 also showed good potency. Carbamate derivative 275 displayed a good membrane Aβ IC_{50} value; however, it showed poor CYP properties. Further modification led to compound 276 with good inhibitory activity and improved CYP properties.

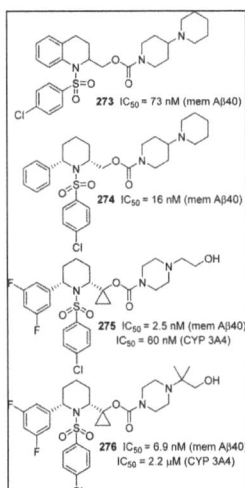

Tetrahydroquinoline and piperidine sulfonamide carbamate-derived γ-secretase inhibitors.

Bergstrom and co-workers reported a series of carbamate-appended *N*-alkyl sulfonamides as γ-secretase inhibitors. Figure depicts selected examples that show potent Aβ inhibitory activity. Sulfonamide derivative 277 was identified as a potent γ-secretase inhibitor. Exploration of carbamate-appended *N*-alkylsulfonamides resulted in potent inhibitors such as 278–280. Tertiary carbamate 280 showed significant reduction of brain Aβ in transgenic mice compared to that of its benzyl derivative. This compound also showed improved brain-to-plasma ratio and good absolute brain concentration.

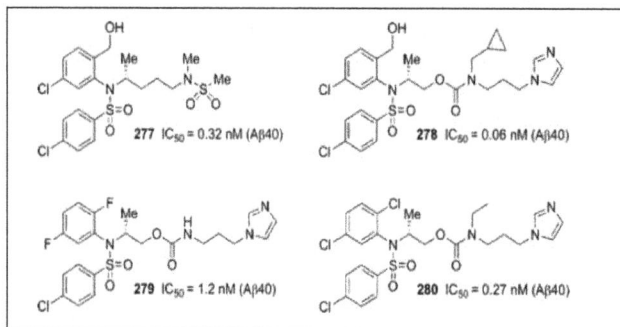

Carbamate-appended sulfonamides as γ-secretase inhibitors.

Carbamate-based HCV Therapeutics

Hepatitis C virus (HCV) is a bloodborne virus that is found worldwide. There are multiple strains or genotypes of the HCV virus. HCV infections lead to progressive liver damage, cirrhosis, and liver cancer. In recent years, there have been a number of new and effective antiviral drugs developed for the treatment of hepatitis C. These include the development of HCV NS3/4A protease inhibitors and inhibitors HCV NS5A.

Carbamate-derived Serine Protease Inhibitors

Serine proteases are a large family of proteolytic enzymes that play a variety of critical roles in many physiological processes. Deregulation of serine proteases has been related to the pathogenesis of diseases such as stroke, inflammation, Alzheimer's disease, cancer, and arthritis. Therefore, significant research efforts have been focused in the discovery of serine protease inhibitors. The active site of all serine proteases consists of a catalytic triad of Ser, His, and Asp. The nucleophilic attack by the hydroxyl group of serine at the carbonyl carbon of the scissile bond of the substrate, via general base catalysis by histidine, leads to the tetrahedral transition state. The tetrahedral intermediate ultimately collapses, leading to cleavage products. These key active residues are conserved in all serine proteases. X-ray structural studies revealed that these residues are superimposable in the majority of serine proteases. Therefore, selectivity over other serine proteases represents a key issue to be taken into consideration during inhibitor design. Most early inhibitors acted via a covalent mechanism in which an electrophilic group formed a covalent bond with the serine hydroxyl of the catalytic triad. The electrophilic groups are commonly referred to as serine traps or warheads. However, covalent inhibitors lack selectivity and specificity against other proteases in the same class or clan. The rational design of covalent serine protease inhibitors usually involves the selection of a good substrate to be linked to a serine trap/warhead. Chloromethyl ketones, diphenyl phosphonate esters, trifluoromethyl ketones, peptidyl boronic acids, α-ketoheterocycles, and β-lactam derivatives are usually employed as warheads. On the basis of these warheads, a variety of irreversible and reversible covalent serine protease inhibitors were designed.

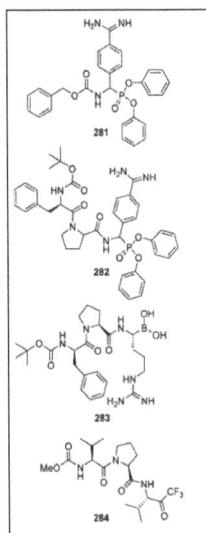

Structures of representative carbamate-containing kallikrein, thrombin, and elastase inhibitors.

Carbamate derivative 281, a diphenyl phosphonate ester containing a Cbz group and bearing a single amino acid side chain, showed very good inhibitory activity against human plasma kallikrein, useful for the treatment of hereditary angioedema. Thrombin is an attractive therapeutic target for drug development against pulmonary embolism, thrombosis, and related diseases. Compound 282 showed good potency and selectivity against human thrombin. It is stable and displayed no activity against acetylcholinesterase and no selectivity over cysteine proteases. Peptidyl boronic acid-based thrombin inhibitors were developed by DuPont-Merck. In particular, N-Boc derived inhibitor 283 is a potent inhibitor (K_i = 0.004 nM). Imperiali and co-workers introduced trifluoromethyl ketones as specific serine protease inhibitors, particularly for chymotrypsin and elastase. Researchers at AstraZeneca designed numerous peptidyl trifluoromethyl ketone derivatives as potent human elastase inhibitors. Further optimization of features resulted in the development of a number of orally active inhibitors. In particular, methyl carbamate derivative inhibitor 284 was shown to be a very potent inhibitor (K_i = 13 nM) with excellent oral bioavailability in laboratory animals. Optically pure compound 284 with an (S)-configuration at the P1 isopropyl side chain became a candidate for clinical development for potential treatment of elastase-implicated respiratory diseases.

Peptidomimetic boronic acid-based hepatitis C virus (HCV) NS3/4A protease inhibitors were designed and synthesized for the treatment of chronic HCV infections. HCV infections can lead to progressive liver damage, cirrhosis, and liver cancer. The NS3/4A serine protease plays a critical role in virus replication and has become an antiviral drug development target. The first specific and potent HCV protease inhibitor with good oral bioavailability was ciluprevir, which contains a carbamate functionality. This noncovalent macrocyclic peptidic inhibitor was the result of a substrate-based approach for the design of active site inhibitors. This inhibitor is very active in enzymatic (IC_{50} = 3 nM) and cell-based replicon assays (IC_{50} = 1.2 nM) of HCV genotype 1. Ciluprevir was later discontinued due to cardiac toxicity in animal models, but its development paved the way to boceprevir (Victrelis, Schering-Plough, approved by FDA in May 2011) and telaprevir (VX-950, Vertex Pharmaceuticals and Johnson & Johnson). In particular, for the development of boceprevir, the introduction of a ketoamide moiety, together with P2 and P3 optimization, led to inhibitor 286 showing a K_i of 66 nM. Its X-ray crystal structure in complex with the enzyme also provided insight for further optimization. Indeed, a cyclopropylalanine residue was found to be optimal at P1, and the resulting carbamate derivative 287 showed a K_i of 15 nM.

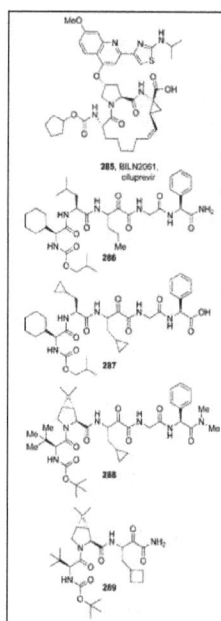

Structural evolution of carbamate-containing HCV NS3/4A protease inhibitors from ciluprevir to the discovery of boceprevir.

Although inhibitors 286 and 287 displayed good enzyme inhibitory potency, they did not display cellular activity in a subgenomic HCV replicon assay, possibly because of their strong peptidic character. The discovery that an *N*-methylated leucine at P2 was critical for both enzymatic potency and cellular activity led to the potential of cyclopropyl-fused proline being envisaged as an optimum, conformationally constrained surrogate for this part of the inhibitor. Combination of the P2-optimized ligand with previously optimized P1 and P3 residues provided carbamate derivative 288 with a K_i = 3.8 nM and IC$_{90}$ = 100 nM. Finally, truncation and P1 optimization, by the employment of a cyclobutyl moiety, led to compound 289 (K_i = 76 nM), the direct boceprevir ancestor.

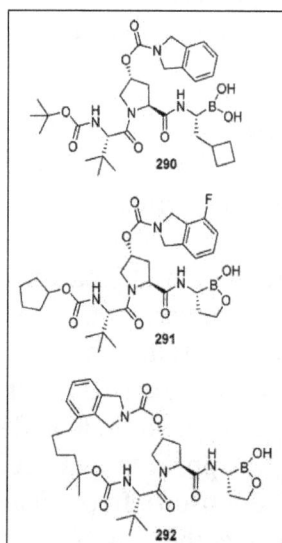

Structure of carbamate-containing HCV NS3/4A protease inhibitors.

Subsequently, compounds 290 and 291 with a carbamate containing P2 proline core showed very potent inhibitory activity (IC_{50} = 2 nM for 290 and 23 nM for 291). Similarly, macrocyclic inhibitor 292 with an α-amino cyclic boronate showed good potency (IC_{50} = 43 nM).

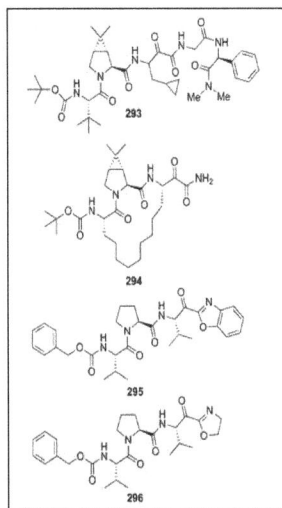

Carbamate-containing α-ketoamide inhibitors of HCV
NS3/4A protease and α-ketoheterocycle inhibitors of HNE.

The electron-withdrawing effect of the ester and amide functionalities was also utilized in the design of α-ketoester- or α-ketoamide-derived transition state inhibitors. A range of HCV NS3/4A protease inhibitors were designed and synthesized, incorporating α-ketoamide templates at the scissile site. Structure-based design led to a variety of potent acyclic and cyclic inhibitors with ketoamide templates, as exemplified in compounds 293 (IC_{50} = 3.8 nM) and 294 (IC_{50} = 30 nM). Edwards et al. developed peptidyl α-ketoheterocycles as a new template for inactivation of elastase. Tripeptidyl α-ketobenzoxazole 295 inhibited human neutrophil elastase (HNE) with an IC_{50} of 3 nM. The ketooxazoline-derived inhibitor 296 displayed very potent activity against HNE (IC_{50} = 0.6 nM).

HCV NS5A Inhibitors

Carbamate derivatives also play a key role as inhibitors of HCV NS5A, which represents a new and promising target for HCV therapy. HCV NS5A is a zinc-binding phosphoprotein, and its role in the HCV virus life cycle is still not clear. However, it plays a critical role in HCV RNA replication. Also, it is involved in virion morphogenesis. Due to the lack of enzymatic function, inhibitors of this viral-encoded protein have been pursued. Researchers at Bristol-Myers Squibb screened a library of compounds for their ability to inhibit HCV RNA replication. This led to the identification of a lead compound specifically interfering with RNA replication and later proving to inhibit the activity of NS5A protein. Subsequent optimization was focused on broadening the genotype specificity and improving pharmacokinetic properties of compounds. Symmetry of the molecule played an important role in inhibitory potency. This finally led to the discovery of daclatasvir a first-in-class inhibitor of the HCV NS5A replication complex. Daclatasvir was approved in Europe in August, 2014. Ledipasvir is another carbamate-containing HCV NS5A inhibitor with potent antiviral activity against HCV genotypes 1a and 1b. Harvoni, a combination of ledipasvir and sofosbuvir (a nucleotide polymerase inhibitor), was approved by the FDA in October 2014 for the treatment of chronic HCV genotype 1 infection. This also represents the first approved regimen that does not require administration with interferon or ribavirin.

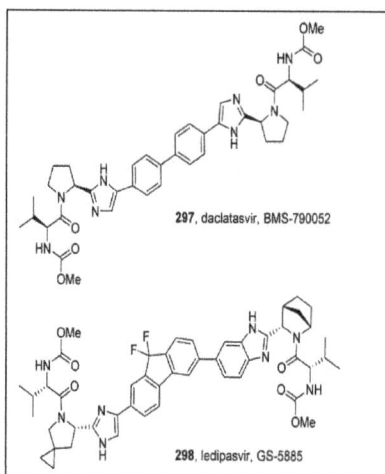

Carbamate-containing HCV NS5A inhibitors daclatasvir and ledipasvir.

Carbamates as Cysteine Protease Inhibitors

Cysteine proteases, also known as thiol proteases, are proteolytic enzymes responsible for the degradation of proteins. These enzymes are divided into three classes based on their sequence homology: the papain, caspase, and picornaviridae families. The papain family of proteases is the most known and studied.

Cysteine proteases have been identified in a variety of diverse organisms, such as bacteria, eukaryotic micro-organisms, plants, and animals and are divided into the clans CA, CD, CE, CF, and CH in the MEROPS peptidase database.

The largest subfamily among the class of cysteine proteases is the papain-like cysteine proteases, originating from papain as the archetype of the cysteine proteases. Clan CA proteases utilize catalytic Cys, His, and Asn residues that are invariably in this order in the primary sequence of the protease. Clan CA, Family C1 (papain-family) cysteine proteases are well-characterized for many eukaryotic organisms. Also, the best characterized Plasmodium cysteine proteases, namely, the falcipains, belong to papain-family (clan CA) enzymes.

Clan CD presents two catalytic residues, His and Cys, in sequence; Clan CE has a triad formed by His, Glu, or Asp and Cys at the C-terminus; in clan CF, the asparagine residue of the catalytic triad is replaced by a glutamate residue and the catalytic triad is ordered as Glu, Cys, and His; clan CG has a dyad of two cysteine residues, and Clan CH presents a Cys, Thr, and His triad with the catalytic cysteine at the N-terminus.

The proteolytic mechanism involves the formation of a thiolate–imidazolium ion pair, which provides a highly nucleophilic cysteine thiol. Over the years, many cysteine protease inhibitors have been designed by appropriately linking electrophilic warheads to the specific recognition sequence of peptide substrates. Reversible inhibitor warheads include aldehydes, α-ketoamides, α-ketoesters, and α-ketoacids. These inhibitors interact with the protease active site, forming the tetrahedral intermediate, but are eventually hydrolyzed, regenerating both the enzyme and the inhibitor in an equilibrium reaction. Irreversible inhibitors of cysteine proteases include epoxides, aziridines, haloketones, vinyl sulfones, and acyloxymethylketones. These inhibitors inactivate the target through alkylation of the active site cysteine thiol, permanently disabling enzyme function.

The occurrence of severe acute respiratory syndrome (SARS) in 2003 and the subsequent identification of a novel coronavirus as the etiological agent recognized cysteine proteases SARS-CoV 3CLpro and SARS-CoV PLpro (papain-like protease) as possible targets for drug design. Subsequent structure-based design based on a previous inhibitor's X-ray co-crystal structure with the enzyme provided carbamate derivative 299 as a potent SARS-CoV 3CLpro inhibitor (IC_{50} = 80 µM).

A wide variety of human rhinovirus 3C (HRV 3C) protease inhibitors were developed by the incorporation of α,β-unsaturated carbonyl moieties as warheads. Hanzlik et al. reported the first HRV 3C protease inhibitors containing a peptide portion and incorporating α,β-unsaturated esters. The peptide parts were selected based on the substrate cleavage site. The representative carbamate-containing inhibitor 300 showed an IC_{50} value of 130 nM.

Human cathepsin K plays a critical role in bone resorption. In an effort to block bone resorption, noncovalent cathepsin K inhibitors were developed. Kim et al. provided carbamate derivative 301 as a noncovalent and reversible cathepsin K (IC_{50} = 0.01 µM) and L inhibitor (IC_{50} = 0.002 µM). GlaxoWellcome scientists developed carbamate-containing ketoamide-based cathepsin K inhibitors such as 302 (IC_{50} = 0.072 nM). Starting from a potent ketone-based inhibitor with unsatisfactory drug-like properties, incorporation of P_2–P_3 elements from the ketoamide-based inhibitor 302 led to a hybrid series of ketone-based cathepsin K inhibitors with improved bioavailability, as exemplified in inhibitor 303 (IC_{50} = 4 nM).

Cathepsin S has been suggested for the development of agents against a range of immune disorders. A new class of nonpeptidic and noncovalent cathepsin S inhibitors was reported in 2007. Subsequent structural optimization resulted in a very potent and competitive noncovalent carbamate-containing inhibitor 304 (IC_{50} = 20 nM).

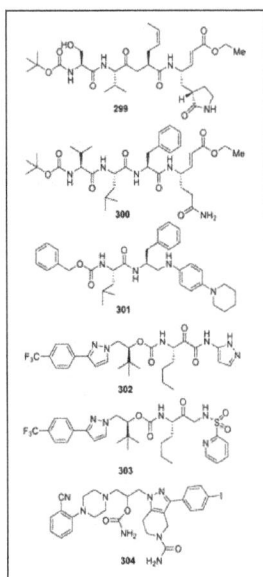

Representative carbamate-containing cysteine protease inhibitors.

Carbamates as Endocannabinoid Metabolizing Enzyme Inhibitors

Carbamates have been employed in the design of serine hydrolase inhibitiors. The endocannabinoid system is known to be a ubiquitous neuromodulatory system with a wide range of action that can be found in every primitive organism. It is composed of cannabinoid receptors (CBRs), endogenous cannabinoids (endocannabinoids, ECs), and the enzymes responsible for their production, transport, and degradation. ECs are a class of signaling lipids, such as N-arachidonoyl ethanolamine (anandamide, AEA), oleamide, and 2-arachidonoyl glycerol (2-AG), that exert their biological actions through the interaction with two G-protein coupled receptors, CB1 and CB2. They modulate a range of responses and processes including pain, inflammation, appetite, motility, sleep, thermoregulation, and cognitive and emotional states. The actions of these signaling lipids are rapidly terminated by cellular reuptake and subsequent hydrolysis operated by a number of enzymes. An attractive approach involved the modulation of the EC system and aimed at eliciting the desirable effects of CBRs activation through the pharmacological inactivation of the main endocannabinoid metabolizing enzymes, namely, monoacylglycerol lipase (MAGL) and α/β-hydrolase domain containing 6 and 12 (ABHD6 and ABHD12). These three serine hydrolases account for approximately 99% of 2-AG hydrolysis in the CNS, whereas fatty acid amide hydrolase (FAAH) is responsible for AEA inactivation. Inactivation of these enzymes would elevate the endogenous concentrations of all of its substrate and consequently prolong and potentiate their beneficial effects on pain and anxiety without evoking the classical CB1R agonists side effects (hypomotility, hypothermia, and catalepsy).

Monoacylglycerol lipase (MAGL) is the primary enzyme responsible for the hydrolysis of 2-AG in the CNS. About 85% of the total 2-AG hydrolysis in the brain is ascribed to MAGL. MAGL is a 33 kDa membrane enzyme belonging to the superfamily of the serine hydrolases with a catalytic triad represented by Ser122, His269, and Asp239. It is ubiquitously present in the brain (cortex, hippocampus, cerebellum, thalamu, and striatum), where it localizes to presynaptic terminals, even if lower levels are found in the brainstem and hypothalamus. A concomitant distribution in membranes as well as in the cytosol has been reported. MAGL shares a common folding motif called the α/β-hydrolase fold. Studies in recent years have shown that MAGL inhibitors elicit antinociceptive, anxiolytic, and antiemetic responses. MAGL inhibitors have also been shown to exert anti-inflammatory action in the brain and protect against neurodegeneration through lowering eicosanoid production. Recently, the potential of MAGL inhibitors for the therapy of Fragile X syndrome has been reported. The early discovered MAGL inhibitors were molecules able to target the cysteine residues present in the active site of the enzyme. Later, the research has been focused on the synthesis of compounds covalently binding to Ser241 of the catalytic triad. Among them, carbamate 305 was the first selective inhibitor of 2-AG degradation, although its potency remained limited (IC_{50} = 28 μM on rat brain). Selective MAGL inhibitors bearing a carbamate scaffold were developed by Cravatt and co-workers. Inhibitor 306 exhibited selectivity toward FAAH in $vitro$ (IC_{50} = 3.9 nM and 4 μM for human recombinant MAGL and FAAH, respectively). More recently, Cravatt and co-workers reported a distinct class of O-hexafluoroisopropyl (HFIP) carbamates bearing a reactive group that is bioisosteric with endocannabinoid substrates. The representative compound, 307(KML29, figure, IC_{50} = 5.9 nM, human MAGL), displays excellent potency and in $vivo$. In comparison to previously described O-aryl carbamates, inhibitor showed enhanced selectivity over FAAH and other serine hydrolases.

ABHD6 gene encodes a ~35 kDa protein containing an N-terminal transmembrane region followed by a catalytic domain that includes the canonical GXSXG active-site motif of serine hydrolases. ABHD6 is a unique and highly conserved enzyme in mammals and is mainly expressed in the brain, liver, kidney, and brown adipose tissue. As a member of the serine hydrolase class, ABHD6 is predicted to hydrolyze esters, amides, or thioester bonds in substrates that could include small molecules, lipids, or peptides. Although, the full range of substrates regulated by this enzyme *in vivo* is currently unknown. Recent studies have also shown that ABHD6 carbamate inhibitors produce anti-inflammatory and neuroprotective effects in a mouse model of traumatic brain injury. Among them, optimized inhibitor 308 displayed an IC_{50} value of 70 nM and notable selectivity.

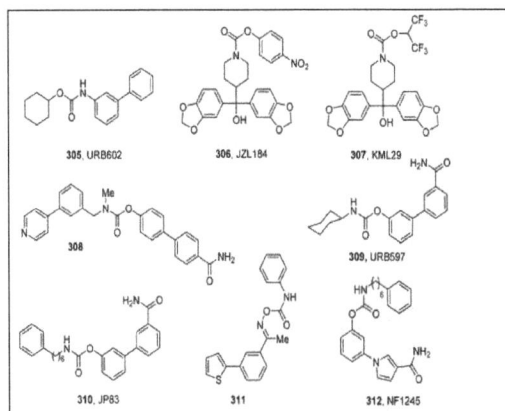

Representative carbamate-containing inhibitors of MAGL, ABHD6, and FAAH.

FAAH is a membrane-bound enzyme belonging to the amidase family. The analysis of its crystal structure revealed a core composed of a characteristic Ser-Ser-Lys catalytic triad. The catalytic residues of FAAH are buried deep within the enzyme and are accessible by two narrow channels. The importance of FAAH was demonstrated by the generation of FAAH knockout mice. FAAH$^{-/-}$ mice showed an elevated resting brain concentration of AEA and manifested (i) an analgesic phenotype in both the carrageenan model of inflammatory pain and in the formalin model of spontaneous pain, (ii) a reduction in inflammatory responses, and (iii) improvements in slow wave sleep and memory acquisition. The URB class of compounds was the first class of inhibitors identified for FAAH, and it is well-represented by 309 (URB597, Figure, IC_{50} = 4.6 nM). The *N*-(6-phenyl)hexylcarbamate analogue 310 (JP83, Figure, IC_{50} = 14 nM) is another very potent compound representative of the biphenyl series of inhibitors. Gattinoni and co-workers developed a series of oxime carbamate inhibitors. Compound 311 (Figure , IC_{50} = 8 nM) displayed good affinity and selectivity toward FAAH. More recently, Butini et al. developed a new class of potent and selective FAAH reversible carbamate inhibitors. Among them, compound 312 (NF1245, Figure, K_i = 0.16 nM on mouse brain FAAH) showed excellent activity. The compound showed impressive selectivity toward all the enzymes and receptors of the endocannabinoid system.

Classification of Medicinal Drugs

- **Drug Classifications based on Chemical Makeup**
- **Drug Classifications based On Effect on CNS**
- **Analgesics**
- **Antibiotic**
- **Antiviral Drug**
- **Antiseptics**
- **Tranquilizer**

Drugs are broadly classified on the basis of their chemical makeup and their effects. Some of the common types of drugs are analgesics, antibiotics, antiviral drugs, antiseptics and tranquilizers. The chapter closely examines these classes of drugs to provide an extensive understanding of the subject.

Drugs are classified chemically according to how they affect the brain and the body. Common classifications include stimulants, depressants, hallucinogens, and opioids. Additionally, the DEA legally classifies drugs into schedules (I, II, III, IV, and V) based on their medical use and potential for abuse and dependence.

Drugs can be categorized in a number of ways. In the world of medicine and pharmacology, a drug can be classified by its chemical activity or by the condition that it treats. Anticonvulsant medications, for example, are used to prevent seizures, while mucolytic drugs break down mucus and relieve congestion.

With regard to addiction treatment and rehabilitation, the drug classifications used most often are the following five classes regulated by the Controlled Substances Act:

- Narcotics

- Depressants

- Stimulants

- Hallucinogens

- Anabolic steroids

All of these drugs, with the exception of anabolic steroids, are considered to be psychoactive – meaning they affect one or more of the mental faculties including mood, feelings, thoughts, perception, memory, cognition, and behavior. Additionally, use of these drugs can be associated with a host of physical, mental health, and personal complications, including alcoholic liver cirrhosis, cannabis-induced psychosis, social problems like stigma, occupational difficulties, financial problems, and even legal problems.

According to the U.S. Drug Enforcement Administration (DEA), substances from any of these classes may lead to the development of chemical dependence in one or both of the following forms:

- Physical dependence to a drug suggests that the body has become habituated to the presence of a drug. Consequently, physical dependence is reflected in both the development of tolerance and the presence of a withdrawal syndrome. Tolerance refers to reduced effects compared to what was experienced with a previous amount of the substance. Withdrawal develops when excessive or prolonged use of a drug is sharply reduced or stopped. The onset of withdrawal often prompts the dependent individual to resume use of the drug (or one similar to it) to avoid withdrawal. For example, withdrawal symptoms such as shaking, sweating, nausea, vomiting, or seizures may occur once alcohol use is stopped after regular or excessive use.

- Psychological dependence is manifested in the form of craving for a drug. A person with psychological dependence has an excessive, irresistible, uncontrollable desire to use the drug. Psychological dependence may not cause physical symptoms, but can lead to drug-seeking behavior.

Chemical Classifications of Drugs

Each of the regulated drugs that act on the central nervous system or alter your feelings and perceptions can be classified according to their physical and psychological effects. The different drug types include the following:

- Depressants: Drugs that suppress or slow the activity of the brain and nerves, acting directly on the central nervous system to create a calming or sedating effect. This category includes barbiturates (phenobarbital, thiopental, butalbital), benzodiazepines (alprazolam, diazepam, clonazepam, lorazepam, midazolam), alcohol, and gamma hydroxybutyrate (GHB). Depressants are taken to relieve anxiety, promote sleep and manage seizure activity.

- Stimulants: Drugs that accelerate the activity of the central nervous system. Stimulants can make you feel energetic, focused, and alert. This class of drugs can also make you feel edgy, angry, or paranoid. Stimulants include drugs such as cocaine, crack cocaine, amphetamine, and methamphetamine. According to the recent World Drug Report published by the United Nations Office on Drugs and Crime, amphetamine-derived stimulants like ecstasy and methamphetamine are the most commonly abused drugs around the world after marijuana.

- Hallucinogens: Also known as psychedelics, these drugs act on the central nervous system to alter your perception of reality, time, and space. Hallucinogens may cause you to hear or see things that don't exist or imagine situations that aren't real. Hallucinogenic drugs include psilocybin (found in magic mushrooms), lysergic acid diethylamide (LSD), peyote, and dimethyltryptamine (DMT).

- Opioids: These are the drugs that act through the opioid receptors. Opioids are one of the most commonly prescribed medicines worldwide and are commonly used to treat pain and cough. These include drugs such as heroin, codeine, morphine, fentanyl, hydrocodone, oxycodone, buprenorphine, and methadone.

- Inhalants: These are a broad class of drugs with the shared trait of being primarily consumed through inhalation. Most of the substances in this class can exist in vapor form at room temperature. As many of these substances can be found as household items, inhalants are frequently abused by children and adolescents. These include substances such as paint, glue, paint thinners, gasoline, marker or pen ink, and others. Though ultimately all of these substances cross through the lungs into the bloodstream, their precise method of abuse may vary but can include sniffing, spraying, huffing, bagging, and inhaling, among other delivery routes.

- Cannabis: Cannabis is a plant-derived drug that is the most commonly used illicit drug worldwide. It acts through the cannabinoid receptors in the brain. Cannabis is abused in various forms including bhang, ganja, charas, and hashish oil.

- New psychoactive substances (NPS): These are drugs designed to evade the existing drug laws. Drugs such as synthetic cannabinoids, synthetic cathinones, ketamine, piperazines, and some plant-based drugs such as khat and kratom are examples of NPS.

Legal Classifications of Drugs

The Controlled Substances Act established five classifications, or schedules, for drugs regulated by law. According to the DEA, these classifications are broken down based on their potential for abuse and if they have a legitimate medical use:

- Schedule I include the drugs that have a high potential for abuse, that have no currently accepted medical use in treatment in the United States, and that there is a lack of accepted safety for use of the drug under medical supervision. Drugs such as cannabis, ecstasy, GHB, heroin, LSD, mescaline, and methaqualone are included in Schedule I.

- Schedule II includes drugs that have a high potential for abuse, have currently accepted medical use in treatment in the United States or currently accepted medical use with severe restrictions, and that the abuse of may lead to severe psychological or physical dependence. Drugs such as amphetamine, cocaine, fentanyl, hydromorphone oxycodone, and hydrocodone are included in Schedule II.

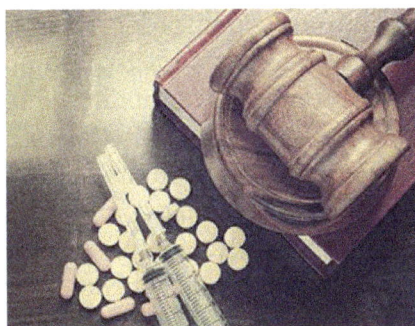

- Schedule III includes drugs that have a potential for abuse less than the drugs or other substances in schedules I and II, have a currently accepted medical use in treatment in the United States, and that the abuse of may lead to moderate or low physical dependence or high psychological dependence. Drugs such as anabolic steroids, buprenorphine, and ketamine are included in Schedule III.

- Schedule IV includes drugs that have a low potential for abuse relative to the drugs or other substances in schedule III, have a currently accepted medical use in treatment in the United States, and that the abuse of may lead to limited physical dependence or psychological dependence relative to the drugs or other substances in schedule III. Drugs such as benzodiazepines, modafinil, and tramadol are included in Schedule IV.

- Schedule V includes drugs that have a low potential for abuse relative to the drugs or other substances in schedule IV, have a currently accepted medical use in treatment in the United States, and that the abuse of may lead to limited physical dependence or psychological dependence relative to the drugs or other substances in schedule IV. Drugs such as diphenoxylate (in combination with atropine), lacosamide, and pregabalin are included in Schedule V.

The legal and personal consequences of misusing controlled substances can be severe. With your doctor's help, you can use these drug classifications as guidelines to help you determine if a medication or substance is both safe and beneficial.

Drug Classifications based on Chemical Makeup

CNS Stimulants and Depressants

Physicians do drug categories according to the effects they have on the human body. Drug recognition experts use seven different drug categories to group them together depending on how they impact the body after use. Some drugs may slow down the body, and other drugs can speed up bodily functions.

Some of the Drug Categories

Central Nervous System Depressants

Central nervous system depressants may also be referred to as tranquilizers or sedatives. A person experiencing anxiety, a panic attack, or a sleep disorder might receive a prescription for a CNS-depressant drug. Benzodiazepines can be highly addictive, so physicians usually prescribe these drugs only for short-term treatment. Examples of benzodiazepines include diazepam, alprazolam, triazolam, and estazolam. Non-benzodiazepine drugs also fall under this category of prescriptions. These medications are not as addictive, but they act on the same brain receptors as the more addictive benzodiazepines do. Examples of non-benzodiazepine drugs include zolpidem, eszopiclone, and zalepon. Barbiturates are another type of CNS depressant. These drugs are used less often due to a potential for overdose. Examples of barbiturates include mephobarbital, phenobarbital, and pentobarbital sodium.

Central Nervous System Stimulants

More than one of the drug categories affect the central nervous system, but these drugs increase the speed of mental and physical processes. CNS stimulants can be addictive due to the feelings of euphoria they create in people. A person under the influence of a CNS stimulant may feel as if the drug enhances and improves performance. However, these drugs typically make the brain and nervous system work harder, not better. The two major CNS stimulants are amphetamines and cocaine. Minor stimulants include caffeine and nicotine.

Hallucinogens

Hallucinogenic drugs can have a powerful impact on the brain. Common hallucinogens include LSD(*lysergic acid diethylamide*), PMA (*paramethoxyamphetamine*), and specific types of mushrooms. Drugs in this category can change how the user perceives reality because they change how nerve cells communicate in the brain. Results of taking hallucinogenic drugs can include reduced coordination, seeing visions, hearing voices, and feeling nonexistent sensations. While hallucinogens can be moderately addictive, the biggest risk with taking these drugs involves injuries and accidents while under the influence of the drug.

Dissociative Anesthetics

The original purpose of dissociative anesthetics involved surgical anesthesia. The effect of these drugs involves distorting perceptions and creating feelings of detachment between the body and the surrounding environment. Dissociative anesthetics affect the brain by changing the distribution of glutamate, which is instrumental in the perception of pain and memory. The two main dissociative anesthetics are PCP and ketamine. Dextromethorphan, an active ingredient in cough suppressants, can also produce dissociative anesthetic results when taken in large quantities.

Narcotic Analgesics

When severe pain occurs, narcotic analgesics can be effective for relieving discomfort. These drugs work by blocking how the central nervous system perceives pain. Common effects of narcotic analgesics include euphoria, drowsiness, and contentedness. Under the influence of narcotics, people also tend to experience slowed respiration and pupil constriction. Narcotic analgesics include morphine, codeine, and heroin. These drugs can result in increased tolerance and physical dependence.

Inhalants

Drugs in the inhalants category require inhalation of chemical vapors. Upon *"huffing,"* or inhalation, these chemicals interrupt the supply of oxygen to the brain. Reduced oxygen changes the way the brain works. Common physical effects include dizziness, distorted perceptions, and effects that mimic alcohol intoxication. The physical effects wear off quickly, which often leads to repeated use of the inhalants. Users might inhale volatile solvents, aerosols, and gases including nitrous oxide. Use of inhalants can cause significant brain damage.

Cannabis (Marijuana)

Cannabis contains *delta-9 tetrahydrocannabinol*, which is a psychoactive chemical. Marijuana comes from the leaves and flowers of the cannabis sativa plant. Marijuana might be smoked or ingested to create physical effects. Common effects of marijuana include increased heart rate, dry mouth, bloodshot eyes, increased appetite, and euphoria. Some users feel paranoia and anxiety while under the effects of marijuana. After the drug wears off, users may feel drowsy.

Cannabinoid

A cannabinoid is one of a class of diverse chemical compounds that acts on cannabinoid receptors, also known as the endocannabinoid system in cells that alter neurotransmitter release in the brain. Ligands for these receptor proteins include the endocannabinoids produced naturally in the body by animals; phytocannabinoids, found in cannabis; and synthetic cannabinoids, manufactured artificially. The most notable cannabinoid is the phytocannabinoid tetrahydrocannabinol (THC), the primary psychoactive compound in cannabis. Cannabidiol (CBD) is another major constituent of the plant. There are at least 113 different cannabinoids isolated from cannabis, exhibiting varied effects.

Synthetic cannabinoids encompass a variety of distinct chemical classes: the classical cannabinoids structurally related to THC, the nonclassical cannabinoids (cannabimimetics) including the aminoalkylindoles, 1,5-diarylpyrazoles, quinolines, and arylsulfonamides as well as eicosanoids related to endocannabinoids.

Uses

Medical uses include the treatment of nausea due to chemotherapy, spasticity, and possibly neuropathic pain. Common side effects include dizziness, sedation, confusion, dissociation and "feeling high".

Cannabinoid Receptors

Before the 1980s, it was often speculated that cannabinoids produced their physiological and behavioral effects via nonspecific interaction with cell membranes, instead of interacting with specific membrane-bound receptors. The discovery of the first cannabinoid receptors in the 1980s helped to resolve this debate. These receptors are common in animals, and have been found in mammals, birds, fish, and reptiles. At present, there are two known types of cannabinoid receptors, termed

CB_1 and CB_2, with mounting evidence of more. The human brain has more cannabinoid receptors than any other G protein-coupled receptor (GPCR) type.

Cannabinoid Receptor Type 1

CB_1 receptors are found primarily in the brain, more specifically in the basal ganglia and in the limbic system, including the hippocampus and the striatum. They are also found in the cerebellum and in both male and female reproductive systems. CB_1 receptors are absent in the medulla oblongata, the part of the brain stem responsible for respiratory and cardiovascular functions. CB1 is also found in the human anterior eye and retina.

Cannabinoid Receptor Type 2

CB_2 receptors are predominantly found in the immune system, or immune-derived cells with the greatest density in the spleen. While found only in the peripheral nervous system, a report does indicate that CB_2 is expressed by a subpopulation of microglia in the human cerebellum. CB_2 receptors appear to be responsible for the anti-inflammatory and possibly other therapeutic effects of cannabis seen in animal models.

Phytocannabinoids

Main classes of natural cannabinoids		
Type	Skeleton	Cyclization
Cannabigerol-type CBG		
Cannabichromene-type CBC		
Cannabidiol-type CBD		
Tetrahydrocannabinol- and Cannabinol-type THC, CBN		
Cannabielsoin-type CBE		

iso- Tetrahydrocannabinol- type iso-THC		
Cannabicyclol-type CBL		
Cannabicitran-type CBT		

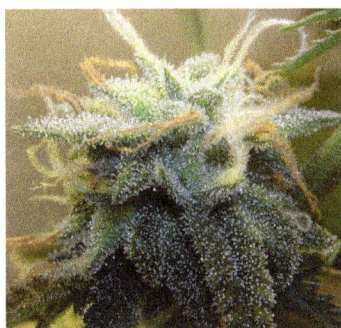

The bracts surrounding a cluster of Cannabis sativa fruits are coated
with cannabinoid-laden trichomes.

Cannabis-derived Cannabinoids

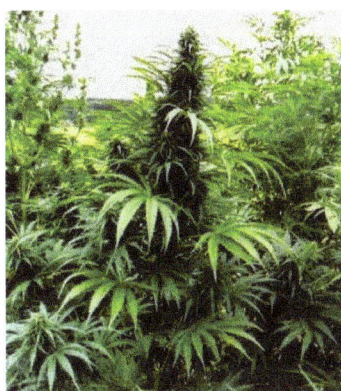

Cannabis indica plant.

The classical cannabinoids are concentrated in a viscous resin produced in structures known
as glandular trichomes. At least 113 different cannabinoids have been isolated from the *Cannabis* plant To the right, the main classes of cannabinoids from *Cannabis* are shown. The best
studied cannabinoids include tetrahydrocannabinol (THC), cannabidiol (CBD) and cannabinol (CBN).

Types

All classes derive from cannabigerol-type (CBG) compounds and differ mainly in the way this precursor is cyclized. The classical cannabinoids are derived from their respective 2-carboxylic acids (2-COOH) by decarboxylation (catalyzed by heat, light, or alkaline conditions).

- THC (tetrahydrocannabinol).

- THCA (tetrahydrocannabinolic acid).

- CBD (cannabidiol).

- CBDA (cannabidiolic acid).

- CBN (cannabinol).

- CBG (cannabigerol).

- CBC (cannabichromene).

- CBL (cannabicyclol).

- CBV (cannabivarin).

- THCV (tetrahydrocannabivarin).

- CBDV (cannabidivarin).

- CBCV (cannabichromevarin).

- CBGV (cannabigerovarin).

- CBGM (cannabigerol monomethyl ether).

- CBE (cannabielsoin).

- CBT (cannabicitran).

Tetrahydrocannabinol

Tetrahydrocannabinol (THC) is the primary psychoactive component of the Cannabis plant. *Delta*-9-tetrahydrocannabinol (Δ^9-THC, THC) and *delta*-8-tetrahydrocannabinol (Δ^8-THC), through intracellular CB_1 activation, induce anandamide and 2-arachidonoylglycerol synthesis produced naturally in the body and brain. These cannabinoids produce the effects associated with cannabis by binding to the CB_1 cannabinoid receptors in the brain.

Cannabidiol

Cannabidiol (CBD) is non-psychotropic. Recent evidence shows that the compound counteracts cognitive impairment associated with the use of cannabis. Cannabidiol has little affinity for CB_1 and CB_2 receptors but acts as an indirect antagonist of cannabinoid agonists. It was found to be an antagonist at the putative new cannabinoid receptor, GPR55, a GPCR expressed in the caudate nucleus and putamen. Cannabidiol has also been shown to act as a $5\text{-}HT_{1A}$ receptor agonist. CBD can interfere with the uptake of adenosine, which plays an important role in biochemical processes, such as energy transfer. It may play a role in promoting sleep and suppressing arousal.

CBD shares a precursor with THC and is the main cannabinoid in CBD-dominant *Cannabis* strains. CBD has been shown to play a role in preventing the short-term memory loss associated with THC.

There is tentative evidence that CBD had an anti-psychotic effect, but research in this area is limited.

Cannabinol

Cannabinol (CBN) is the primary product of THC degradation, and there is usually little of it in a fresh plant. CBN content increases as THC degrades in storage, and with exposure to light and air. It is only mildly psychoactive. Its affinity to the CB_2 receptor is higher than for the CB_1 receptor.

Cannabigerol

Cannabigerol (CBG) is non-psychoactive but still contributes to the overall effects of Cannabis.

Tetrahydrocannabivarin

Tetrahydrocannabivarin (THCV) is prevalent in certain central Asian and southern African strains of *Cannabis*. It is an antagonist of THC at CB_1 receptors and lessens the psychoactive effects of THC.

Cannabidivarin

Although cannabidivarin (CBDV) is usually a minor constituent of the cannabinoid profile, enhanced levels of CBDV have been reported in feral cannabis plants from the northwest Himalayas, and in hashish from Nepal.

Cannabichromene

Cannabichromene (CBC) is non-psychoactive and does not affect the psychoactivity of THC. CBC acts on the TRPV1 and TRPA1 receptors, interfering with their ability to break down endocannabinoids (chemicals such as anandamide and 2-AG that the body creates naturally). CBC has shown antitumor effects in breast cancer xenoplants in mice. More common in tropical cannabis varieties.

Biosynthesis

Cannabinoid production starts when an enzyme causes geranyl pyrophosphate and olivetolic acid to combine and form CBGA. Next, CBGA is independently converted to either CBG, THCA, CBDA or CBCA by four separate synthase, FAD-dependent dehydrogenase enzymes. There is no evidence for enzymatic conversion of CBDA or CBD to THCA or THC. For the propyl homologues (THCVA, CBDVA and CBCVA), there is an analogous pathway that is based on CBGVA from divarinolic acid instead of olivetolic acid.

Double Bond Position

In addition, each of the compounds above may be in different forms depending on the position of the double bond in the alicyclic carbon ring. There is potential for confusion because there are different numbering systems used to describe the position of this double bond. Under the dibenzopyran numbering system widely used today, the major form of THC is called Δ^9-THC, while the minor form is called Δ^8-THC. Under the alternate terpene numbering system, these same compounds are called Δ^1-THC and Δ^6-THC, respectively.

Length

Most classical cannabinoids are 21-carbon compounds. However, some do not follow this rule, primarily because of variation in the length of the side-chain attached to the aromatic ring. In THC, CBD, and CBN, this side-chain is a pentyl (5-carbon) chain. In the most common homologue, the pentyl chain is replaced with a propyl (3-carbon) chain. Cannabinoids with the propyl side chain are named using the suffix *varin*, and are designated, for example, THCV, CBDV, or CBNV.

Cannabinoids in other Plants

Phytocannabinoids are known to occur in several plant species besides cannabis. These include Echinacea purpurea, Echinacea angustifolia, Acmella oleracea, Helichrysum umbraculigerum, and Radula marginata. The best-known cannabinoids that are not derived from Cannabis are the lipophilic alkamides (alkylamides) from Echinacea species, most notably the cis/trans isomers dodeca-2E,4E,8Z,10E/Z-tetraenoic-acid-isobutylamide. At least 25 different alkylamides have been identified, and some of them have shown affinities to the CB_2-receptor. In some *Echinacea* species, cannabinoids are found throughout the plant structure, but are most concentrated in the roots and flowers. Yangonin found in the Kava plant has significant affinity to the CB1 receptor. Tea (Camellia sinensis) catechins have an affinity for human cannabinoid receptors. A widespread dietary terpene, beta-caryophyllene, a component from the essential oil of cannabis and other medicinal plants, has also been identified as a selective agonist of peripheral CB_2-receptors, *in vivo*. Black truffles contain anandamide. Perrottetinene, a moderately psychoactive cannabinoid, has been isolated from different *Radula* varieties.

Most of the phytocannabinoids are nearly insoluble in water but are soluble in lipids, alcohols, and other non-polar organic solvents.

Cannabis Plant Profile

Cannabis plants can exhibit wide variation in the quantity and type of cannabinoids they produce. The mixture of cannabinoids produced by a plant is known as the plant's cannabinoid profile. Selective breeding has been used to control the genetics of plants and modify the cannabinoid profile. For example, strains that are used as fiber (commonly called hemp) are bred such that they are low in psychoactive chemicals like THC. Strains used in medicine are often bred for high CBD content, and strains used for recreational purposes are usually bred for high THC content or for a specific chemical balance.

Quantitative analysis of a plant's cannabinoid profile is often determined by gas chromatography (GC), or more reliably by gas chromatography combined with mass spectrometry (GC/MS). Liquid chromatography (LC) techniques are also possible and, unlike GC methods, can differentiate between the acid and neutral forms of the cannabinoids. There have been systematic attempts to monitor the cannabinoid profile of cannabis over time, but their accuracy is impeded by the illegal status of the plant in many countries.

Pharmacology

Cannabinoids can be administered by smoking, vaporizing, oral ingestion, transdermal patch, intravenous injection, sublingual absorption, or rectal suppository. Once in the body, most cannabinoids are metabolized in the liver, especially by cytochrome P450 mixed-function oxidases, mainly CYP 2C9. Thus supplementing with CYP 2C9 inhibitors leads to extended intoxication.

Some is also stored in fat in addition to being metabolized in the liver. Δ^9-THC is metabolized to 11-hydroxy-Δ^9-THC, which is then metabolized to 9-carboxy-THC. Some cannabis metabolites can be detected in the body several weeks after administration. These metabolites are the chemicals recognized by common antibody-based "drug tests"; in the case of THC or others, these loads do not represent intoxication (compare to ethanol breath tests that measure instantaneous blood alcohol levels), but an integration of past consumption over an approximately month-long window. This is because they are fat-soluble, lipophilic molecules that accumulate in fatty tissues.

Research shows the effect of cannabinoids might be modulated by aromatic compounds produced by the cannabis plant, called terpenes. This interaction would lead to the entourage effect.

Cannabinoid-based Pharmaceuticals

Nabiximols (brand name Sativex) is an aerosolized mist for oral administration containing a near 1:1 ratio of CBD and THC. Also included are minor cannabinoids and terpenoids, ethanol and propylene glycol excipients, and peppermint flavoring. The drug, made by GW Pharmaceuticals, was first approved by Canadian authorities in 2005 to alleviate pain associated with multiple sclerosis, making it the first cannabis-based medicine. It is marketed by Bayer in Canada. Sativex has been approved in 25 countries; clinical trials are underway in the United States to gain FDA approval. In 2007, it was approved for treatment of cancer pain. In Phase III trials, the most common adverse effects were dizziness, drowsiness and disorientation; 12% of subjects stopped taking the drug because of the side effects.

Dronabinol (brand name Marinol) is a THC drug used to treat poor appetite, nausea, and sleep apnea. It is approved by the FDA for treating HIV/AIDS induced anorexia and chemotherapy induced nausea and vomiting.

The CBD drug Epidiolex has been approved by the Food and Drug Administration for treatment of two rare and severe forms of epilepsy, Dravet and Lennox-Gastaut syndromes.

Separation

Cannabinoids can be separated from the plant by extraction with organic solvents. Hydrocarbons and alcohols are often used as solvents. However, these solvents are flammable and many are toxic. Butane may be used, which evaporates extremely quickly. Supercritical solvent extraction with carbon dioxide is an alternative technique. Once extracted, isolated components can be separated using wiped film vacuum distillation or other distillation techniques. Also, techniques such as SPE or SPME are found useful in the extraction of this compounds.

The first discovery of an individual cannabinoid was made, when British chemist Robert S. Cahn reported the partial structure of Cannabinol (CBN), which he later identified as fully formed in 1940.

Two years later, in 1942, American chemist, Roger Adams, made history when he discovered Cannabidiol (CBD). Progressing from Adams research, in 1963 Israeli professor Raphael Mechoulam later identified the stereochemistry of CBD. The following year, in 1964, Mechoulam and his team identified the stereochemistry of Tetrahydrocannabinol (THC).

Due to molecular similarity and ease of synthetic conversion, CBD was originally believed to be a natural precursor to THC. However, it is now known that CBD and THC are produced independently in the cannabis plant from the precursor CBG.

Endocannabinoids

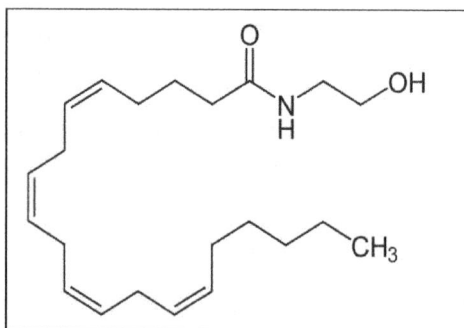

Anandamide, an endogenous ligand of CB_1 and CB_2.

Endocannabinoids are substances produced from within the body that activate cannabinoid receptors. After the discovery of the first cannabinoid receptor in 1988, scientists began searching for an endogenous ligand for the receptor.

Types of Endocannabinoid Ligands

Arachidonoylethanolamine (Anandamide or AEA)

Anandamide was the first such compound identified as arachidonoyl ethanolamine. The name is derived from the Sanskrit word for bliss and -*amide*. It has a pharmacology similar to THC, although its structure is quite different. Anandamide binds to the central (CB_1) and, to a lesser extent, peripheral (CB_2) cannabinoid receptors, where it acts as a partial agonist. Anandamide is about as potent as THC at the CB_1 receptor. Anandamide is found in nearly all tissues in a wide range of animals. Anandamide has also been found in plants, including small amounts in chocolate.

Two analogs of anandamide, 7,10,13,16-docosatetraenoylethanolamide and *homo*-γ-linolenoyletha-nolamine, have similar pharmacology. All of these compounds are members of a family of signalling lipids called *N*-acylethanolamines, which also includes the noncannabimimetic palmitoylethanol-amide and oleoylethanolamide, which possess anti-inflammatory and anorexigenic effects, respectively. Many *N*-acylethanolamines have also been identified in plant seeds and in molluscs.

2-Arachidonoylglycerol (2-AG)

Another endocannabinoid, 2-arachidonoylglycerol, binds to both the CB_1 and CB_2 receptors with similar affinity, acting as a full agonist at both. 2-AG is present at significantly higher concentrations in the brain than anandamide, and there is some controversy over whether 2-AG rather than anandamide is chiefly responsible for endocannabinoid signalling *in vivo*. In particular, one *in vitro* study suggests that 2-AG is capable of stimulating higher G-protein activation than anandamide, although the physiological implications of this finding are not yet known.

2-Arachidonyl Glyceryl Ether (Noladin Ether)

In 2001, a third, ether-type endocannabinoid, 2-arachidonyl glyceryl ether (noladin ether), was isolated from porcine brain. Prior to this discovery, it had been synthesized as a stable analog of 2-AG; indeed, some controversy remains over its classification as an endocannabinoid, as another group failed to detect the substance at "any appreciable amount" in the brains of several different mammalian species. It binds to the CB_1 cannabinoid receptor (K_i = 21.2 nmol/L) and causes sedation, hypothermia, intestinal immobility, and mild antinociception in mice. It binds primarily to the CB_1 receptor, and only weakly to the CB_2 receptor.

N-Arachidonoyl Dopamine (Nada)

Discovered in 2000, NADA preferentially binds to the CB_1 receptor. Like anandamide, NADA is also an agonist for the vanilloid receptor subtype 1 (TRPV1), a member of the vanilloid receptor family.

Virodhamine (OAE)

A fifth endocannabinoid, virodhamine, or *O*-arachidonoyl-ethanolamine (OAE), was discovered in June 2002. Although it is a full agonist at CB_2 and a partial agonist at CB_1, it behaves as a CB_1 antagonist *in vivo*. In rats, virodhamine was found to be present at comparable or slightly lower concentrations than anandamide in the brain, but 2- to 9-fold higher concentrations peripherally.

Lysophosphatidylinositol (LPI)

Recent evidence has highlighted lysophosphatidylinositol as the endogenous ligand to novel endocannabinoid receptor GPR55, making it a strong contender as the sixth endocannabinoid.

Function

Endocannabinoids serve as intercellular 'lipid messengers', signaling molecules that are released from one cell and activating the cannabinoid receptors present on other nearby cells. Although in this intercellular signaling role they are similar to the well-known monoamine neurotransmitters such as dopamine, endocannabinoids differ in numerous ways from them. For instance, they are used in retrograde signaling between neurons. Furthermore, endocannabinoids are lipophilic molecules that are not very soluble in water. They are not stored in vesicles and exist as integral constituents of the membrane bilayers that make up cells. They are believed to be synthesized 'on-demand' rather than made and stored for later use. The mechanisms and enzymes underlying the biosynthesis of endocannabinoids remain elusive and continue to be an area of active research. The endocannabinoid 2-AG has been found in bovine and human maternal milk.

A review by Matties et al. (1994) summed up the phenomenon of gustatory enhancement by certain cannabinoids. Recently, a paper by Yoshida et al. showed a selective stimulation of sweet receptor (Tlc1) by indirectly increasing its expression and suppressing the activity of leptin, the Tlc1 antagonist. It is proposed that the competition of leptin and cannabinoids for Tlc1 is implicated in energy homeostasis.

Retrograde Signal

Conventional neurotransmitters are released from a 'presynaptic' cell and activate appropriate receptors on a 'postsynaptic' cell, where presynaptic and postsynaptic designate the sending and receiving sides of a synapse, respectively. Endocannabinoids, on the other hand, are described as retrograde transmitters because they most commonly travel 'backward' against the usual synaptic transmitter flow. They are, in effect, released from the postsynaptic cell and act on the presynaptic cell, where the target receptors are densely concentrated on axonal terminals in the zones from which conventional neurotransmitters are released. Activation of cannabinoid receptors temporarily reduces the amount of conventional neurotransmitter released. This endocannabinoid-mediated system permits the postsynaptic cell to control its own incoming synaptic traffic. The ultimate effect on the endocannabinoid-releasing cell depends on the nature of the conventional transmitter being controlled. For instance, when the release of the inhibitory transmitter GABA is reduced, the net effect is an increase in the excitability of the endocannabinoid-releasing cell. On the converse, when release of the excitatory neurotransmitter glutamate is reduced, the net effect is a decrease in the excitability of the endocannabinoid-releasing cell.

Range

Endocannabinoids are hydrophobic molecules. They cannot travel unaided for long distances in the aqueous medium surrounding the cells from which they are released and therefore act locally on nearby target cells. Hence, although emanating diffusely from their source cells, they have much more restricted spheres of influence than do hormones, which can affect cells throughout the body.

Synthetic Cannabinoids

Historically, laboratory synthesis of cannabinoids was often based on the structure of herbal cannabinoids, and a large number of analogs have been produced and tested, especially in a group led by Roger Adams as early as 1941 and later in a group led by Raphael Mechoulam. Newer compounds are no longer related to natural cannabinoids or are based on the structure of the endogenous cannabinoids.

Synthetic cannabinoids are particularly useful in experiments to determine the relationship between the structure and activity of cannabinoid compounds, by making systematic, incremental modifications of cannabinoid molecules.

When synthetic cannabinoids are used recreationally, they present significant health dangers to users. In the period of 2012 through 2014, over 10,000 contacts to poison control centers in the United States were related to use of synthetic cannabinoids.

Medications containing natural or synthetic cannabinoids or cannabinoid analogs:

- Dronabinol (Marinol), is Δ^9-tetrahydrocannabinol (THC), used as an appetite stimulant, anti-emetic, and analgesic.

- Nabilone (Cesamet, Canemes), a synthetic cannabinoid and an analog of Marinol. It is Schedule II unlike Marinol, which is Schedule III.

- Rimonabant (SR141716), a selective cannabinoid (CB_1) receptor inverse agonist once used as an anti-obesity drug under the proprietary name Acomplia. It was also used for smoking cessation.

Other notable synthetic cannabinoids include:

- JWH-018, a potent synthetic cannabinoid agonist discovered by John W. Huffman at Clemson University. It is being increasingly sold in legal smoke blends collectively known as "spice". Several countries and states have moved to ban it legally.

- JWH-073.

- CP-55940, produced in 1974, this synthetic cannabinoid receptor agonist is many times more potent than THC.

- Dimethylheptylpyran.

- HU-210, about 100 times as potent as THC.

- HU-331 a potential anti-cancer drug derived from cannabidiol that specifically inhibits to-poisomerase II.

- SR144528, a CB_2 receptor antagonist.

- WIN 55,212-2, a potent cannabinoid receptor agonist.

- JWH-133, a potent selective CB_2 receptor agonist.

- Levonantradol (Nantrodolum), an anti-emetic and analgesic but not currently in use in medicine.

- AM-2201, a potent cannabinoid receptor agonist.

Barbiturate

A barbiturate is a drug that acts as a central nervous system depressant, and can therefore produce a wide range of effects, from mild sedation to death. Barbiturates are effective as anxiolytics, hypnotics, and anticonvulsants, but have physical and psychological addiction potential as well as overdose potential among other possible adverse effects. They have largely been replaced by benzodiazepines and nonbenzodiazepines ("Z-drugs") in routine medical practice, particularly in the treatment of anxiety and insomnia, due to the significantly lower risk of addiction and overdose and the lack of an antidote for barbiturate overdose. Despite this, barbiturates are still in use for various purposes: in general anesthesia, epilepsy, treatment of acute migraines or cluster headaches, euthanasia, capital punishment, and assisted suicide.

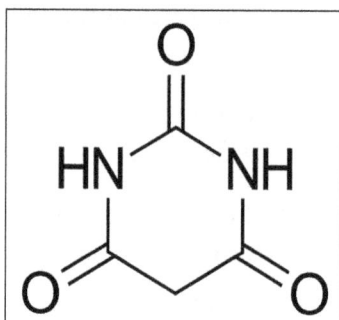

Barbituric acid, the parent structure of all barbiturates.

The name barbiturate originates from the fact that they are all chemical derivatives of barbituric acid.

Uses

Medicine

Barbiturates such as phenobarbital were long used as anxiolytics and hypnotics, but today have been largely replaced by benzodiazepines for these purposes because the latter are less toxic in drug overdose. However, barbiturates are still used as anticonvulsants (e.g., phenobarbital and primidone) and general anesthetics (e.g., sodium thiopental).

Barbiturates in high doses are used for physician-assisted suicide, and in combination with a muscle relaxant for euthanasia and for capital punishment by lethal injection. Barbiturates are frequently employed as euthanizing agents in small-animal veterinary medicine.

Interrogation

Sodium thiopental is an ultra-short-acting barbiturate that is marketed under the name Sodium Pentothal. It is often mistaken for "truth serum", or sodium amytal, an intermediate-acting barbiturate that is used for sedation and to treat insomnia, but was also used in so-called sodium amytal "interviews" where the person being questioned would be much more likely to provide the truth whilst under the influence of this drug. When dissolved in water, sodium amytal can be swallowed, or it can be administered by intravenous injection. The drug does not itself force people to tell the truth, but is thought to decrease inhibitions and slow creative thinking, making subjects more likely to be caught off guard when questioned, and increasing the possibility of the subject revealing information through emotional outbursts. Lying is somewhat more complex than telling the truth, especially under the influence of a sedative-hypnotic drug.

The memory-impairing effects and cognitive impairments induced by sodium thiopental are thought to reduce a subject's ability to invent and remember lies. This practice is no longer considered legally admissible in court due to findings that subjects undergoing such interrogations may form false memories, putting the reliability of all information obtained through such methods into question. Nonetheless, it is still employed in certain circumstances by defense and law enforcement agencies as a "humane" alternative to torture interrogation when the subject is believed to have information critical to the security of the state or agency employing the tactic.

Chemistry

In 1988, the synthesis and binding studies of an artificial receptor binding barbiturates by six complementary hydrogen bonds was published. Since this first article, different kind of receptors were designed, as well as different barbiturates and cyanurates, not for their efficiencies as drugs but for applications in supramolecular chemistry, in the conception of materials and molecular devices.

Sodium barbital and barbital have also been used as pH buffers for biological research, e.g., in immunoelectrophoresis or in fixative solutions.

Side Effects

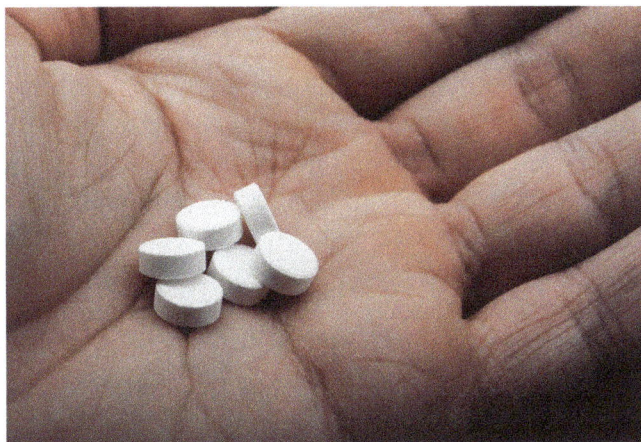

Addiction experts in psychiatry, chemistry, pharmacology, forensic science, epidemiology, and the police and legal services engaged in delphic analysis regarding 20 popular recreational drugs. Barbiturates were ranked 5th in dependence, 3rd in physical harm, and 4th in social harm.

There are special risks to consider for older adults, women who are pregnant, and babies. When a person ages, the body becomes less able to rid itself of barbiturates. As a result, people over the age of sixty-five are at higher risk of experiencing the harmful effects of barbiturates, including drug dependence and accidental overdose. When barbiturates are taken during pregnancy, the drug passes through the placenta to the fetus. After the baby is born, it may experience withdrawal symptoms and have trouble breathing. In addition, nursing mothers who take barbiturates may transmit the drug to their babies through breast milk. A rare adverse reaction to barbiturates is Stevens–Johnson syndrome, which primarily affects the mucous membranes.

Tolerance and Dependence

With regular use, tolerance to the effects of barbiturates develops. Research shows that tolerance can develop with even one administration of a barbiturate. As with all GABAergic drugs, barbiturate withdrawal produces potentially fatal effects such as seizures in a manner reminiscent of delirium tremens and benzodiazepine withdrawal although its more direct mechanism of GABA agonism makes barbiturate withdrawal even more severe than that of alcohol or benzodiazepines (subsequently making it one of the most dangerous withdrawals of any known addictive substance). Similarly to benzodiazepines, the longer acting barbiturates produce a less severe withdrawal syndrome than short acting and ultra-short acting barbiturates. Withdrawal symptoms are dose-dependent with heavier users being more affected than lower-dose addicts.

The pharmacological treatment of barbiturate withdrawal is an extended process often consisting of converting the patient to a long-acting benzodiazepine (i.e. Valium), followed by slowly tapering off the benzodiazepine. Mental cravings for barbiturates can last for months or years in some cases and counselling/support groups are highly encouraged by addiction specialists. Patients should never try to tackle the task of discontinuing barbiturates without consulting a doctor due to the high lethality and relatively sudden onset of the withdrawal. Attempting to quit "cold turkey" may result in serious neurological damage, severe physical injuries received during convulsions, and even death via glutamatergic excitotoxicity.

Overdose

Some symptoms of an overdose typically include sluggishness, incoordination, difficulty in thinking, slowness of speech, faulty judgement, drowsiness, shallow breathing, staggering, and, in severe cases, coma or death. The lethal dosage of barbiturates varies greatly with tolerance and from one individual to another. The lethal dose is highly variable among different members of the class with superpotent barbiturates such as pentobarbital being potentially fatal in considerably lower doses than the low-potency barbiturates such as butalbital. Even in inpatient settings the development of tolerance is still a problem, as dangerous and unpleasant withdrawal symptoms can result when the drug is stopped after dependence has developed. Tolerance to the anxiolytic and sedative effects of barbiturates tends to develop faster than tolerance to their effects on smooth muscle, respiration, and heart rate, making them generally unsuitable for a long time psychiatric use. Tolerance to the anticonvulsant effects tends to correlate more with tolerance to physiological effects, however, meaning that they are still a viable option for long-term epilepsy treatment.

Barbiturates in overdose with other CNS (central nervous system) depressants (e.g. alcohol, opiates, benzodiazepines) are even more dangerous due to additive CNS and respiratory depressant effects. In the case of benzodiazepines, not only do they have additive effects, barbiturates also increase the binding affinity of the benzodiazepine binding site, leading to exaggerated benzodiazepine effects. (ex. If a benzodiazepine increases the frequency of channel opening by 300%, and a barbiturate increases the duration of their opening by 300%, then the combined effects of the drugs increase the channels overall function by 900%, not 600%).

The longest-acting barbiturates have half-lives of a day or more, and subsequently result in bioaccumulation of the drug in the system. The therapeutic and recreational effects of long-acting barbiturates wear off significantly faster than the drug can be eliminated, allowing the drug to reach toxic concentrations in the blood following repeated administration (even when taken at the therapeutic or prescribed dose) despite the user feeling little or no effects from the plasma-bound concentrations of the drug. Users who consume alcohol or other sedatives after the drugs effects have worn but before it has cleared the system may experience a greatly exaggerated effect from the other sedatives which can be incapacitating or even fatal.

Barbiturates induce a number of hepatic CYP enzymes (most notably CYP2C9, CYP2C19, and CYP3A4), leading to exaggerated effects from many prodrugs and decreased effects from drugs which are metabolized by these enzymes to inactive metabolites. This can result in fatal overdoses from drugs such as codeine, tramadol, and carisoprodol, which become considerably more potent after being metabolized by CYP enzymes. Although all known members of the class possess relevant enzyme induction capabilities the degree of inhibition overall as well as the impact on each specific enzyme span a broad range with phenobarbital and secobarbital being the most potent enzyme inducers and butalbital and talbutal being among the weakest enzyme inducers in the class.

People who are known to have killed themselves with a barbiturate overdose include the members of Heaven's Gate cult, Charles Boyer, Dalida, Felix Hausdorff, Abbie Hoffman, Phyllis Hyman, Carole Landis, Helen Palmer, C. P. Ramanujam, Jean Seberg, Donald Sinclair, and Lupe Velez. Others who have died as a result of barbiturate overdose include Pier Angeli, Brian Epstein, Judy Garland, Jimi Hendrix, Dorothy Kilgallen, Thalia Massie, Edie Sedgwick, Inger Stevens, Ellen Wilkinson, Kenneth Williams, and Alan Wilson; in some cases these have been speculated to be suicides as well. Dorothy Dandridge died of either an overdose or an unrelated embolism. Ingeborg Bachmann may have died of the consequences of barbiturate withdrawal (she was hospitalized with burns, the doctors treating her not being aware of her barbiturate addiction).

Mechanism of Action

Barbiturates act as positive allosteric modulators and, at higher doses, as agonists of $GABA_A$ receptors. GABA is the principal inhibitory neurotransmitter in the mammalian central nervous system (CNS). Barbiturates bind to the $GABA_A$ receptor at multiple homologous transmembrane pockets located at subunit interfaces, which are binding sites distinct from GABA itself and also distinct from the benzodiazepine binding site. Like benzodiazepines, barbiturates potentiate the effect of GABA at this receptor. In addition to this GABAergic effect, barbiturates also block AMPA and kainate receptors, subtypes of ionotropic glutamate receptor. Glutamate is the principal excitatory neurotransmitter in the mammalian CNS. Taken together, the findings that barbiturates potentiate inhibitory $GABA_A$ receptors and inhibit excitatory AMPA receptors can explain the superior CNS-depressant effects of these agents to alternative GABA potentiating agents such as benzodiazepines and quinazolinones. At higher concentration, they inhibit the Ca^{2+}-dependent release of neurotransmitters such as glutamate via an effect on P/Q-type voltage-dependent calcium channels. Barbiturates produce their pharmacological effects by increasing the duration of chloride ion channel opening at the $GABA_A$ receptor (pharmacodynamics: This increases the efficacy of GABA), whereas benzodiazepines increase the frequency of the chloride ion channel opening at the $GABA_A$ receptor (pharmacodynamics: This increases the potency of GABA). The direct gating or opening of the chloride ion channel is the reason for the increased toxicity of barbiturates compared to benzodiazepines in overdose.

Further, barbiturates are relatively non-selective compounds that bind to an entire superfamily of ligand-gated ion channels, of which the $GABA_A$ receptor channel is only one of several representatives. This Cys-loop receptor superfamily of ion channels includes the neuronal nACh receptor channel, the $5\text{-}HT_3$ receptor channel, and the glycine receptor channel. However, while $GABA_A$ receptor currents are increased by barbiturates (and other general anaesthetics), ligand-gated ion channels that are predominantly permeable for cationic ions are blocked by these compounds. For example, neuronal nAChR channels are blocked by clinically relevant anaesthetic concentrations of both thiopental and pentobarbital. Such findings implicate (non-GABA-ergic) ligand-gated ion channels, e.g. the neuronal nAChR channel, in mediating some of the (side) effects of barbiturates. This is the mechanism responsible for the (mild to moderate) anesthetic effect of barbiturates in high doses when used in anesthetic concentration.

Barbituric acid was first synthesized November 27, 1864, by German chemist Adolf von Baeyer. This was done by condensing urea (an animal waste product) with diethyl malonate (an ester derived from the acid of apples). There are several stories about how the substance got its name. The most likely story is that Baeyer and his colleagues went to celebrate their discovery in a tavern where the town's artillery garrison were also celebrating the feast of Saint Barbara – the patron saint of artillerymen. An artillery officer is said to have christened the new substance by amalgamating *Barbara* with *urea*. Another story was barbiturate was invented on the feast day of St.Barbara. Another story holds that Baeyer synthesized the substance from the collected urine of a Munich waitress named Barbara. No substance of medical value was discovered, however, until 1903 when two German scientists working at Bayer, Emil Fischer and Joseph von Mering, discovered that barbital was very effective in putting dogs to sleep. Barbital was then marketed by Bayer under the trade name Veronal. It is said that Mering proposed this name because the most peaceful place he knew was the Italian city of Verona.

It was not until the 1950s that the behavioural disturbances and physical dependence potential of barbiturates became recognized.

Barbituric acid itself does not have any direct effect on the central nervous system and chemists have derived over 2,500 compounds from it that possess pharmacologically active qualities. The broad class of barbiturates is further broken down and classified according to speed of onset and duration of action. Ultrashort-acting barbiturates are commonly used for anesthesia because their extremely short duration of action allows for greater control. These properties allow doctors to rapidly put a patient "under" in emergency surgery situations. Doctors can also bring a patient out of anesthesia just as quickly, should complications arise during surgery. The middle two classes of barbiturates are often combined under the title "short/intermediate-acting." These barbiturates are also employed for anesthetic purposes, and are also sometimes prescribed for anxiety or insomnia. This is not a common practice anymore, however, owing to the dangers of long-term use of barbiturates; they have been replaced by the benzodiazepines for these purposes. The final class of barbiturates are known as long-acting barbiturates (the most notable one being phenobarbital, which has a half-life of roughly 92 hours). This class of barbiturates is used almost exclusively as anticonvulsants, although on rare occasions they are prescribed for daytime sedation. Barbiturates in this class are not used for insomnia, because, owing to their extremely long half-life, patients would awake with a residual "hang-over" effect and feel groggy.

Barbiturates can in most cases be used either as the free acid or as salts of sodium, calcium, potassium, magnesium, lithium, etc. Codeine- and Dionine-based salts of barbituric acid have been developed. In 1912, Bayer introduced another barbituric acid derivative, phenobarbital, under the trade name Luminal, as a sedative–hypnotic.

Society and Culture

Legal Status

During World War II, military personnel in the Pacific region were given "goofballs" to allow them to tolerate the heat and humidity of daily working conditions. Goofballs were distributed to reduce the demand on the respiratory system, as well as maintaining blood pressure, to combat the extreme conditions. Many soldiers returned with addictions that required several months of rehabilitation before discharge. This led to growing dependency problems, often exacerbated by indifferent doctors prescribing high doses to unknowing patients through the 1950s and 1960s.

In the late 1950s and 1960s, an increasing number of published reports of barbiturate overdoses and dependence problems led physicians to reduce their prescription, particularly for spurious requests. This eventually led to the scheduling of barbiturates as controlled drugs.

In the Netherlands, the Opium Law classifies all barbiturates as List II drugs, with the exception of secobarbital, which is on List I.

There is a small group of List II drugs for which doctors have to write the prescriptions according to the same, tougher guidelines as those for List I drugs (writing the prescription in full in letters, listing the patients name, and have to contain the name and initials, address, city and telephone number of the licensed prescriber issuing the prescriptions, as well as the name and initials, address and city of the person the prescription is issued to). Among that group of drugs are the barbiturates amobarbital, butalbital, cyclobarbital, and pentobarbital.

In the United States, the Controlled Substances Act of 1970 classified most barbiturates as controlled substances—and they remain so as of September 2015. Barbital, methylphenobarbital (also known as mephobarbital), and phenobarbital are designated schedule IV drugs, and "Any substance which contains any quantity of a derivative of barbituric acid, or any salt of a derivative of barbituric acid" (all other barbiturates) were designated as being schedule III. Under the original CSA, no barbiturates were placed in schedule I, II, or V, however amobarbital, pentobarbital, and secobarbital are schedule II controlled substances unless they are in a suppository dosage form.

In 1971, the Convention on Psychotropic Substances was signed in Vienna. Designed to regulate amphetamines, barbiturates, and other synthetics, the 34th version of the treaty, as of 25 January 2014, regulates secobarbital as schedule II, amobarbital, butalbital, cyclobarbital, and pentobarbital as schedule III, and allobarbital, barbital, butobarbital, mephobarbital, phenobarbital, butabarbital, and vinylbital as schedule IV on its "Green List". The combination medication Fioricet, consisting of butalbital, caffeine, and paracetamol (acetaminophen), however, is specifically exempted from controlled substance status, while its sibling Fiorinal, which contains aspirin instead of paracetamol and may contain codeine phosphate, remains a schedule III drug.

Recreational Use

Recreational users report that a barbiturate high gives them feelings of relaxed contentment and euphoria. Physical and psychological dependence may also develop with repeated use. Chronic misuse of barbiturates is associated with significant morbidity. One study found that 11% of males and 23% of females with a sedative-hypnotic misuse die by suicide. Other effects of barbiturate intoxication include drowsiness, lateral and vertical nystagmus, slurred speech and ataxia, decreased anxiety, and loss of inhibitions. Barbiturates are also used to alleviate the adverse or withdrawal effects of illicit drug use, in a manner similar to long-acting benzodiazepines such as diazepam and clonazepam. Often poly drug abuse occurs: Barbiturates are consumed with or substituted by other available substances, most commonly alcohol.

Drug users tend to prefer short-acting and intermediate-acting barbiturates. The most commonly used are amobarbital (Amytal), pentobarbital (Nembutal), and secobarbital (Seconal). A combination of amobarbital and secobarbital (called Tuinal) is also highly used. Short-acting and intermediate-acting barbiturates are usually prescribed as sedatives and sleeping pills. These pills begin acting fifteen to forty minutes after they are swallowed, and their effects last from five to six hours.

Slang terms for barbiturates include barbs, barbies, bluebirds, dolls, wallbangers, yellows, downers, goofballs, sleepers, 'reds & blues', and tooties.

Examples:

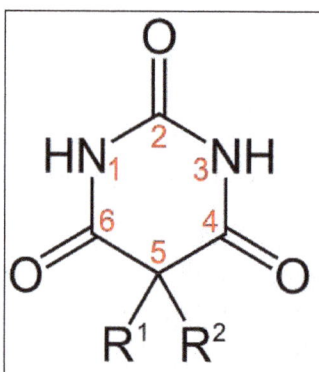

Generic structure of a barbiturate, including numbering scheme

Barbiturates			
Short Name	R^1	R^2	IUPAC Name
allobarbital	CH_2CHCH_2	CH_2CHCH_2	5,5-diallylbarbiturate
amobarbital	CH_2CH_3	$(CH_2)_2CH(CH_3)_2$	5-ethyl-5-isopentyl-barbiturate
aprobarbital	CH_2CHCH_2	$CH(CH_3)_2$	5-allyl-5-isopropyl-barbiturate
alphenal	CH_2CHCH_2	C_6H_5	5-allyl-5-phenyl-barbiturate
barbital	CH_2CH_3	CH_2CH_3	5,5-diethylbarbiturate
brallobarbital	CH_2CHCH_2	CH_2CBrCH_2	5-allyl-5-(2-bromo-allyl)-barbiturate
pentobarbital	CH_2CH_3	$CHCH_3(CH_2)_2CH_3$	5-ethyl-5-(1-methylbutyl)-barbiturate
phenobarbital	CH_2CH_3	C_6H_5	5-ethyl-5-phenylbarbiturate
secobarbital	CH_2CHCH_2	$CHCH_3(CH_2)_2CH_3$	5-[(2R)-pentan-2-yl]-5-prop-2-enyl-barbiturate; 5-allyl-5-[(2R)-pentan-2-yl]-barbiturate

Thiopental is a barbiturate with one of the C-O double bonds (with the carbon being labelled 2 in the adjacent diagram) replaced with a C-S double bond, R^1 being CH_2CH_3 and R^2 being $CH(CH_3)CH_2CH_2CH_3$.

Benzodiazepine

Benzodiazepines (BZD, BDZ, BZs), sometimes called "benzos", are a class of psychoactive drugs whose core chemical structure is the fusion of a benzene ring and a diazepine ring. The first such drug, chlordiazepoxide (Librium), was discovered accidentally by Leo Sternbach in 1955, and made available in 1960 by Hoffmann–La Roche, which, since 1963, has also marketed the benzodiazepine diazepam (Valium). In 1977 benzodiazepines were globally the most prescribed medications. They are in the family of drugs commonly known as minor tranquilizers.

Benzodiazepines enhance the effect of the neurotransmitter gamma-aminobutyric acid (GABA) at the $GABA_A$ receptor, resulting in sedative, hypnotic (sleep-inducing), anxiolytic (anti-anxiety), anticonvulsant, and muscle relaxant properties. High doses of many shorter-acting benzodiazepines may also cause anterograde amnesia and dissociation. These properties make benzodiazepines useful in treating anxiety, insomnia, agitation, seizures, muscle spasms, alcohol withdrawal and as a premedication for medical or dental procedures. Benzodiazepines are categorized as either short, intermediary, or long-acting. Short- and intermediate-acting benzodiazepines are preferred for the treatment of insomnia; longer-acting benzodiazepines are recommended for the treatment of anxiety.

Benzodiazepines are generally viewed as safe and effective for short-term use, although cognitive impairment and paradoxical effects such as aggression or behavioral disinhibition occasionally occur. A minority of people can have paradoxical reactions such as worsened agitation or panic. Benzodiazepines are also associated with increased risk of suicide. Long-term use is controversial because of concerns about decreasing effectiveness, physical dependence, withdrawal, and an increased risk of dementia. Stopping benzodiazepines often leads to improved physical and mental health. The elderly are at an increased risk of both short- and long-term adverse effects, and as a result, all benzodiazepines are listed in the Beers List of inappropriate medications for older adults. There is controversy concerning the safety of benzodiazepines in pregnancy. While they are not major teratogens, uncertainty remains as to whether they cause cleft palate in a small number of babies and whether neurobehavioural effects occur as a result of prenatal exposure; they are known to cause withdrawal symptoms in the newborn.

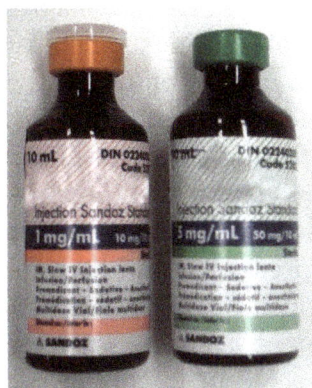

Midazolam 1 & 5 mg/mL injections (Canada).

Benzodiazepines can be taken in overdoses and can cause dangerous deep unconsciousness. However, they are less toxic than their predecessors, the barbiturates, and death rarely results when a benzodiazepine is the only drug taken. When combined with other central nervous system (CNS) depressants such as alcoholic drinks and opioids, the potential for toxicity and fatal overdose increases. Benzodiazepines are commonly misused and taken in combination with other drugs of abuse.

Benzodiazepines possess psycholeptic, sedative, hypnotic, anxiolytic, anticonvulsant, muscle relaxant, and amnesic actions, which are useful in a variety of indications such as alcohol dependence, seizures, anxiety disorders, panic, agitation, and insomnia. Most are administered orally; however, they can also be given intravenously, intramuscularly, or rectally. In general, benzodiazepines are well-tolerated and are safe and effective drugs in the short term for a wide range of conditions. Tolerance can develop to their effects and there is also a risk of dependence, and upon discontinuation a withdrawal syndrome may occur. These factors, combined with other possible secondary effects after prolonged use such as psychomotor, cognitive, or memory impairments, limit their long-term applicability. The effects of long-term use or misuse include the tendency to cause or worsen cognitive deficits, depression, and anxiety. The College of Physicians and Surgeons of British Columbia recommends discontinuing the usage of benzodiazepines in those on opioids and those who have used them long term. Benzodiazepines can have serious adverse health outcomes, and these findings support clinical and regulatory efforts to reduce usage, especially in combination with non-benzodiazepine receptor agonists.

Panic Disorder

Because of their effectiveness, tolerability, and rapid onset of anxiolytic action, benzodiazepines are frequently used for the treatment of anxiety associated with panic disorder. However, there is disagreement among expert bodies regarding the long-term use of benzodiazepines for panic disorder. The views range from those that hold that benzodiazepines are not effective long-term and that they should be reserved for treatment-resistant cases to those that hold that they are as effective in the long term as selective serotonin reuptake inhibitors.

The American Psychiatric Association (APA) guidelines note that, in general, benzodiazepines are well tolerated, and their use for the initial treatment for panic disorder is strongly supported by numerous controlled trials. APA states that there is insufficient evidence to recommend any of the established panic disorder treatments over another. The choice of treatment between benzodiazepines, SSRIs, serotonin–norepinephrine reuptake inhibitors, tricyclic antidepressants, and psychotherapy should be based on the patient's history, preference, and other individual characteristics. Selective serotonin reuptake inhibitors are likely to be the best choice of pharmacotherapy for many patients with panic disorder, but benzodiazepines are also often used, and some studies suggest that these medications are still used with greater frequency than the SSRIs. One advantage of benzodiazepines is that they alleviate the anxiety symptoms much faster than antidepressants, and therefore may be preferred in patients for whom rapid symptom control is critical. However, this advantage is offset by the possibility of developing benzodiazepine dependence. APA does not recommend benzodiazepines for persons with depressive symptoms or a recent history of substance abuse. The APA guidelines state that, in general, pharmacotherapy of panic disorder should be continued for at least a year, and that clinical experience supports continuing benzodiazepine treatment to prevent recurrence. Although major concerns about benzodiazepine tolerance and withdrawal have been raised, there is no evidence for significant dose escalation in patients using benzodiazepines long-term. For many such patients, stable doses of benzodiazepines retain their efficacy over several years.

Guidelines issued by the UK-based National Institute for Health and Clinical Excellence (NICE), carried out a systematic review using different methodology and came to a different conclusion. They questioned the accuracy of studies that were not placebo-controlled. And, based on the findings of placebo-controlled studies, they do not recommend use of benzodiazepines beyond two to four weeks, as tolerance and physical dependence develop rapidly, with withdrawal symptoms including rebound anxiety occurring after six weeks or more of use. Nevertheless, benzodiazepines are still prescribed for long-term treatment of anxiety disorders, although specific antidepressants and psychological therapies are recommended as the first-line treatment options with the anticonvulsant drug pregabalin indicated as a second- or third-line treatment and suitable for long-term use. NICE stated that long-term use of benzodiazepines for panic disorder with or without agoraphobia is an unlicensed indication, does not have long-term efficacy, and is, therefore, not recommended by clinical guidelines. Psychological therapies such as cognitive behavioural therapy are recommended as a first-line therapy for panic disorder; benzodiazepine use has been found to interfere with therapeutic gains from these therapies.

Benzodiazepines are usually administered orally; however, very occasionally lorazepam or diazepam may be given intravenously for the treatment of panic attacks.

Generalized Anxiety Disorder

Benzodiazepines have robust efficacy in the short-term management of generalized anxiety disorder (GAD), but were not shown effective in producing long-term improvement overall. According to National Institute for Health and Clinical Excellence (NICE), benzodiazepines can be used in the immediate management of GAD, if necessary. However, they should not usually be given for longer than 2–4 weeks. The only medications NICE recommends for the longer term management of GAD are antidepressants.

Likewise, Canadian Psychiatric Association (CPA) recommends benzodiazepines alprazolam, bromazepam, lorazepam, and diazepam only as a second-line choice, if the treatment with two different antidepressants was unsuccessful. Although they are second-line agents, benzodiazepines can be used for a limited time to relieve severe anxiety and agitation. CPA guidelines note that after 4–6 weeks the effect of benzodiazepines may decrease to the level of placebo, and that benzodiazepines are less effective than antidepressants in alleviating ruminative worry, the core symptom of GAD. However, in some cases, a prolonged treatment with benzodiazepines as the add-on to an antidepressant may be justified.

A 2015 review found a larger effect with medications than talk therapy. Medications with benefit include serotonin-noradrenaline reuptake inhibitors, benzodiazepines, and selective serotonin reuptake inhibitors.

Insomnia

Benzodiazepines can be useful for short-term treatment of insomnia. Their use beyond 2 to 4 weeks is not recommended due to the risk of dependence. The Committee on Safety of Medicines report recommended that where long-term use of benzodiazepines for insomnia is indicated then treatment should be intermittent wherever possible. It is preferred that benzodiazepines be taken intermittently and at the lowest effective dose. They improve sleep-related problems by shortening the time spent in bed before falling asleep, prolonging the sleep time, and, in general, reducing wakefulness. However, they worsen sleep quality by increasing light sleep and decreasing deep sleep. Other drawbacks of hypnotics, including benzodiazepines, are possible tolerance to their effects, rebound insomnia, and reduced slow-wave sleep and a withdrawal period typified by rebound insomnia and a prolonged period of anxiety and agitation.

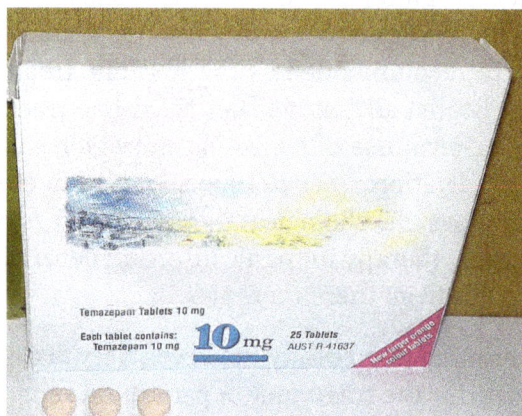

Temazepam (Normison) 10 mg tablets.

The list of benzodiazepines approved for the treatment of insomnia is fairly similar among most countries, but which benzodiazepines are officially designated as first-line hypnotics prescribed for the treatment of insomnia varies between countries. Longer-acting benzodiazepines such as nitrazepam and diazepam have residual effects that may persist into the next day and are, in general, not recommended.

Since the release of non benzodiazepines in 1992 in response to safety concerns, individuals with insomnia and other sleep disorders have increasingly been prescribed nonbenzodiazepines (2.3% in 1993 to 13.7% of Americans in 2010), less often prescribed benzodiazepines (23.5% in 1993 to 10.8% in 2010). It is not clear as to whether the new non benzodiazepine hypnotics (Z-drugs) are better than the short-acting benzodiazepines. The efficacy of these two groups of medications is similar. According to the US Agency for Healthcare Research and Quality, indirect comparison indicates that side-effects from benzodiazepines may be about twice as frequent as from nonbenzodiazepines. Some experts suggest using nonbenzodiazepines preferentially as a first-line long-term treatment of insomnia. However, the UK National Institute for Health and Clinical Excellence did not find any convincing evidence in favor of Z-drugs. NICE review pointed out that short-acting Z-drugs were inappropriately compared in clinical trials with long-acting benzodiazepines. There have been no trials comparing short-acting Z-drugs with appropriate doses of short-acting benzodiazepines. Based on this, NICE recommended choosing the hypnotic based on cost and the patient's preference.

Older adults should not use benzodiazepines to treat insomnia unless other treatments have failed. When benzodiazepines are used, patients, their caretakers, and their physician should discuss the increased risk of harms, including evidence that shows twice the incidence of traffic collisions among driving patients, and falls and hip fracture for older patients.

Seizures

Prolonged convulsive epileptic seizures are a medical emergency that can usually be dealt with effectively by administering fast-acting benzodiazepines, which are potent anticonvulsants. In a hospital environment, intravenous clonazepam, lorazepam, and diazepam are first-line choices. In the community, intravenous administration is not practical and so rectal diazepam or buccal midazolam are used, with a preference for midazolam as its administration is easier and more socially acceptable.

When benzodiazepines were first introduced, they were enthusiastically adopted for treating all forms of epilepsy. However, drowsiness and tolerance become problems with continued use and none are now considered first-line choices for long-term epilepsy therapy. Clobazam is widely used by specialist epilepsy clinics worldwide and clonazepam is popular in the Netherlands, Belgium and France. Clobazam was approved for use in the United States in 2011. In the UK, both clobazam and clonazepam are second-line choices for treating many forms of epilepsy. Clobazam also has a useful role for very short-term seizure prophylaxis and in catamenial epilepsy. Discontinuation after long-term use in epilepsy requires additional caution because of the risks of rebound seizures. Therefore, the dose is slowly tapered over a period of up to six months or longer.

Alcohol Withdrawal

Chlordiazepoxide is the most commonly used benzodiazepine for alcohol detoxification, but diazepam may be used as an alternative. Both are used in the detoxification of individuals who are motivated to stop drinking, and are prescribed for a short period of time to reduce the risks of developing tolerance and dependence to the benzodiazepine medication itself. The benzodiazepines with a longer half-life make detoxification more tolerable, and dangerous (and potentially lethal) alcohol withdrawal effects are less likely to occur. On the other hand, short-acting benzodiazepines may lead to breakthrough seizures, and are, therefore, not recommended for detoxification in an outpatient setting. Oxazepam and lorazepam are often used in patients at risk of drug accumulation, in particular, the elderly and those with cirrhosis, because they are metabolized differently from other benzodiazepines, through conjugation.

Benzodiazepines are the preferred choice in the management of alcohol withdrawal syndrome, in particular, for the prevention and treatment of the dangerous complication of seizures and in subduing severe delirium. Lorazepam is the only benzodiazepine with predictable intramuscular absorption and it is the most effective in preventing and controlling acute seizures.

Anxiety

Benzodiazepines are sometimes used in the treatment of acute anxiety, as they bring about rapid and marked or moderate relief of symptoms in most individuals; however, they are not recommended beyond 2–4 weeks of use due to risks of tolerance and dependence and a lack of long-term effectiveness. As for insomnia, they may also be used on an irregular/"as-needed" basis, such as in cases where said anxiety is at its worst. Compared to other pharmacological treatments, benzodiazepines are twice as likely to lead to a relapse of the underlying condition upon discontinuation. Psychological therapies and other pharmacological therapies are recommended for the long-term treatment of generalized anxiety disorder. Antidepressants have higher remission rates and are, in general, safe and effective in the short and long term.

Other Indications

Benzodiazepines are often prescribed for a wide range of conditions:

- They can sedate patients receiving mechanical ventilation or those in extreme distress. Caution is exercised in this situation due to the risk of respiratory depression, and it is recommended that benzodiazepine overdose treatment facilities should be available.

- Benzodiazepines are indicated in the management of breathlessness (shortness of breath) in advanced diseases, in particular where other treatments have failed to adequately control symptoms.

- Benzodiazepines are effective as medication given a couple of hours before surgery to relieve anxiety. They also produce amnesia, which can be useful, as patients may not remember unpleasantness from the procedure. They are also used in patients with dental phobia as well as some ophthalmic procedures like refractive surgery; although such use is controversial and only recommended for those who are very anxious. Midazolam is the most commonly prescribed for this use because of its strong sedative actions and fast recovery time, as well as its water solubility, which reduces pain upon injection. Diazepam and lorazepam are sometimes used. Lorazepam has particularly marked amnesic properties that may make it more effective when amnesia is the desired effect.

- Benzodiazepines are well known for their strong muscle-relaxing properties and can be useful in the treatment of muscle spasms, although tolerance often develops to their muscle relaxant effects. Baclofen or tizanidine are sometimes used as an alternative to benzodiazepines. Tizanidine has been found to have superior tolerability compared to diazepam and baclofen.

- Benzodiazepines are also used to treat the acute panic caused by hallucinogen intoxication. Benzodiazepines are also used to calm the acutely agitated individual and can, if required, be given via an intramuscular injection. They can sometimes be effective in the short-term treatment of psychiatric emergencies such as acute psychosis as in schizophrenia or mania, bringing about rapid tranquillization and sedation until the effects of lithium or neuroleptics (antipsychotics) take effect. Lorazepam is most commonly used but clonazepam is sometimes prescribed for acute psychosis or mania; their long-term use is not recommended due to risks of dependence. Further research investigating the use of benzodiazepines alone and in combination with antipsychotic medications for treating acute psychosis is warranted.

- Clonazepam, a benzodiazepine is used to treat many forms of parasomnia. Rapid eye movement behavior disorder responds well to low doses of clonazepam. Restless legs syndrome can be treated using clonazepam as a third line treatment option as the use of clonazepam is still investigational.

- Benzodiazepines are sometimes used for obsessive–compulsive disorder (OCD), although they are generally believed ineffective for this indication. Effectiveness was, however, found in one small study. Benzodiazepines can be considered as a treatment option in treatment resistant cases.

- Antipsychotics are generally a first-line treatment for delirium; however, when delirium is caused by alcohol or sedative hypnotic withdrawal, benzodiazepines are a first-line treatment.

- There is some evidence that low doses of benzodiazepines reduce adverse effects of electro-convulsive therapy.

Contraindications

Because of their muscle relaxant action, benzodiazepines may cause respiratory depression in susceptible individuals. For that reason, they are contraindicated in people with myasthenia gravis, sleep apnea, bronchitis, and COPD. Caution is required when benzodiazepines are used in people with personality disorders or intellectual disability because of frequent paradoxical reactions. In major depression, they may precipitate suicidal tendencies and are sometimes used for suicidal overdoses. Individuals with a history of alcohol, opioid and barbiturate abuse should avoid benzodiazepines, as there is a risk of life-threatening interactions with these drugs.

Pregnancy

In the United States, the Food and Drug Administration has categorized benzodiazepines into either category D or X meaning potential for harm in the unborn has been demonstrated.

Exposure to benzodiazepines during pregnancy has been associated with a slightly increased (from 0.06 to 0.07%) risk of cleft palate in newborns, a controversial conclusion as some studies find no association between benzodiazepines and cleft palate. Their use by expectant mothers shortly before the delivery may result in a floppy infant syndrome, with the newborns suffering from hypotonia, hypothermia, lethargy, and breathing and feeding difficulties. Cases of neonatal withdrawal syndrome have been described in infants chronically exposed to benzodiazepines in utero. This syndrome may be hard to recognize, as it starts several days after delivery, for example, as late as 21 days for chlordiazepoxide. The symptoms include tremors, hypertonia, hyperreflexia, hyperactivity, and vomiting and may last for up to three to six months. Tapering down the dose during pregnancy may lessen its severity. If used in pregnancy, those benzodiazepines with a better and longer safety record, such as diazepam or chlordiazepoxide, are recommended over potentially more harmful benzodiazepines, such as temazepam or triazolam. Using the lowest effective dose for the shortest period of time minimizes the risks to the unborn child.

Elderly

The benefits of benzodiazepines are least and the risks are greatest in the elderly. They are listed as a potentially inappropriate medication for older adults by the American Geriatrics Society. The elderly are at an increased risk of dependence and are more sensitive to the adverse effects such as memory problems, daytime sedation, impaired motor coordination, and increased risk of motor vehicle accidents and falls, and an increased risk of hip fractures. The long-term effects of benzodiazepines and benzodiazepine dependence in the elderly can resemble dementia, depression, or anxiety syndromes, and progressively worsens over time. Adverse effects on cognition can be mistaken for the effects of old age. The benefits of withdrawal include improved cognition, alertness, mobility, reduced risk incontinence, and a reduced risk of falls and fractures. The success of gradual-tapering benzodiazepines is as great in the elderly as in younger people. Benzodiazepines should be prescribed to the elderly only with caution and only for a short period at low doses. Short to intermediate-acting benzodiazepines are preferred in the elderly such as oxazepam and temazepam. The high potency benzodiazepines alprazolam and triazolam and long-acting benzodiazepines are not recommended in the elderly due to increased adverse effects. Nonbenzodiazepines such as zaleplon and zolpidem and low doses of sedating antidepressants are sometimes used as alternatives to benzodiazepines.

Long-term use of benzodiazepines is associated with increased risk of cognitive impairment and dementia, and reduction in prescribing levels is likely to reduce dementia risk. The association of a past history of benzodiazepine use and cognitive decline is unclear, with some studies reporting a lower risk of cognitive decline in former users, some finding no association and some indicating an increased risk of cognitive decline.

Benzodiazepines are sometimes prescribed to treat behavioral symptoms of dementia. However, like antidepressants, they have little evidence of effectiveness, although antipsychotics have shown some benefit. Cognitive impairing effects of benzodiazepines that occur frequently in the elderly can also worsen dementia.

Adverse Effects

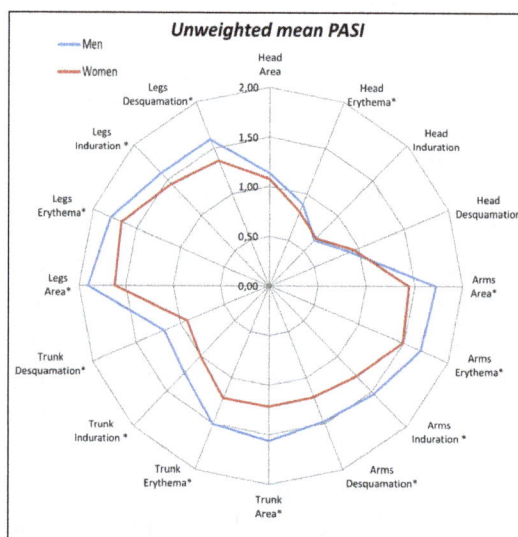

The most common side-effects of benzodiazepines are related to their sedating and muscle-relaxing action. They include drowsiness, dizziness, and decreased alertness and concentration. Lack of coordination may result in falls and injuries, in particular, in the elderly. Another result is impairment of driving skills and increased likelihood of road traffic accidents. Decreased libido and erection problems are a common side effect. Depression and disinhibition may emerge. Hypotension and suppressed breathing (hypoventilation) may be encountered with intravenous use. Less common side effects include nausea and changes in appetite, blurred vision, confusion, euphoria, depersonalization and nightmares. Cases of liver toxicity have been described but are very rare.

The long-term effects of benzodiazepine use can include cognitive impairment as well as affective and behavioural problems. Feelings of turmoil, difficulty in thinking constructively, loss of sex-drive, agoraphobia and social phobia, increasing anxiety and depression, loss of interest in leisure pursuits and interests, and an inability to experience or express feelings can also occur. Not everyone, however, experiences problems with long-term use. Additionally, an altered perception of self, environment and relationships may occur.

Compared to other sedative-hypnotics, visits to the hospital involving benzodiazepines had a 66% greater odds of a serious adverse health outcome. This included hospitalization, patient transfer, or death, and visits involving a combination of benzodiazepines and non-benzodiapine receptor agonists had almost four-times increased odds of a serious health outcome.

Cognitive Effects

The short-term use of benzodiazepines adversely affects multiple areas of cognition, the most notable one being that it interferes with the formation and consolidation of memories of new material and may induce complete anterograde amnesia. However, researchers hold contrary opinions regarding the effects of long-term administration. One view is that many of the short-term effects continue into the long-term and may even worsen, and are not resolved after stopping benzodiazepine usage. Another view maintains that cognitive deficits in chronic benzodiazepine users occur only for a short period after the dose, or that the anxiety disorder is the cause of these deficits.

While the definitive studies are lacking, the former view received support from a 2004 meta-analysis of 13 small studies. This meta-analysis found that long-term use of benzodiazepines was associated with moderate to large adverse effects on all areas of cognition, with visuospatial memory being the most commonly detected impairment. Some of the other impairments reported were decreased IQ, visiomotor coordination, information processing, verbal learning and concentration. The authors of the meta-analysis and a later reviewer noted that the applicability of this meta-analysis is limited because the subjects were taken mostly from withdrawal clinics; the coexisting drug, alcohol use, and psychiatric disorders were not defined; and several of the included studies conducted the cognitive measurements during the withdrawal period.

Paradoxical Effects

Paradoxical reactions, such as increased seizures in epileptics, aggression, violence, impulsivity, irritability and suicidal behavior sometimes occur. These reactions have been explained as consequences of disinhibition and the subsequent loss of control over socially unacceptable behavior. Paradoxical reactions are rare in the general population, with an incidence rate below 1% and similar to placebo. However, they occur with greater frequency in recreational abusers, individuals with borderline personality disorder, children, and patients on high-dosage regimes. In these groups, impulse control problems are perhaps the most important risk factor for disinhibition; learning disabilities and neurological disorders are also significant risks. Most reports of disinhibition involve high doses of high-potency benzodiazepines. Paradoxical effects may also appear after chronic use of benzodiazepines.

Long-term Worsening of Psychiatric Symptoms

While benzodiazepines may have short-term benefits for anxiety, sleep and agitation in some patients, long-term (i.e., greater than 2–4 weeks) use can result in a worsening of the very symptoms the medications are meant to treat. Potential explanations include exacerbating cognitive problems that are already common in anxiety disorders, causing or worsening depression and suicidality, disrupting sleep architecture by inhibiting deep stage sleep, withdrawal symptoms or rebound symptoms in between doses mimicking or exacerbating underlying anxiety or sleep disorders, inhibiting the benefits of psychotherapy by inhibiting memory consolidation and reducing fear extinction, and reducing coping with trauma/stress and increasing vulnerability to future stress. Anxiety, insomnia and irritability may be temporarily exacerbated during withdrawal, but psychiatric symptoms after discontinuation are usually less than even while taking benzodiazepines. Functioning significantly improves within 1 year of discontinuation.

Reinforcement Disorders

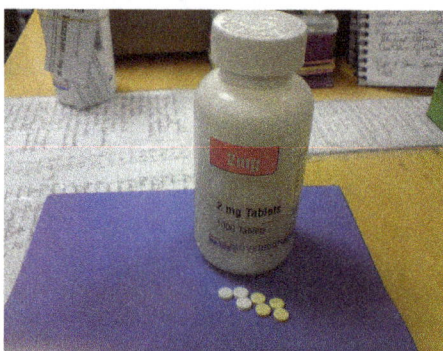

Diazepam 2 mg and 5 mg diazepam tablets, which are commonly used in the treatment of benzodiazepine withdrawal.

Tolerance

The main problem of the chronic use of benzodiazepines is the development of tolerance and dependence. Tolerance manifests itself as diminished pharmacological effect and develops relatively quickly to the sedative, hypnotic, anticonvulsant, and muscle relaxant actions of benzodiazepines. Tolerance to anti-anxiety effects develops more slowly with little evidence of continued effectiveness beyond four to six months of continued use. In general, tolerance to the amnesic effects does not occur. However, controversy exists as to tolerance to the anxiolytic effects with some evidence that benzodiazepines retain efficacy and opposing evidence from a systematic review of the literature that tolerance frequently occurs and some evidence that anxiety may worsen with long-term use. The question of tolerance to the amnesic effects of benzodiazepines is, likewise, unclear. Some evidence suggests that partial tolerance does develop, and that, "memory impairment is limited to a narrow window within 90 minutes after each dose".

A major disadvantage of benzodiazepines that tolerance to therapeutic effects develops relatively quickly while many adverse effects persist. Tolerance develops to hypnotic and myorelaxant effects within days to weeks, and to anticonvulsant and anxiolytic effects within weeks to months. Therefore, benzodiazepines are unlikely to be effective long-term treatments for sleep and anxiety. While BZD therapeutic effects disappear with tolerance, depression and impulsivity with high suicidal risk commonly persist. Several studies have confirmed that long-term benzodiazepines are not significantly different from placebo for sleep or anxiety. This may explain why patients commonly increase doses over time and many eventually take more than one type of benzodiazepine after the first loses effectiveness. Additionally, because tolerance to benzodiazepine sedating effects develops more quickly than does tolerance to brainstem depressant effects, those taking more benzodiazepines to achieve desired effects may suffer sudden respiratory depression, hypotension or death. Most patients with anxiety disorders and PTSD have symptoms that persist for at least several months, making tolerance to therapeutic effects a distinct problem for them and necessitating the need for more effective long-term treatment (e.g., psychotherapy, serotonergic antidepressants).

Withdrawal Symptoms and Management

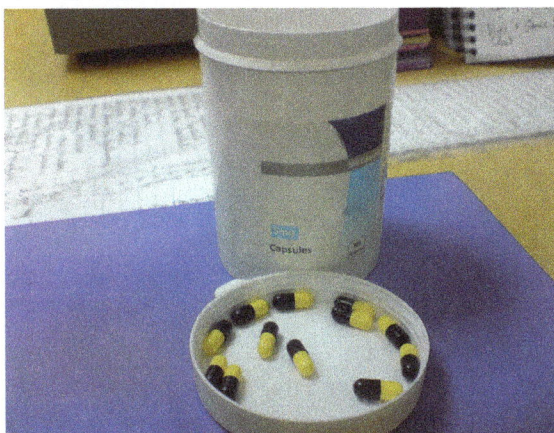

Chlordiazepoxide 5 mg capsules, which are sometimes used as an alternative to diazepam for benzodiazepine withdrawal. Like diazepam it has a long elimination half-life and long-acting active metabolites.

Discontinuation of benzodiazepines or abrupt reduction of the dose, even after a relatively short course of treatment (two to four weeks), may result in two groups of symptoms—rebound and withdrawal. Rebound symptoms are the return of the symptoms for which the patient was treated but worse than before. Withdrawal symptoms are the new symptoms that occur when the benzodiazepine is stopped. They are the main sign of physical dependence.

The most frequent symptoms of withdrawal from benzodiazepines are insomnia, gastric problems, tremors, agitation, fearfulness, and muscle spasms. The less frequent effects are irritability, sweating, depersonalization, derealization, hypersensitivity to stimuli, depression, suicidal behavior, psychosis, seizures, and delirium tremens. Severe symptoms usually occur as a result of abrupt or over-rapid withdrawal. Abrupt withdrawal can be dangerous, therefore a gradual reduction regimen is recommended.

Symptoms may also occur during a gradual dosage reduction, but are typically less severe and may persist as part of a protracted withdrawal syndrome for months after cessation of benzodiazepines. Approximately 10% of patients experience a notable protracted withdrawal syndrome, which can persist for many months or in some cases a year or longer. Protracted symptoms tend to resemble those seen during the first couple of months of withdrawal but usually are of a sub-acute level of severity. Such symptoms do gradually lessen over time, eventually disappearing altogether.

Benzodiazepines have a reputation with patients and doctors for causing a severe and traumatic withdrawal; however, this is in large part due to the withdrawal process being poorly managed. Over-rapid withdrawal from benzodiazepines increases the severity of the withdrawal syndrome and increases the failure rate. A slow and gradual withdrawal customised to the individual and, if indicated, psychological support is the most effective way of managing the withdrawal. Opinion as to the time needed to complete withdrawal ranges from four weeks to several years. A goal of less than six months has been suggested, but due to factors such as dosage and type of benzodiazepine, reasons for prescription, lifestyle, personality, environmental stresses, and amount of available support, a year or more may be needed to withdraw.

Withdrawal is best managed by transferring the physically dependent patient to an equivalent dose of diazepam because it has the longest half-life of all of the benzodiazepines, is metabolised into long-acting active metabolites and is available in low-potency tablets, which can be quartered for smaller doses. A further benefit is that it is available in liquid form, which allows for even smaller reductions. Chlordiazepoxide, which also has a long half-life and long-acting active metabolites, can be used as an alternative.

Nonbenzodiazepines are contraindicated during benzodiazepine withdrawal as they are cross tolerant with benzodiazepines and can induce dependence. Alcohol is also cross tolerant with benzodiazepines and more toxic and thus caution is needed to avoid replacing one dependence with another. During withdrawal, fluoroquinolone-based antibiotics are best avoided if possible; they displace benzodiazepines from their binding site and reduce GABA function and, thus, may aggravate withdrawal symptoms. Antipsychotics are not recommended for benzodiazepine withdrawal (or other CNS depressant withdrawal states) especially clozapine, olanzapine or low potency phenothiazines e.g. chlorpromazine as they lower the seizure threshold and can worsen withdrawal effects; if used extreme caution is required.

Withdrawal from long term benzodiazepines is beneficial for most individuals. Withdrawal of benzodiazepines from long-term users, in general, leads to improved physical and mental health particularly in the elderly; although some long term users report continued benefit from taking benzodiazepines, this may be the result of suppression of withdrawal effects.

Controversial Associations

Beyond the well established link between benzodiazepines and psychomotor impairment resulting in motor vehicle accidents and falls leading to fracture; research in the 2000s and 2010s has raised the association between benzodiazepines (and Z-Drugs) and other, as of yet unproven, adverse effects including dementia, cancer, infections, pancreatitis and respiratory disease exacerbations.

Dementia

A number of studies have drawn an association between long-term benzodiazepine use and neuro-degenerative disease, particularly Alzheimer's disease. It has been determined that long-term use of benzodiazepines is associated with increased dementia risk, even after controlling for protopathic bias.

Infections

Some observational studies have detected significant associations between benzodiazepines and respiratory infections such as pneumonia where others have not. A large meta-analysis of pre-marketing randomized controlled trials on the pharmacologically related Z-Drugs suggest a small increase in infection risk as well. An immunodeficiency effect from the action of benzodiazepines on GABA-A receptors has been postulated from animal studies.

Cancer

A Meta-analysis of observational studies has determined an association between benzodiazepine use and cancer, though the risk across different agents and different cancers varied significantly. Furthermore, most of these studies were unable to control for confounding variables that may have influenced the relationship such as lifestyle exposures (i.e. tobacco, alcohol). In terms of experimental basic science evidence, an analysis of carcinogenetic and genotoxicity data for various benzodiazepines has suggested a small possibility of carcinogenesis for a small number of benzodiazepines. A large, properly designed randomized controlled trial with appropriate follow-up in addition to further pharmacologic/toxicologic investigation is needed to confirm these preliminary findings.

Pancreatitis

The evidence suggesting a link between benzodiazepines (and Z-Drugs) and pancreatic inflammation is very sparse and limited to a few observational studies from Taiwan. A criticism of confounding can be applied to these findings as with the other controversial associations above. Further well-designed research from other populations as well as a biologically plausible mechanism is required to confirm this association.

Overdose

Although benzodiazepines are much safer in overdose than their predecessors, the barbiturates, they can still cause problems in overdose. Taken alone, they rarely cause severe complications in overdose; statistics in England showed that benzodiazepines were responsible for 3.8% of all deaths by poisoning from a single drug. However, combining these drugs with alcohol, opiates or tricyclic antidepressants markedly raises the toxicity. The elderly are more sensitive to the side effects of benzodiazepines, and poisoning may even occur from their long-term use. The various benzodiazepines differ in their toxicity; temazepam appears most toxic in overdose and when used with other drugs. The symptoms of a benzodiazepine overdose may include; drowsiness, slurred speech, nystagmus, hypotension, ataxia, coma, respiratory depression, and cardiorespiratory arrest.

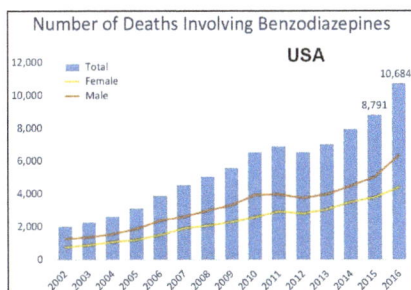

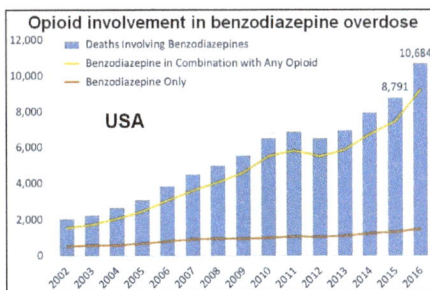

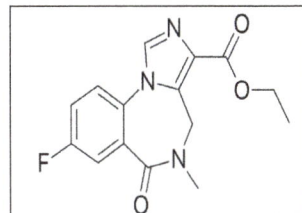

Left: US yearly overdose deaths involving benzodiazepines. Center: The top line represents the number of benzodiazepine deaths that also involved opioids in the US. The bottom line represents benzodiazepine deaths that did not involve opioids.. Right: Chemical structure of the benzodiazepine flumazenil, whose use is controversial following benzodiazepine overdose.

A reversal agent for benzodiazepines exists, flumazenil (Anexate). Its use as an antidote is not routinely recommended because of the high risk of resedation and seizures. In a double-blind, placebo-controlled trial of 326 people, 4 people had serious adverse events and 61% became resedated following the use of flumazenil. Numerous contraindications to its use exist. It is contraindicated in people with a history of long-term use of benzodiazepines, those having ingested a substance that lowers the seizure threshold or may cause an arrhythmia, and in those with abnormal vital signs. One study found that only 10% of the people presenting with a benzodiazepine overdose are suitable candidates for treatment with flumazenil.

Interactions

Individual benzodiazepines may have different interactions with certain drugs. Depending on their metabolism pathway, benzodiazepines can be divided roughly into two groups. The largest group consists of those that are metabolized by cytochrome P450 (CYP450) enzymes and possess significant potential for interactions with other drugs. The other group comprises those that are metabolized through glucuronidation, such as lorazepam, oxazepam, and temazepam, and, in general, have few drug interactions.

Many drugs, including oral contraceptives, some antibiotics, antidepressants, and antifungal agents, inhibit cytochrome enzymes in the liver. They reduce the rate of elimination of the benzodiazepines that are metabolized by CYP450, leading to possibly excessive drug accumulation and increased side-effects. In contrast, drugs that induce cytochrome P450 enzymes, such as St John's wort, the antibiotic rifampicin, and the anticonvulsants carbamazepine and phenytoin, accelerate elimination of many benzodiazepines and decrease their action. Taking benzodiazepines with alcohol, opioids and other central nervous system depressants potentiates their action. This often results in increased sedation, impaired motor coordination, suppressed breathing, and other adverse effects that have potential to be lethal. Antacids can slow down absorption of some benzodiazepines; however, this effect is marginal and inconsistent.

Pharmacology

Pharmacodynamics

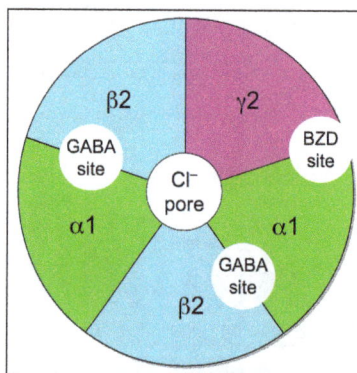

Schematic diagram of the $(\alpha 1)_2(\beta 2)_2(\gamma 2)$ GABA$_A$ receptor complex that depicts the five-protein subunits that form the receptor, the chloride (Cl⁻) ion channel pore at the center, the two GABA active binding sites at the α1 and β2 interfaces and the benzodiazepine (BZD) allosteric binding site at the α1 and γ2 interface.

Benzodiazepines work by increasing the effectiveness of the endogenous chemical, GABA, to decrease the excitability of neurons . This reduces the communication between neurons and, therefore, has a calming effect on many of the functions of the brain.

GABA controls the excitability of neurons by binding to the $GABA_A$ receptor. The $GABA_A$ receptor is a protein complex located in the synapses between neurons. All $GABA_A$ receptors contain an ion channel that conducts chloride ions across neuronal cell membranes and two binding sites for the neurotransmitter gamma-aminobutyric acid (GABA), while a subset of $GABA_A$ receptor complexes also contain a single binding site for benzodiazepines. Binding of benzodiazepines to this receptor complex does not alter binding of GABA. Unlike other positive allosteric modulators that increases ligand binding, benzodiazepine binding acts as a positive allosteric modulator by increasing the total conduction of chloride ions across the neuronal cell membrane when GABA is already bound to its receptor. This increased chloride ion influx hyperpolarizes the neuron's membrane potential. As a result, the difference between resting potential and threshold potential is increased and firing is less likely. Different $GABA_A$ receptor subtypes have varying distributions within different regions of the brain and, therefore, control distinct neuronal circuits. Hence, activation of different $GABA_A$ receptor subtypes by benzodiazepines may result in distinct pharmacological actions. In terms of the mechanism of action of benzodiazepines, their similarities are too great to separate them into individual categories such as anxiolytic or hypnotic. For example, a hypnotic administered in low doses produces anxiety-relieving effects, whereas a benzodiazepine marketed as an anti-anxiety drug at higher doses induces sleep.

The subset of $GABA_A$ receptors that also bind benzodiazepines are referred to as benzodiazepine receptors (BzR). The $GABA_A$ receptor is a heteromer composed of five subunits, the most common ones being two αs, two βs, and one γ ($\alpha_2\beta_2\gamma1$). For each subunit, many subtypes exist (α_{1-6}, β_{1-3}, and γ_{1-3}). $GABA_A$ receptors that are made up of different combinations of subunit subtypes have different properties, different distributions in the brain and different activities relative to pharmacological and clinical effects. Benzodiazepines bind at the interface of the α and γ subunits on the $GABA_A$ receptor. Binding also requires that alpha subunits contain a histidine amino acid residue, (i.e., α_1, α_2, α_3, and α_5 containing $GABA_A$ receptors). For this reason, benzodiazepines show no affinity for $GABA_A$ receptors containing α_4 and α_6 subunits with an arginine instead of a histidine residue. Once bound to the benzodiazepine receptor, the benzodiazepine ligand locks the benzodiazepine receptor into a conformation in which it has a greater affinity for the GABA neurotransmitter. This increases the frequency of the opening of the associated chloride ion channel and hyperpolarizes the membrane of the associated neuron. The inhibitory effect of the available GABA is potentiated, leading to sedative and anxiolytic effects. For instance, those ligands with high activity at the α_1 are associated with stronger hypnotic effects, whereas those with higher affinity for $GABA_A$ receptors containing α_2 and/or α_3 subunits have good anti-anxiety activity.

The benzodiazepine class of drugs also interact with peripheral benzodiazepine receptors. Peripheral benzodiazepine receptors are present in peripheral nervous system tissues, glial cells, and to a lesser extent the central nervous system. These peripheral receptors are not structurally related or coupled to $GABA_A$ receptors. They modulate the immune system and are involved in the body response to injury. Benzodiazepines also function as weak adenosine reuptake inhibitors. It has been suggested that some of their anticonvulsant, anxiolytic, and muscle relaxant effects may be in part mediated by this action. It also should be noted Benzodiazepines have binding sites in the periphery, however their effects on muscle tone is not mediated through these peripheral receptors. The peripheral binding sites for benzodiazepines are present in immune cells and gastrointestinal tract.

Pharmacokinetics

Benzodiazepine	Half-life (range, hours)	Speed of Onset
Alprazolam	12–15	Intermediate
Flunitrazepam	18-26	Fast
Chlordiazepoxide	10–30	Intermediate
Clonazepam	19–60	Slow
Diazepam	20–80	Fast
Lorazepam	10–20	Intermediate
Midazolam	1.5-2.5	Fast
Oxazepam	5–10	Slow
Prazepam	50–200	Slow

A benzodiazepine can be placed into one of three groups by its elimination half-life, or time it takes for the body to eliminate half of the dose. Some benzodiazepines have long-acting active metabolites, such as diazepam and chlordiazepoxide, which are metabolised into desmethyldiazepam. Desmethyldiazepam has a half-life of 36–200 hours, and flurazepam, with the main active metabolite of desalkylflurazepam, with a half-life of 40–250 hours. These long-acting metabolites are partial agonists.

- Short-acting compounds have a median half-life of 1–12 hours. They have few residual effects if taken before bedtime, rebound insomnia may occur upon discontinuation, and they might cause daytime withdrawal symptoms such as next day rebound anxiety with prolonged usage. Examples are brotizolam, midazolam, and triazolam.

- Intermediate-acting compounds have a median half-life of 12–40 hours. They may have some residual effects in the first half of the day if used as a hypnotic. Rebound insomnia, however, is more common upon discontinuation of intermediate-acting benzodiazepines than longer-acting benzodiazepines. Examples are alprazolam, estazolam, flunitrazepam, clonazepam, lormetazepam, lorazepam, nitrazepam, and temazepam.

- Long-acting compounds have a half-life of 40–250 hours. They have a risk of accumulation in the elderly and in individuals with severely impaired liver function, but they have a reduced severity of rebound effects and withdrawal. Examples are diazepam, clorazepate, chlordiazepoxide, and flurazepam.

Chemistry

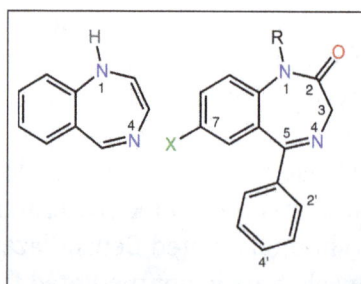

Left: The 1,4-benzodiazepine ring system. Right: 5-phenyl-1*H*-benzo[*e*] [1,4]diazepin-2(3*H*)-one forms the skeleton of many of the most common benzodiazepine pharmaceuticals, such as diazepam (7-chloro-1-methyl substituted).

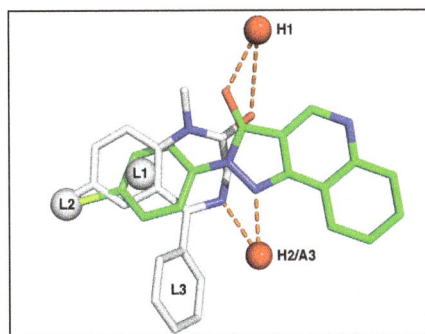

A pharmacophore model of the benzodiazepine binding site on the GABA$_A$ receptor. White sticks represent the carbon atoms of the benzodiazepine diazepam, while green represents carbon atoms of the nonbenzodiazepine CGS-9896. Red and blue sticks are oxygen and nitrogen atoms that are present in both structures. The red spheres labeled H1 and H2/A3 are, respectively, hydrogen bond donating and accepting sites in the receptor, while L1, L2, and L3 denote lipophilic binding sites.

Benzodiazepines share a similar chemical structure, and their effects in humans are mainly produced by the allosteric modification of a specific kind of neurotransmitter receptor, the GABA$_A$ receptor, which increases the overall conductance of these inhibitory channels; this results in the various therapeutic effects as well as adverse effects of benzodiazepines. Other less important modes of action are also known.

The term *benzodiazepine* is the chemical name for the heterocyclic ring system, which is a fusion between the benzene and diazepine ring systems. Under Hantzsch–Widman nomenclature, a diazepine is a heterocycle with two nitrogen atoms, five carbon atom and the maximum possible number of cumulative double bonds. The "benzo" prefix indicates the benzene ring fused onto the diazepine ring.

Benzodiazepine drugs are substituted 1,4-benzodiazepines, although the chemical term can refer to many other compounds that do not have useful pharmacological properties. Different benzodiazepine drugs have different side groups attached to this central structure. The different side groups affect the binding of the molecule to the GABA$_A$ receptor and so modulate the pharmacological properties. Many of the pharmacologically active "classical" benzodiazepine drugs contain the 5-phenyl-1*H*-benzo[*e*] [1,4]diazepin-2(3*H*)-one substructure. Benzodiazepines have been found to mimic protein reverse turns structurally, which enable them with their biological activity in many cases.

Nonbenzodiazepines also bind to the benzodiazepine binding site on the GABA$_A$ receptor and possess similar pharmacological properties. While the nonbenzodiazepines are by definition structurally unrelated to the benzodiazepines, both classes of drugs possess a common pharmacophore, which explains their binding to a common receptor site.

Common Types

- 2-keto compounds:
  - Clorazepate, diazepam, flurazepam, halazepam, prazepam, and others.
- 3-hydroxy compounds:
  - Lorazepam, lormetazepam, oxazepam, temazepam.

- 7-nitro compounds:
  - Clonazepam, flunitrazepam, nimetazepam, nitrazepam.
- Triazolo compounds:
  - Adinazolam, alprazolam, estazolam, triazolam.
- Imidazo compounds:
  - Climazolam, loprazolam, midazolam.

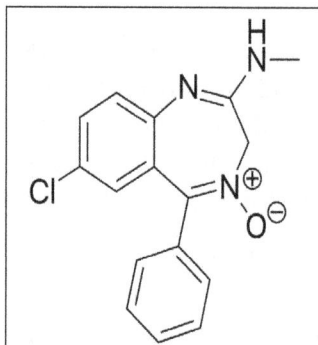

The molecular structure of chlordiazepoxide, the first benzodiazepine. It was marketed by Hoffmann–La Roche from 1960 branded as *Librium*.

The first benzodiazepine, chlordiazepoxide (*Librium*), was synthesized in 1955 by Leo Stern-bach while working at Hoffmann–La Roche on the development of tranquilizers. The pharmacological properties of the compounds prepared initially were disappointing, and Sternbach abandoned the project. Two years later, in April 1957, co-worker Earl Reeder noticed a "nicely crystalline" compound left over from the discontinued project while spring-cleaning in the lab. This compound, later named chlordiazepoxide, had not been tested in 1955 because of Sternbach's focus on other issues. Expecting pharmacology results to be negative, and hoping to publish the chemistry-related findings, researchers submitted it for a standard battery of animal tests. The compound showed very strong sedative, anticonvulsant, and muscle relaxant effects. These impressive clinical findings led to its speedy introduction throughout the world in 1960 under the brand name *Librium*. Following chlordiazepoxide, diazepam marketed by Hoffmann–La Roche under the brand name *Valium* in 1963, and for a while the two were the most commercially successful drugs. The introduction of benzodiazepines led to a decrease in the prescription of barbiturates, and by the 1970s they had largely replaced the older drugs for sedative and hypnotic uses.

The new group of drugs was initially greeted with optimism by the medical profession, but gradually concerns arose; in particular, the risk of dependence became evident in the 1980s. Benzodiazepines have a unique history in that they were responsible for the largest-ever class-action lawsuit against drug manufacturers in the United Kingdom, involving 14,000 patients and 1,800 law firms that alleged the manufacturers knew of the dependence potential but intentionally withheld this information from doctors. At the same time, 117 general practitioners and 50 health authorities were sued by patients to recover damages for the harmful effects of dependence and withdrawal. This led some doctors to require a signed consent form from their patients and to recommend that all patients be adequately warned of the risks of dependence and withdrawal before starting treatment with benzodiazepines. The court case against the drug manufacturers never reached a verdict; legal aid had been withdrawn and there were allegations that the consultant psychiatrists, the expert witnesses, had a conflict of interest. This litigation led to changes in the British law, making class action lawsuits more difficult.

Although antidepressants with anxiolytic properties have been introduced, and there is increasing awareness of the adverse effects of benzodiazepines, prescriptions for short-term anxiety relief have not significantly dropped. For treatment of insomnia, benzodiazepines are now less popular than nonbenzodiazepines, which include zolpidem, zaleplon and eszopiclone. Nonbenzodiazepines are molecularly distinct, but nonetheless, they work on the same benzodiazepine receptors and produce similar sedative effects.

Society and Culture

Legal Status

In the United States, benzodiazepines are Schedule IV drugs under the Federal Controlled Substances Act, even when not on the market (for example, nitrazepam and bromazepam). Flunitrazepam is subject to more stringent regulations in certain states and temazepam prescriptions require specially coded pads in certain states.

In Canada, possession of benzodiazepines is legal for personal use. All benzodiazepines are categorized as Schedule IV substances under the Controlled Drugs and Substances Act. Since 2000, benzodiazepines have been classed as *targeted substances*, meaning that additional regulations exist especially affecting pharmacists' records. Since approximately 2014, Health Canada, the Canadian Medical Association and provincial Colleges of Physicians and Surgeons have been issuing progressively stricter guidelines for the prescription of benzodiazepines, especially for the elderly (e.g. College of Physicians and Surgeons of British Columbia). Many of these guidelines are not readily available to the public.

In the United Kingdom, the benzodiazepines are Class C controlled drugs, carrying the maximum penalty of 7 years imprisonment, an unlimited fine or both for possession and a maximum penalty of 14 years imprisonment an unlimited fine or both for supplying benzodiazepines to others.

In the Netherlands, since October 1993, benzodiazepines, including formulations containing less than 20 mg of temazepam, are all placed on List 2 of the Opium Law. A prescription is needed for possession of all benzodiazepines. Temazepam formulations containing 20 mg or greater of the drug are placed on List 1, thus requiring doctors to write prescriptions in the List 1 format.

In East Asia and Southeast Asia, temazepam and nimetazepam are often heavily controlled and restricted. In certain countries, triazolam, flunitrazepam, flutoprazepam and midazolam are also restricted or controlled to certain degrees. In Hong Kong, all benzodiazepines are regulated under Schedule 1 of Hong Kong's Chapter 134 *Dangerous Drugs Ordinance*. Previously only brotizolam, flunitrazepam and triazolam were classed as dangerous drugs.

Internationally, benzodiazepines are categorized as Schedule IV controlled drugs, apart from flunitrazepam, which is a Schedule III drug under the Convention on Psychotropic Substances.

Recreational Use

Benzodiazepines are considered major drugs of abuse. Benzodiazepine abuse is mostly limited to individuals who abuse other drugs, i.e., poly-drug abusers. On the international scene, benzodiazepines are categorized as Schedule IV controlled drugs by the INCB, apart from flunitrazepam, which is a Schedule III drug under the Convention on Psychotropic Substances. Some variation in drug scheduling exists in individual countries; for example, in the United Kingdom, midazolam and temazepam are Schedule III controlled drugs.

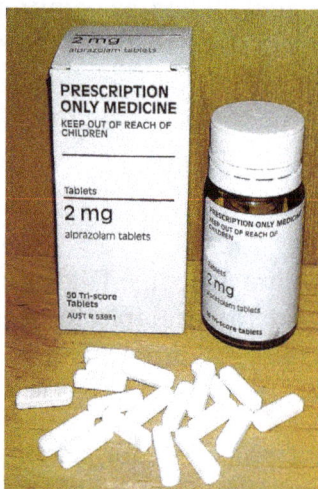

Xanax (alprazolam) 2 mg tri-score tablets.

British law requires that temazepam (but *not* midazolam) be stored in safe custody. Safe custody requirements ensures that pharmacists and doctors holding stock of temazepam must store it in securely fixed double-locked steel safety cabinets and maintain a written register, which must be bound and contain separate entries for temazepam and must be written in ink with no use of correction fluid (although a written register is not required for temazepam in the United Kingdom). Disposal of expired stock must be witnessed by a designated inspector (either a local drug-enforcement police officer or official from health authority). Benzodiazepine abuse ranges from occasional binges on large doses, to chronic and compulsive drug abuse of high doses.

Benzodiazepines are used recreationally and by problematic drug misusers. Mortality is higher among poly-drug misusers that also use benzodiazepines. Heavy alcohol use also increases mortality among poly-drug users. Dependence and tolerance, often coupled with dosage escalation, to benzodiazepines can develop rapidly among drug misusers; withdrawal syndrome may appear after as little as three weeks of continuous use. Long-term use has the potential to cause both physical and psychological dependence and severe withdrawal symptoms such as depression, anxiety (often to the point of panic attacks), and agoraphobia. Benzodiazepines and, in particular, temazepam are sometimes used intravenously, which, if done incorrectly or in an unsterile manner, can lead to medical complications including abscesses, cellulitis, thrombophlebitis, arterial puncture, deep vein thrombosis, and gangrene. Sharing syringes and needles for this purpose also brings up the possibility of transmission of hepatitis, HIV, and other diseases. Benzodiazepines are also misused intranasally, which may have additional health consequences. Once benzodiazepine dependence has been established, a clinician usually converts the patient to an equivalent dose of diazepam before beginning a gradual reduction program.

A 1999–2005 Australian police survey of detainees reported preliminary findings that self-reported users of benzodiazepines were less likely than non-user detainees to work full-time and more likely to receive government benefits, use methamphetamine or heroin, and be arrested or imprisoned. Benzodiazepines are sometimes used for criminal purposes; they serve to incapacitate a victim in cases of drug assisted rape or robbery.

Overall, anecdotal evidence suggests that temazepam may be the most psychologically habit-forming (addictive) benzodiazepine. Temazepam abuse reached epidemic proportions in some parts of the world, in particular, in Europe and Australia, and is a major drug of abuse in many Southeast Asian countries. This led authorities of various countries to place temazepam under a more restrictive legal status. Some countries, such as Sweden, banned the drug outright. Temazepam also has certain pharmacokinetic properties of absorption, distribution, elimination, and clearance that make it more apt to abuse compared to many other benzodiazepines.

Veterinary Use

Benzodiazepines are used in veterinary practice in the treatment of various disorders and conditions. As in humans, they are used in the first-line management of seizures, status epilepticus, and tetanus, and as maintenance therapy in epilepsy (in particular, in cats). They are widely used in small and large animals (including horses, swine, cattle and exotic and wild animals) for their anxiolytic and sedative effects, as pre-medication before surgery, for induction of anesthesia and as adjuncts to anesthesia.

Drug Classifications based on Effect on CNS

Central nervous system agents are medicines that affect the central nervous system (CNS). The CNS is responsible for processing and controlling most of our bodily functions, and consists of the nerves in the brain and spinal cord.

There are many different types of drugs that work on the CNS, including anesthetics, anticonvulsants, antiemetics, antiparkinson agents, CNS stimulants, muscle relaxants, narcotic analgesics (pain relievers), nonnarcotic analgesics (such as acetaminophen and NSAIDs), and sedatives.

Depressant

A depressant, or central depressant, is a drug that lowers neurotransmission levels, which is to depress or reduce arousal or stimulation, in various areas of the brain. Depressants are also occasionally referred to as "downers" as they lower the level of arousal when taken. Stimulants or "uppers" increase mental and/or physical function, hence the opposite drug class of depressants is stimulants, not antidepressants.

Depressants are widely used throughout the world as prescription medicines and as illicit substances. Alcohol is a very prominent depressant. Alcohol can be and is more likely to be a large problem among teenagers and young adults. When depressants are used, effects often include ataxia, anxiolysis, pain relief, sedation or somnolence, and cognitive/memory impairment, as well as in some instances euphoria, dissociation, muscle relaxation, lowered blood pressure or heart rate, respiratory depression, and anticonvulsant effects, and even similar effects of General Anaesthesia and/or death at high doses. Cannabis may sometimes be considered a depressant. THC may slow brain function to a small degree, while reducing reaction to stimuli. Cannabis may also treat insomnia, anxiety and muscle spasms similar to other depressive drugs. Other depressants can include drugs like Xanax (a benzodiazepine) and a number of opiates.

Depressants exert their effects through a number of different pharmacological mechanisms, the most prominent of which include facilitation of GABA, and inhibition of glutamatergic or monoaminergic activity. Other examples are chemicals that modify the electrical signaling inside the body. The most prominent of these being bromides and channel blockers.

Indications

Depressants are used medicinally to relieve the following symptoms:

- Anxiety
  - ◦ Generalized anxiety
  - ◦ Social anxiety
  - ◦ Panic attacks
- Insomnia
- Obsessive–compulsive disorder
- Seizures
- Convulsions
- Depression

Types

Alcohol

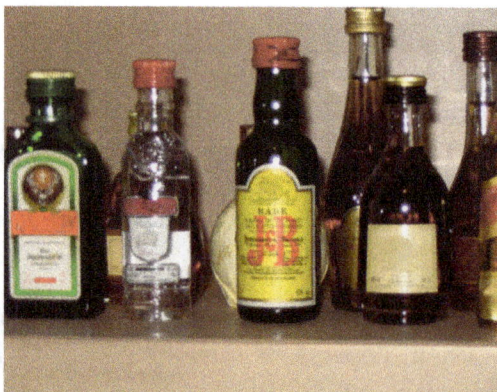

Distilled (concentrated) alcoholic beverages, often called "hard liquor", roughly eight times more alcoholic than beer.

An alcoholic beverage is a drink that contains alcohol (also known formally as ethanol), an anesthetic that has been used as a psychoactive drug for several millennia. Ethanol is the oldest recreational drug still used by humans. Ethanol can cause alcohol intoxication when consumed. Alcoholic beverages are divided into three general classes for taxation and regulation of production: beers, wines, and spirits (distilled beverages). They are legally consumed in most countries around the world. More than 100 countries have laws regulating their production, sale, and consumption.

The most common way to measure intoxication for legal or medical purposes is through blood alcohol content (also called blood alcohol concentration or blood alcohol level). It is usually expressed as a percentage of alcohol in the blood in units of mass of alcohol per volume of blood, or mass of alcohol per mass of blood, depending on the country. For instance, in North America a blood alcohol content of "0.10" or more correctly 0.10 g/dL means that there are 0.10 g of alcohol for every dL of blood (i.e., mass per volume is used there).

Barbiturates

Barbiturates are effective in relieving the conditions that they are designed to address (insomnia, seizures). They are also commonly used for unapproved purposes, physically addictive, and have serious potential for overdose. In the late 1950s, when many thought that the social cost of barbiturates was beginning to outweigh the medical benefits, a serious search began for a replacement drug. Most people still using barbiturates today do so in the prevention of seizures or in mild form for relief from the symptoms of migraines.

Benzodiazepines

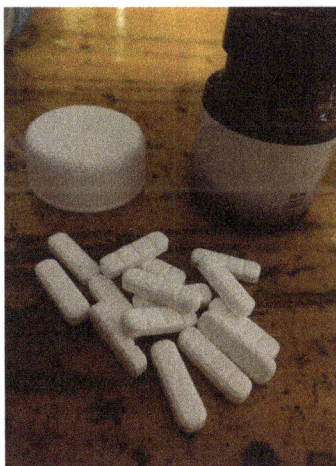

Xanax (alprazolam) 2 mg tri-score tablets.

A benzodiazepine (sometimes colloquially "benzo"; often abbreviated "BZD") is a drug whose core chemical structure is the fusion of a benzene ring and a diazepine ring. The first such drug, chlordiazepoxide (Librium), was discovered accidentally by Leo Sternbach in 1955, and made available in 1960 by Hoffmann–La Roche, which has also marketed the benzodiazepine diazepam (Valium) since 1963.

Benzodiazepines enhance the effect of the neurotransmitter gamma-aminobutyric acid (GABA) at the $GABA_A$ receptor, resulting in sedative, hypnotic (sleep-inducing), anxiolytic (anti-anxiety), anticonvulsant, and muscle relaxant properties; also seen in the applied pharmacology of high doses of many shorter-acting benzodiazepines are amnesic-dissociative actions. These properties make benzodiazepines useful in treating anxiety, insomnia, agitation, seizures, muscle spasms, alcohol withdrawal and as a premedication for medical or dental procedures. Benzodiazepines are categorized as either short-, intermediate-, or long-acting. Short- and intermediate-acting benzodiazepines are preferred for the treatment of insomnia; longer-acting benzodiazepines are recommended for the treatment of anxiety.

In general, benzodiazepines are safe and effective in the short term, although cognitive impairments and paradoxical effects such as aggression or behavioral disinhibition occasionally occur. A minority react reverse and contrary to what would normally be expected. For example, a state of panic may worsen considerably following intake of a benzodiazepine. Long-term use is controversial due to concerns about adverse psychological and physical effects, increased questioning of effectiveness, and, because benzodiazepines are prone to cause tolerance, physical dependence, and, upon cessation of use after long-term use, a withdrawal syndrome. Due to adverse effects associated with the long-term use of benzodiazepines, withdrawal from benzodiazepines, in general, leads to improved physical and mental health. The elderly are at an increased risk of suffering from both short- and long-term adverse effects.

There is controversy concerning the safety of benzodiazepines in pregnancy. While they are not major teratogens, uncertainty remains as to whether they cause cleft palate in a small number of babies and whether neurobehavioural effects occur as a result of prenatal exposure; they are known to cause withdrawal symptoms in the newborn. Benzodiazepines can be taken in overdoses and can cause dangerous deep unconsciousness. However, they are much less toxic than their predecessors, the barbiturates, and death rarely results when a benzodiazepine is the only drug taken; however, when combined with other central nervous system depressants such as alcohol and opiates, the potential for toxicity and fatal overdose increases. Benzodiazepines are commonly misused and taken in combination with other drugs of abuse. In addition, all benzodiazepines are listed in Beers List, which is significant in clinical practice.

Cannabis

Cannabis is often considered either in its own unique category or as a mild psychedelic. The chemical compound tetrahydrocannabidiol (THC), which is found in cannabis, has many depressant effects such as muscle relaxation, sedation, decreased alertness, and less tiredness. Contrary to the previous statement, activation of the CB1 receptor by cannabinoids causes an inhibition of GABA, the exact opposite of what central nervous system depressants do.

Opioids

Contrary to popular misconception, opioids are not depressants in the classical sense. They do produce central nervous system depression, however, they also excite certain areas of the central nervous system. To remain true to the term 'depressant' – opioids cannot be classified as such. For opioid agonists and opium derivatives, these are classified differently. Analgesic or narcotic correctly identifies these drugs. However, they do have depressant actions nonetheless.

- Morphine
- Heroin
- Codeine
- Hydrocodone
- Oxycodone
- Methadone

Miscellaneous

- Alpha and beta blockers (Carvedilol, Propranolol, atenolol, etc.)
- Anticholinergics (Atropine, hyoscyamine, scopolamine, etc.)
- Anticonvulsants (Topiramate, carbamazepine, lamotrigine, etc.)
- Antihistamines (Diphenhydramine, doxylamine, promethazine, etc.)
- Antipsychotics (Haloperidol, chlorpromazine, clozapine, etc.)
- Hypnotics (Zolpidem, zopiclone, chloral hydrate, eszopiclone, etc.)
- Muscle relaxants (Baclofen, phenibut, carisoprodol, cyclobenzaprine, etc.)
- Sedatives (Gamma-hydroxybutyrate, etc.)

Methods of Intake

Combining multiple depressants can be very dangerous because the central nervous system's depressive properties have been proposed to increase exponentially instead of linearly. This characteristic makes depressants a common choice for deliberate overdoses in the case of suicide. The use of alcohol or benzodiazepines along with the usual dose of heroin is often the cause of overdose deaths in opiate addicts.

Hallucinogen

A hallucinogen is a psychoactive agent which can cause hallucinations, perceptual anomalies, and other substantial subjective changes in thoughts, emotion, and consciousness. The common types of hallucinogens are psychedelics, dissociatives and deliriants. Although hallucinations are a common symptom of amphetamine psychosis, amphetamines are not considered hallucinogens as they are not a primary effect of the drugs themselves. While hallucinations can occur when abusing stimulants, the nature of stimulant psychosis is not unlike delirium.

Nomenclature

A debate persists on criteria which would easily differentiate a substance which is 'psychedelic' from one 'hallucinogenic'. Sir Thomas Browne in 1646 coined the term 'hallucination' from the Latin word "alucinari" meaning "to wander in the mind".

A 'hallucinogen' and a 'psychedelic' may refer correctly to the same substance. Psychedelics are considered by many to be the 'traditional' or 'classical hallucinogens'. A 'hallucinogen' in this sense broadly refers to any substance which causes changes in perception or hallucinations, while psychedelics also carry a connotation of psychedelic culture.

Psychedelics (Classical Hallucinogens)

The word psychedelic was coined to express the idea of a drug that makes manifest a hidden but real aspect of the mind. It is commonly applied to any drug with perception-altering effects such as LSD and other ergotamine derivatives, DMT and other tryptamines including the alkaloids of *Psilocybe spp.*, mescaline and other phenethylamines.

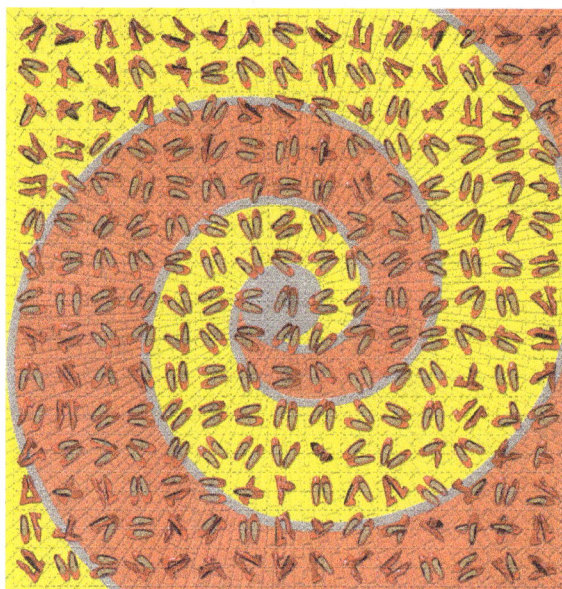

One "Blotter" sheet of 900 LSD doses.

The term "psychedelic" is applied somewhat interchangeably with "psychotomimetic" and "hallucinogen", The classical hallucinogens are considered to be the representative psychedelics and LSD is generally considered the prototypical psychedelic. In order to refer to the LSD-like psychedelics, scientific authors have used the term "classical hallucinogen" in the sense defined by Glennon (1999): "The classical hallucinogens are agents that meet Hollister's original definition, but are also agents that: (a) bind at 5-HT2 serotonin receptors, and (b) are recognized by animals trained to discriminate 1-(2,5-dimethoxy-4-methylphenyl)-2-aminopropane (DOM) from vehicle. Otherwise, when the term 'psychedelic' is used to refer only to the LSD-like psychedelics (a.k.a. the classical hallucinogens), authors explicitly point that they intend 'psychedelic' to be understood according to this more restrictive interpretation.

One explanatory model for the experiences provoked by psychedelics is the "reducing valve" concept, first articulated in Aldous Huxley's book *The Doors of Perception*. In this view, the drugs disable the brain's "filtering" ability to selectively prevent certain perceptions, emotions, memories and thoughts from ever reaching the conscious mind. This effect has been described as *mind expanding*, or *consciousness expanding*, for the drug "expands" the realm of experience available to conscious awareness.

While possessing a unique mechanism of action, cannabis or marijuana has historically been regarded alongside the classic psychedelics.

Research Chemicals and Designer Drugs

A designer drug is a structural or functional analog of a controlled substance that has been designed to mimic the pharmacological effects of the original drug while at the same time avoid being classified as illegal (by specification as a research chemical) and/or avoid detection in standard drug tests. Many designer drugs and research chemicals are hallucinogenic in nature, such as those in the 2C and 25-NB (NBOMe) families.

Dissociatives

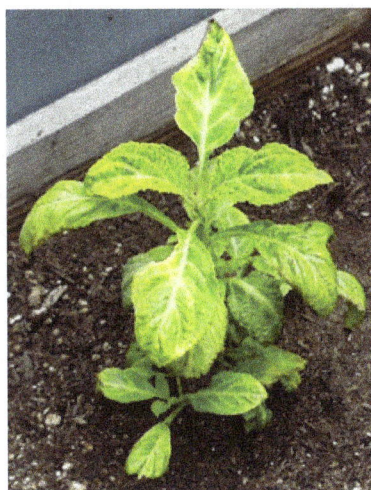

Salvia divinorum.

Dissociatives produce analgesia, amnesia and catalepsy at anesthetic doses. They also produce a sense of detachment from the surrounding environment, hence "the state has been designated as dissociative anesthesia since the patient truly seems disassociated from his environment." Dissociative symptoms include the disruption or compartmentalization of "the usually integrated functions of consciousness, memory, identity or perception." Dissociation of sensory input can cause derealization, the perception of the outside world as being dream-like or unreal. Other dissociative experiences include depersonalization, which includes feeling detached from one's body; feeling unreal; feeling able to observe one's actions but not actively take control; being unable to recognize one's self in the mirror while maintaining rational awareness that the image in the mirror is the same person. Simeon (2004) offered "common descriptions of depersonalisation experiences: watching oneself from a distance (similar to watching a movie); candid out-of-body experiences; a sense of just going through the motions; one part of the self acting/participating while the other part is observing."

The classical dissociatives achieve their effect through blocking the signals received by the NMDA receptor set (NMDA receptor antagonism) and include ketamine, methoxetamine (MXE), phencyclidine (PCP), dextromethorphan (DXM), and nitrous oxide. However, dissociation is also remarkably administered by salvinorin A's (the active constituent in *Salvia divinorum* shown to the left) potent κ-opioid receptor agonism, though sometimes described as an atypical psychedelic.

Some dissociatives can have CNS depressant effects, thereby carrying similar risks as opioids, which can slow breathing or heart rate to levels resulting in death (when using very high doses). DXM in higher doses can increase heart rate and blood pressure and still depress respiration. Inversely, PCP can have more unpredictable effects and has often been classified as a stimulant and a depressant in some texts along with being as a dissociative. While many have reported that they "feel no pain" while under the effects of PCP, DXM and Ketamine, this does not fall under the usual classification of anesthetics in recreational doses (anesthetic doses of DXM may be dangerous). Rather, true to their name, they process pain as a kind of "far away" sensation; pain, although present, becomes a disembodied experience and there is much less emotion associated with it. As for probably the most common dissociative, nitrous oxide, the principal risk seems to be due to oxygen deprivation. Injury from falling is also a danger, as nitrous oxide may cause sudden loss of consciousness, an effect of oxygen deprivation. Because of the high level of physical activity and relative imperviousness to pain induced by PCP, some deaths have been reported due to the release of myoglobin from ruptured muscle cells. High amounts of myoglobin can induce renal shutdown.

Many users of dissociatives have been concerned about the possibility of NMDA antagonist neurotoxicity (NAN). This concern is partly due to William E. White, the author of the DXM FAQ, who claimed that dissociatives definitely cause brain damage. The argument was criticized on the basis of lack of evidence and White retracted his claim. White's claims and the ensuing criticism surrounded original research by John Olney.

In 1989, John Olney discovered that neuronal vacuolation and other cytotoxic changes ("lesions") occurred in brains of rats administered NMDA antagonists, including PCP and ketamine. Repeated doses of NMDA antagonists led to cellular tolerance and hence continuous exposure to NMDA antagonists did not lead to cumulative neurotoxic effects. Antihistamines such as diphenhydramine, barbiturates and even diazepam have been found to prevent NAN. LSD and DOB have also been found to prevent NAN.

Deliriants

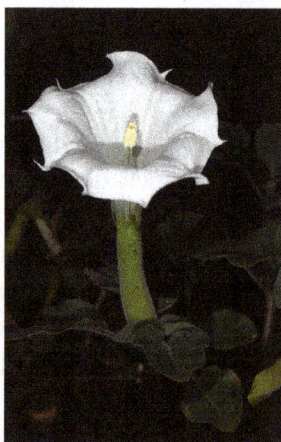

Datura

Deliriants, as their name implies, induce a state of delirium in the user, characterized by extreme confusion and an inability to control one's actions. They are called deliriants because their subjective effects are similar to the experiences of people with delirious fevers. The term was introduced by David F. Duncan and Robert S. Gold to distinguish these drugs from psychedelics and dissociatives, such as LSD and ketamine respectively, due to their primary effect of causing delirium, as opposed to the more lucid states produced by the other hallucinogens.

Despite the fully legal status of several common deliriant plants, deliriants are largely unpopular as recreational drugs due to the severe and sometimes unpleasant nature of the hallucinations produced.

Typical or classical deliriants are those which block the muscarinic acetylcholine receptors (antagonism). These are said to be anticholinergic. Many of these compounds are produced naturally in the nightshade plants, family Solanaceae. These tropane alkaloids are poisonous and can cause death due to tachycardia-induced heart failure and hyperthermia even in small doses. Additionally, over-the-counter antihistamines such as diphenhydramine (brand name Benadryl) and dimenhydrinate (brand name Dramamine) also have an anticholinergic effect. Uncured tobacco is also a deliriant due to its intoxicatingly high levels of nicotine.

The fly agaric mushroom, *Amanita muscaria*, is often informally lumped with the nightshade plants as a *deliriant*, though regarded as a *dissociative* with some regularity as well. This may be explained by the familiarity of both *A. muscaria* and *Atropa belladonna* to European culture, their formal statuses as deadly poisons, and their generally undesirable, unpleasant, and dangerous nature, with the potential for death from physical and behavioral toxicity a possibility even when dosages are carefully considered.

Nutmeg has deliriant and hallucinogenic effects as well due to some of its psychoactive chemicals, such as myristicin, which may be anticholinergic like the tropane alkaloids of the nightshade plants, or as suggested by Alexander Shulgin, partially metabolized into the *empathogen-entactogen* MMDA.

Use

Psychedelics, dissociatives, and deliriants have a long history of use within medicinal and religious traditions around the world including shamanic forms of ritual healing and divination, initiation rites, and rituals of syncretistic movements such as União do Vegetal, Santo Daime, and the Native American Church.

In the context of religious practice, psychedelic drug use, as well as other substances such as tobacco (hypnotic), are referred to as entheogens. In some places peyote is classified as 'sacrament' for part of religious ceremonies, and is legally condoned for such use.

Hallucinogenic substances are among the oldest drugs used by human kind, as hallucinogenic substances naturally occur in mushrooms, cacti and a variety of other plants. Numerous cultures worldwide have endorsed the use of hallucinogens in medicine, religion and recreation, to varying extents, while some cultures have regulated or outright prohibited their use. In most developed countries today, the possession of many hallucinogens, even those found commonly in nature, is considered a crime punishable by fines, imprisonment or even death. In some countries, such as the United States and the Netherlands, partial deference may be granted to traditional religious use by members of indigenous ethnic minorities such as the Native American Church and the Santo Daime Church. Recently the União do Vegetal, a Christian-based religious sect whose composition is not primarily ethnicity-based, won a United States Supreme Court decision authorizing its use of ayahuasca. However, in Brazil, ayahuasca use in a religious context has been legal since 1987. In fact, it is a common belief among members of the União do Vegetal that ayahuasca presents no risk for adolescents within the church, as long as they take it within a religious context.

Traditional Religious and Shamanic Use

Historically, hallucinogens have been commonly used in religious or shamanic rituals. In this context they are referred to as entheogens, and are used to facilitate healing, divination, communication with spirits, and coming-of-age ceremonies. Evidence exists for the use of entheogens in prehistoric times, as well as in numerous ancient cultures, including Ancient Egyptian, Mycenaean, Ancient Greek, Vedic, Maya, Inca and Aztec cultures. The Upper Amazon is home to the strongest extant entheogenic tradition; the Urarina of the Peruvian Amazon, for instance, continue to practice an elaborate system of ayahuasca shamanism, coupled with an animistic belief system.

Shamans consume hallucinogenic substances in order to induce a trance. Once in this trance, shamans believe that they are able to communicate with the spirit world, and can see what is causing their patients' illness. The Aguaruna of Peru believe that many illnesses are caused by the darts of sorcerers. Under the influence of yaji, a hallucinogenic drink, Aguaruna shamans try to discover and remove the darts from their patients.

Concerning lycanthropy (werewolves) and the use of hallucinogenic drugs, Frida G. Surawicz and Richard Banta wrote "In the first case, this was brought on by LSD and strychnine and continued casual marijuana use. Concerning drugs as causative agents, it is interesting to note that opium has been mentioned in a dual capacity, namely as a drug which can cause lycanthropy as well as a drug for its treatment."

Early Scientific Investigations

Although natural hallucinogenic drugs have been known to mankind for millennia, it was not until the early 20th century that they received extensive attention from Western science. Earlier beginnings include scientific studies of nitrous oxide in the late 18th century, and initial studies of the constituents of the peyote cactus in the late 19th century. Starting in 1927 with Kurt Beringer's *Der Meskalinrausch* (The Mescaline Intoxication), more intensive effort began to be focused on studies of psychoactive plants. Around the same time, Louis Lewin published his extensive survey of psychoactive plants, *Phantastica*. Important developments in the years that followed included the re-discovery of Mexican psilocybin mushrooms (in 1936 by Robert J. Weitlaner) and Christmas vine (in 1939 by Richard Evans Schultes). Arguably the most important pre-World War II development was by Albert Hofmann's 1938 discovery of the semi-synthetic drug LSD, which was later discovered to produce hallucinogenic effects in 1943.

Hallucinogens After World War II

After World War II there was an explosion of interest in hallucinogenic drugs in psychiatry, owing mainly to the invention of LSD. Interest in the drugs tended to focus on either the potential for psychotherapeutic applications of the drugs, or on the use of hallucinogens to produce a "controlled psychosis", in order to understand psychotic disorders such as schizophrenia. By 1951, more than 100 articles on LSD had appeared in medical journals, and by 1961, the number had increased to more than 1000 articles. Hallucinogens were also researched in several countries for their potential as agents of chemical warfare. Most famously, several incidents associated with the CIA's MK-ULTRA mind control research project have been the topic of media attention and lawsuits.

At the beginning of the 1950s, the existence of hallucinogenic drugs was virtually unknown to the general public in the West. However this soon changed as several influential figures were introduced to the hallucinogenic experience. Aldous Huxley's 1953 essay *The Doors of Perception*, describing his experiences with mescaline, and R. Gordon Wasson's 1957 Life magazine article brought the topic into the public limelight. In the early 1960s, counterculture icons such as Jerry Garcia, Timothy Leary, Allen Ginsberg and Ken Kesey advocated the drugs for their psychedelic effects, and a large subculture of psychedelic drug users was spawned. Psychedelic drugs played a major role in catalyzing the vast social changes initiated in the 1960s. As a result of the growing popularity of LSD and disdain for the hippies with whom it was heavily associated, LSD was banned in the United States in 1967. This greatly reduced the clinical research about LSD, although limited experiments continued to take place, such as those conducted by Reese Jones in San Francisco.

As early as the 1960s, research into the medicinal properties of LSD was being conducted. It has been found that LSD is a fairly effective treatment for mental disorders such as obsessive compulsive disorder (OCD). "Savage et al. provided the earliest report of efficacy for a hallucinogen in OCD, where after two doses of LSD, a patient who suffered from depression and violent obsessive sexual thoughts experienced dramatic and permanent improvement."

Starting in the mid-20th century, psychedelic drugs has been the object of extensive attention in the Western world. They have been and are being explored as potential therapeutic agents in treating depression, posttraumatic stress disorder, obsessive–compulsive disorder, alcoholism, drug addiction, cluster headaches, and other ailments. Early military research focused on their use as incapacitating agents. Intelligence agencies tested these drugs in the hope that they would provide an effective means of interrogation, with little success.

Yet the most popular, and at the same time most stigmatized, use of psychedelics in Western culture has been associated with the search for direct religious experience, enhanced creativity, personal development, and "mind expansion". The use of psychedelic drugs was a major element of the 1960s counterculture, where it became associated with various social movements and a general atmosphere of rebellion and strife between generations.

Despite prohibition, the recreational, spiritual, and medical use of psychedelics continues today. Organizations, such as MAPS and the Heffter Research Institute, have arisen to foster research into their safety and efficacy, while advocacy groups such as the Center for Cognitive Liberty and Ethics push for their legalization. In addition to this activity by proponents, hallucinogens are also widely used in basic science research to understand the mind and brain. However, ever since hallucinogenic experimentation was discontinued in the late 1960s, research into the therapeutic applications of such drugs have been almost nonexistent, that is until this last decade where research has finally been allowed to resume.

Legal Status and Attitudes

In Canada, mescaline is listed as prohibited under schedule III of the Controlled Drugs and Substances Acts, but peyote is specifically exempt and legally available.

As of 2008, most well-known hallucinogens (aside from dextromethorphan, diphenhydramine and dimenhydrinate) are illegal in most Western countries. In the United States hallucinogens are classified as a schedule 1 drug. The 3-pronged test for schedule 1 drugs is as follows: the drug has no currently accepted medical use, there is a lack of safety for the use of the drug under medical supervision, and the substance has a high potential for abuse. One notable exception to the current criminalization trend is in parts of Western Europe, especially in the Netherlands, where cannabis is considered to be a "soft drug". Previously included were hallucinogenic mushrooms, but as of October 2007 the Netherlands officials have moved to ban their sale following several widely publicized incidents involving tourists. While the possession of soft drugs is technically illegal, the Dutch government has decided that using law enforcement to combat their use is largely a waste of resources. As a result, public "coffeeshops" in the Netherlands openly sell cannabis for personal use, and "smart shops" sell drugs like *Salvia divinorum*, and until the ban of psilocybin mushrooms took effect, they were still available for purchase in smartshops as well.

Despite being scheduled as a controlled substance in the mid-1980s, MDMA's popularity has been growing since that time in western Europe and in the United States.

Attitudes towards hallucinogens other than cannabis have been slower to change. Several attempts to change the law on the grounds of freedom of religion have been made. Some of these have been successful, for example the Native American Church in the United States, and Santo Daime in Brazil. Some people argue that a religious setting should not be necessary for the legitimacy of hallucinogenic drug use, and for this reason also criticize the euphemistic use of the term "entheogen". Non-religious reasons for the use of hallucinogens including spiritual, introspective, psychotherapeutic, recreational and even hedonistic motives, each subject to some degree of social disapproval, have all been defended as the legitimate exercising of civil liberties and freedom of thought.

Several medical and scientific experts, including the late Albert Hofmann, advocate the drugs should not be banned, but should be strongly regulated and warn they can be dangerous without proper psychological supervision.

Psychedelics and Mental Illnesses in Long-term Users

Most psychedelics are not known to have long-term physical toxicity. However, entactogens such as MDMA that release neurotransmitters may stimulate increased formation of free radicals possibly formed from neurotransmitters released from the synaptic vesicle. Free radicals are associated with cell damage in other contexts, and have been suggested to be involved in many types of mental conditions including Parkinson's disease, senility, schizophrenia, and Alzheimer's. Research on this question has not reached a firm conclusion. The same concerns do not apply to psychedelics that do not release neurotransmitters, such as LSD, nor to dissociatives or deliriants.

No clear connection has been made between psychedelic drugs and organic brain damage. However, hallucinogen persisting perception disorder (HPPD) is a diagnosed condition wherein certain visual effects of drugs persist for a long time, sometimes permanently, although science and medicine have yet to determine what causes the condition.

A large epidemiological study in the U.S. found that other than personality disorders and other substance use disorders, lifetime hallucinogen use was not associated with other mental disorders, and that risk of developing a hallucinogen use disorder was very low.

How Hallucinogens affect the Brain

LSD, mescaline, psilocybin, and PCP are drugs that cause hallucinations, which can alter a person's perception of reality. LSD, mescaline, and psilocybin cause their effects by initially disrupting the interaction of nerve cells and the neurotransmitter serotonin. It is distributed throughout the brain and spinal cord, where the serotonin system is involved with controlling of the behavioral, perceptual, and regulatory systems. This also includes mood, hunger, body temperature, sexual behavior, muscle control, and sensory perception. Certain hallucinogens, such as PCP, act through a glutamate receptor in the brain which is important for perception of pain, responses to the environment, and learning and memory. Thus far, there have been no properly controlled research studies on the specific effects of these drugs on the human brain, but smaller studies have shown some of the documented effects associated with the use of hallucinogens.

Naming and Taxonomy

Psychedelic Nomenclature

The class of drugs described in this topic has been described by a profusion of names, most of which are associated with a particular theory of their nature.

Louis Lewin started out in 1928 by using the word phantastica as the title of his ground-breaking monograph about plants that, in his words, "bring about evident cerebral excitation in the form of hallucinations, illusions and visions followed by unconsciousness or other symptoms of altered cerebral functioning". But no sooner had the term been invented, or Lewin complained that the word "does not cover all that I should wish it to convey", and indeed with the proliferation of research following the discovery of LSD came numerous attempts to improve on it, such as hallucinogen, phanerothyme, psychedelic, psychotomimetic, psychogenic, schizophrenogenic, cataleptogenic, mysticomimetic, psychodysleptic, and entheogenic.

The word *psychotomimetic*, meaning "mimicking psychosis", reflects the hypothesis of early researchers that the effects of psychedelic drugs are similar to naturally occurring symptoms of schizophrenia, though it has since been discovered that some psychedelics resemble endogenous psychoses better than others. PCP and ketamine are known to better resemble endogenous psychoses because they reproduce both positive and negative symptoms of psychoses, while psilocybin and related hallucinogens typically produce effects resembling only the positive symptoms of schizophrenia. While the serotonergic psychedelics (LSD, psilocybin, mescaline, etc.) do produce subjective effects distinct from NMDA antagonist dissociatives (PCP, ketamine, dextrorphan), there is obvious overlap in the mental processes that these drugs affect and research has discovered that there is overlap in the mechanisms by which both types of psychedelics mimic psychotic symptoms. One double-blind study examining the differences between DMT and ketamine hypothesized that *classically psychedelic* drugs most resemble paranoid schizophrenia while *dissociative* drugs best mimicked catatonic subtypes or otherwise undifferentiated schizophrenia. The researchers expressed the view that "a heterogeneous disorder like schizophrenia is unlikely to be modeled accurately by a single pharmacological agent."

The word *psychedelic* was coined by Humphrey Osmond and has the rather mysterious but at least somewhat value-neutral meaning of "mind manifesting". The word *entheogen*, on the other hand, which is often used to describe the religious and ritual use of psychedelic drugs in anthropological studies, is associated with the idea that it could be relevant to religion. The words *entactogen*, *empathogen*, *dissociative* and *deliriant*, at last, have all been coined to refer to classes of drugs similar to the classical psychedelics that seemed deserving of a name of their own.

Many different names have been proposed over the years for this drug class. The famous German toxicologist Louis Lewin used the name phantastica earlier in this century, and as we shall see later, such a descriptor is not so farfetched. The most popular names—hallucinogen, psychotomimetic, and psychedelic ("mind manifesting")—have often been used interchangeably. *Hallucinogen* is now, however, the most common designation in the scientific literature, although it is an inaccurate descriptor of the actual effects of these drugs. In the lay press, the term *psychedelic* is still the most popular and has held sway for nearly four decades. Most recently, there has been a movement in nonscientific circles to recognize the ability of these substances to provoke mystical experiences and evoke feelings of spiritual significance. This term suggests that these substances reveal or allow a connection to the "divine within". Although it seems unlikely that this name will ever be accepted in formal scientific circles, its use has dramatically increased in the popular media and on internet sites. Indeed, in much of the counterculture that uses these substances, entheogen has replaced psychedelic as the name of choice and we may expect to see this trend continue.

Taxonomy

Hallucinogens can be classified by their subjective effects, mechanisms of action, and chemical structure. These classifications often correlate to some extent. They are classified as psychedelics, dissociatives, and deliriants, preferably entirely to the exclusion of the inaccurate word hallucinogen, but the reader is well advised to consider that this particular classification is not universally accepted. The taxonomy used here attempts to blend these three approaches in order to provide as clear and accessible an overview as possible.

Almost all hallucinogens contain nitrogen and are therefore classified as alkaloids. THC and salvinorin A are exceptions. Many hallucinogens have chemical structures similar to those of human neurotransmitters, such as serotonin, and temporarily modify the action of neurotransmitters and/or receptor sites.

Leo Hollister's five criteria for establishing that a drug is hallucinogenic are as follows:

- In proportion to other effects, changes in thought, perception, and mood should predominate;

- Intellectual or memory impairment should be minimal;

- Stupor, narcosis, or excessive stimulation should not be an integral effect;

- Autonomic nervous system side effects should be minimal;

- Addictive craving should be absent.

Lewin's Classes

A classical classification, mainly of historical interest, is that of Lewin: *Class I Phantastica* roughly correspond to the psychedelics, which is a more modern term usually used as synonym to "hallucinogen" by people with positive attitudes towards them. Here the term is used a bit differently to discriminate one particular class of hallucinogens which it seems to describe best. They typically have no sedative effects (sometimes the opposite) and there is usually a clearcut memory to their effects. These drugs have also been referred to as the "classical" hallucinogens.

Class II Phantastica correspond to the other classes in our scheme. They tend to sedate in addition to their hallucinogenic properties and there often is an impaired memory trace after the effects wear off.

Pharmacological Classes of Hallucinogens

One possible way of classifying the hallucinogens is by their chemical structure and that of the receptors they act on. In this vein, the following categories are often used:

Psychedelics: Serotonergics (5-HT2A receptor agonists or classical psychedelics) such as mescaline from peyote *(Lophophora williamsii)*:

- Indoles / Tryptamines such as psilocybin from "magic" mushrooms (*Psilocybe*).

  ○ Ergolines such as lysergol from morning glory (Convolvulaceae).

  ○ Lysergamides such as LSD ("acid"), derived from ergot (*Claviceps purpurea*).

  ○ Beta-carbolines (monoamine oxidase inhibitors or MAOIs, specifically reversible inhibitors of monoamine oxidase A or RIMAs) such as harmala alkaloids such as norharman from ayahuasca (*Banisteriopsis caapi*).

  ○ Complexly substituted tryptamines such as ibogaine from iboga (*Tabernanthe iboga*).

  ○ Phenethylamines such as mescaline.

  ○ *Empathogen–entactogens* such as MDA.

  ○ Substituted methylenedioxyphenethylamines (serotonin releasing agents) such as MDMA ("ecstasy").

- Cannabinoidergics (CB-1 receptor agonists or atypical psychedelics) such as THC from cannabis (*Cannabis*).

- *Dissociatives*:

  ◦ Antiglutamatergics (NMDA receptor antagonists or classical dissociatives) such as "laughing gas" (nitrous oxide) and ketamine.

  ◦ Opioidergics (sometimes regarded as atypical psychedelics) (κ-Opioid receptor agonists or atypical dissociatives) such as salvinorin A from *Salvia divinorum* and pentazocine.

- *Deliriants*

  ◦ Anticholinergics (muscarinic acetylcholine receptor antagonists or classical deliriants) such as tropane alkaloids such as atropine from deadly nightshade (*Atropa belladonna*) and diphenhydramine (Benadryl).

  ◦ GABAergics (sometimes regarded as atypical dissociatives) ($GABA_A$ receptor agonists, and some positive allosteric modulators of the $GABA_A$ receptor, or atypical deliriants) such as muscimol from fly agaric (*Amanita muscaria*) and zolpidem (Ambien).

Problems with structure-based frameworks is that the same structural motif can include a wide variety of drugs which have substantially different effects. For example, both methamphetamine and MDMA are substituted amphetamines, but methamphetamine has a much stronger stimulant action than MDMA, with none of the latter's empathogenic effects. Also, drugs commonly act on more than one receptor; DXM, for instance, is primarily dissociative in high doses, but also acts as a serotonin reuptake inhibitor, similar to many phenethylamines.

Even so, in many cases structure-based frameworks are still very useful, and the identification of a biologically active pharmacophore and synthesis of analogues of known active substances remains an integral part of modern medicinal chemistry.

Inhalant

Inhalants are a broad range of household and industrial chemicals whose volatile vapors or pressurized gases can be concentrated and breathed in via the nose or mouth to produce intoxication (called "getting high" in slang), in a manner not intended by the manufacturer. They are inhaled at room temperature through volatilization (in the case of gasoline or acetone) or from a pressurized container (e.g., nitrous oxide or butane), and do not include drugs that are sniffed after burning or heating. For example, amyl nitrite (poppers), nitrous oxide and toluene – a solvent widely used in contact cement, permanent markers, and certain types of glue – are considered inhalants, but smoking tobacco, cannabis, and crack are not, even though these drugs are inhaled as smoke.

While a small number of inhalants are prescribed by medical professionals and used for medical purposes, as in the case of inhaled anesthetics and nitrous oxide (an anxiolytic and pain relief agent prescribed by dentists), this topic focuses on inhalant use of household and industrial propellants, glues, fuels and other products in a manner not intended by the manufacturer, to produce intoxication or other psychoactive effects. These products are used as recreational drugs for their intoxicating effect. According to a 1995 report by the National Institute on Drug Abuse, the most serious inhalant abuse occurs among homeless children and teens who "live on the streets completely without family ties." Inhalants are the only substance which is used more by younger teens than by older teens. Inhalant users inhale vapor or aerosol propellant gases using plastic bags held over the mouth or by breathing from a solvent-soaked rag or an open container. The practices are known colloquially as "sniffing", "huffing" or "bagging".

The effects of inhalants range from an alcohol-like intoxication and intense euphoria to vivid hallucinations, depending on the substance and the dose. Some inhalant users are injured due to the harmful effects of the solvents or gases or due to other chemicals used in the products that they are inhaling. As with any recreational drug, users can be injured due to dangerous behavior while they are intoxicated, such as driving under the influence. In some cases, users have died from hypoxia (lack of oxygen), pneumonia, cardiac failure or arrest, or aspiration of vomit. Brain damage is typically seen with chronic long-term use of solvents as opposed to short-term exposure.

Even though many inhalants are legal, there have been legal actions taken in some jurisdictions to limit access by minors. While solvent glue is normally a legal product, a Scottish court has ruled that supplying glue to children is illegal if the store knows the children intend to abuse the glue. In the US, thirty-eight of 50 states have enacted laws making various inhalants unavailable to those under the age of 18, or making inhalant use illegal.

Classification

Inhalants can be classified by the intended function. Most inhalant drugs that are used non-medically are ingredients in household or industrial chemical products that are not intended to be concentrated and inhaled. A small number of recreational inhalant drugs are pharmaceutical products that are used illicitly.

Product Category

Another way to categorize inhalants is by their product category. There are three main product categories: solvents; gases; and medical drugs which are used illicitly.

Solvents

A wide range of volatile solvents intended for household or industrial use are inhaled as recreational drugs. This includes petroleum products (gasoline and kerosene), toluene (used in paint thinner, permanent markers, contact cement and model glue), and acetone (used in nail polish remover). These solvents vaporize at room temperature. Ethanol (the alcohol which is normally drunk) is sometimes inhaled, but this cannot be done at room temperature. The ethanol must be converted from liquid into gaseous state (vapor) or aerosol (mist), in some cases using a nebulizer, a machine that agitates the liquid into an aerosol. The sale of nebulizers for inhaling ethanol was banned in some US states due to safety concerns.

Gases

A number of gases intended for household or industrial use are inhaled as recreational drugs. This includes chlorofluorocarbons used in aerosols and propellants (e.g., aerosol hair spray, aerosol deodorant). A gas used as a propellant in whipped cream aerosol containers, nitrous oxide, is used as a recreational drug. Pressurized canisters of propane and butane gas, both of which are intended for use as fuels, are used as inhalants.

Medical Anesthetics

Several medical anesthetics are used as recreational drugs, including diethyl ether (a drug that is no longer used medically, due to its high flammability and the development of safer alternatives) and nitrous oxide, which is widely used in the 2010s by dentists as an anti-anxiety drug during dental procedures. Diethyl ether has a long history of use as a recreational drug. The effects of ether intoxication are similar to those of alcohol intoxication, but more potent. Also, due to NMDA antagonism, the user may experience all the psychedelic effects present in classical dissociatives such as ketamine in forms of thought loops and feeling of mind being disconnected from one's body. Nitrous oxide is a dental anesthetic which is used as a recreational drug, either by users who have access to medical-grade gas canisters (e.g., dental hygienists or dentists) or by using the gas contained in whipped cream aerosol containers. Nitrous oxide inhalation can cause pain relief, depersonalisation, derealisation, dizziness, euphoria, and some sound distortion.

Classification by Effect

It is also possible to classify inhalants by the effect they have on the body. Solvents such as toluene and gasoline act as depressants, causing users to feel relaxed and sleepy. Many inhalants act primarily as asphyxiant gases, with their primary effect due to oxygen deprivation. Nitrous oxide can be categorized as a dissociative drug, as it can cause visual and auditory hallucinations. Other agents may have more direct effects at receptors, as inhalants exhibit a variety of mechanisms of action. The mechanisms of action of many non-medical inhalants have not been well elucidated. Anesthetic gases used for surgery, such as nitrous oxide or enflurane, are believed to induce anesthesia primarily by acting as NMDA receptor antagonists, open channel blockers that bind to the inside of the calcium channels on the outer surface of the neuron, and provide high levels of NMDA receptor blockade for a short period of time.

This makes inhaled anesthetic gases different from other NMDA antagonists, such as ketamine, which bind to a regulatory site on the NMDA-sensitive calcium transporter complex and provide slightly lower levels of NMDA blockade, but for a longer and much more predictable duration. This makes a deeper level of anesthesia achievable more easily using anesthetic gases but can also make them more dangerous than other drugs used for this purpose.

Chemical Structure

Table: Inhalants can also be classified by chemical structure.

Category	ICD-10	Examples	Example image
aliphatic hydrocarbons	T52.0	petroleum products (gasoline and kerosene), propane, butane	
aromatic hydrocarbons	T52.1-T52.2	toluene (used in paint thinner and model glue), xylene	

ketones	T52.4	acetone (used in nail polish remover)	
haloalkanes	T53	hydrofluorocarbons, chlorofluorocarbons (including many aerosols and propellants), 1,1,1-Trichloroethane, trichloroethylene, chloroform (the latter two being antiquated inhalational anaesthetics)	
nitrites	T65.3, T65.5	alkyl nitrites (poppers such as amyl nitrite)	
nitrous oxide	T59.0	nitrous oxide (found in whipped cream canisters)	

Administration and Effects

Inhalant users inhale vapors or aerosol propellant gases using plastic bags held over the mouth or by breathing from an open container of solvents, such as gasoline or paint thinner. Nitrous oxide gases from whipped cream aerosol cans, aerosol hairspray or non-stick frying spray are sprayed into plastic bags. Some nitrous oxide users spray the gas into balloons. When inhaling non-stick cooking spray or other aerosol products, some users may filter the aerosolized particles out with a rag. Some gases, such as propane and butane gases, are inhaled directly from the canister. Once these solvents or gases are inhaled, the extensive capillary surface of the lungs rapidly absorb the solvent or gas, and blood levels peak rapidly. The intoxication effects occur so quickly that the effects of inhalation can resemble the intensity of effects produced by intravenous injection of other psychoactive drugs. Some harm reduction experts encourage glue sniffers to use paper bags rather than thin plastic bags, because plastic bags greatly increase the risk of suffocation, as plastic bags are more likely to stick to the users' nose and mouth while she or he is intoxicated.

Ethanol is also inhaled, either by vaporizing it by pouring it over dry ice in a narrow container and inhaling with a straw or by pouring alcohol in a corked bottle with a pipe, and then using a bicycle pump to make a spray. Alcohol can be vaporized using a simple container and open-flame heater. Medical devices such as asthma nebulizers and inhalers were also reported as means of application. The practice gained popularity in 2004, with marketing of the device dubbed AWOL (Alcohol without liquid), a play on the military term AWOL (Absent Without Leave). AWOL, created by British businessman Dominic Simler, was first introduced in Asia and Europe, and then in United States in August 2004. AWOL was used by nightclubs, at gatherings and parties, and it garnered attraction as a novelty, as people 'enjoyed passing it around in a group'. AWOL uses a nebulizer, a machine that agitates the liquid into an aerosol. AWOL's official website states that "AWOL and AWOL 1 are powered by *Electrical Air Compressors* while AWOL 2 and AWOL 3 are powered by *electrical oxygen generators*", which refer to a couple of mechanisms used by the nebulizer drug delivery device for inhalation. Although the AWOL machine is marketed as having no downsides, such as the lack of calories or hangovers, Amanda Shaffer of *Slate* describes these claims as "dubious at best". Although inhaled alcohol does reduce the caloric content, the savings are minimal. After expressed safety and health concerns, sale or use of AWOL machines was banned in a number of American states.

The effects of solvent intoxication can vary widely depending on the dose and what type of solvent or gas is inhaled. A person who has inhaled a small amount of rubber cement or paint thinner vapor may be impaired in a manner resembling alcohol inebriation. A person who has inhaled a larger quantity of solvents or gases, or a stronger chemical, may experience stronger effects such as distortion in perceptions of time and space, hallucinations, and emotional disturbances. The effects of inhalant use are also modified by the combined use of inhalants and alcohol or other drugs.

In the short term, many users experience headache, nausea and vomiting, slurred speech, loss of motor coordination, and wheezing. A characteristic "glue sniffer's rash" around the nose and mouth is sometimes seen after prolonged use. An odor of paint or solvents on clothes, skin, and breath is sometimes a sign of inhalant abuse, and paint or solvent residues can sometimes emerge in sweat.

According to NIH, even a single session of inhalant abuse "can disrupt heart rhythms and lower oxygen levels", which can lead to death. "Regular abuse can result in serious harm to the brain, heart, kidneys

Dangers and Health Problems

Statistics on deaths caused by inhalant abuse are difficult to determine. It may be severely under-reported, because death is often attributed to a discrete event such as a stroke or a heart attack, even if the event happened because of inhalant abuse. Inhalant use or abuse was mentioned on 144 death certificates in Texas during the period 1988–1998 and was reported in 39 deaths in Virginia between 1987 and 1996 from acute voluntary exposure to abused inhalants.

General Risks

Regardless of which inhalant is used, inhaling vapours or gases can lead to injury or death. One major risk is hypoxia (lack of oxygen), which can occur due to inhaling fumes from a plastic bag, or from using proper inhalation mask equipment (e.g., a medical mask for nitrous oxide) but not adding oxygen or room air. Another danger is freezing the throat. When a gas that was stored under high pressure is released, it cools abruptly and can cause frostbite if it is inhaled directly from the container. This can occur, for example, with inhaling nitrous oxide. When nitrous oxide is used as an automotive power adder, its cooling effect is used to make the fuel-air charge denser. In a person, this effect is potentially lethal. Many inhalants are volatile organic chemicals and can catch fire or explode, especially when combined with smoking. As with many other drugs, users may also injure themselves due to loss of coordination or impaired judgment, especially if they attempt to drive.

Solvents have many potential risks in common, including pneumonia, cardiac failure or arrest, and aspiration of vomit. The inhaling of some solvents can cause hearing loss, limb spasms, and damage to the central nervous system and brain. Serious but potentially reversible effects include liver and kidney damage and blood-oxygen depletion. Death from inhalants is generally caused by a very high concentration of fumes. Deliberately inhaling solvents from an attached paper or plastic bag or in a closed area greatly increases the chances of suffocation. Brain damage is typically seen with chronic long-term use as opposed to short-term exposure. Parkinsonism has been associated with huffing.

Female inhalant users who are pregnant may have adverse effects on the fetus, and the baby may be smaller when it is born and may need additional health care (similar to those seen with alcohol

– fetal alcohol syndrome). There is some evidence of birth defects and disabilities in babies born to women who sniffed solvents such as gasoline.

In the short term, death from solvent abuse occurs most commonly from aspiration of vomit while unconscious or from a combination of respiratory depression and hypoxia, the second cause being especially a risk with heavier-than-air vapors such as butane or gasoline vapor. Deaths typically occur from complications related to excessive sedation and vomiting. Actual overdose from the drug does occur, however, and inhaled solvent abuse is statistically more likely to result in life-threatening respiratory depression than intravenous use of opiates such as heroin. Most deaths from solvent abuse could be prevented if individuals were resuscitated quickly when they stopped breathing and their airway cleared if they vomited. However, most inhalant abuse takes place when people inhale solvents by themselves or in groups of people who are intoxicated. Certain solvents are more hazardous than others, such as gasoline.

In contrast, a few inhalants like amyl nitrate and diethyl ether have medical applications and are not toxic in the same sense as solvents, though they can still be dangerous when used recreationally. Nitrous oxide is thought to be particularly non-toxic, though heavy long-term use can lead to a variety of serious health problems linked to destruction of vitamin B12 and folic acid.

Risks of Specific Agents

The hypoxic effect of inhalants can cause damage to many organ systems (particularly the brain, which has a very low tolerance for oxygen deprivation), but there can also be additional toxicity resulting from either the physical properties of the compound itself or additional ingredients present in a product. Organochlorine solvents are particularly hazardous; many of these are now restricted in developed countries due to their environmental impact.

- Methylene chloride, after being metabolized, can cause carbon monoxide poisoning.

- Gasoline sniffing can cause lead poisoning, in locations where leaded gas is not banned.

- Ingestion of alkyl nitrites can cause methemoglobinemia, and by inhalation it has not been ruled out.

- Carbon tetrachloride can cause significant damage to multiple systems, but its association with liver damage is so strong that it is used in animal models to induce liver injury.

- Use of butane, propane, nitrous oxide and other inhalants can create a risk of freezing burns from contact with the extremely cold liquid. The risk of such contact is greatly increased by the impaired judgement and motor coordination brought on by inhalant intoxication.

- Benzene use can cause bone marrow depression. It is also a known carcinogen.

- Toluene can damage myelin.

Toxicity may also result from the pharmacological properties of the drug; excess NMDA antagonism can completely block calcium influx into neurons and provoke cell death through apoptosis, although this is more likely to be a long-term result of chronic solvent abuse than a consequence of short-term use.

Sudden Sniffing Death Syndrome

Inhaling butane gas can cause drowsiness, unconsciousness, asphyxia, and cardiac arrhythmia. Butane is the most commonly misused volatile solvent in the UK and caused 52% of solvent-related deaths in 2000. When butane is sprayed directly into the throat, the jet of fluid can cool rapidly to −20 °C by adiabatic expansion, causing prolonged laryngospasm. Sudden sniffing death syndrome is commonly known as SSDS. Some inhalants can also indirectly cause sudden death by cardiac arrest, in a syndrome known as "sudden sniffing death". The anaesthetic gases present in the inhalants appear to sensitize the user to adrenaline and, in this state, a sudden surge of adrenaline (e.g., from a frightening hallucination or run-in with aggressors), may cause fatal cardiac arrhythmia.

Furthermore, the inhalation of any gas that is capable of displacing oxygen in the lungs (especially gases heavier than oxygen) carries the risk of hypoxia as a result of the very mechanism by which breathing is triggered. Since reflexive breathing is prompted by elevated carbon dioxide levels (rather than diminished blood oxygen levels), breathing a concentrated, relatively inert gas (such as computer-duster tetrafluoroethane or nitrous oxide) that removes carbon dioxide from the blood without replacing it with oxygen will produce no outward signs of suffocation even when the brain is experiencing hypoxia. Once full symptoms of hypoxia appear, it may be too late to breathe without assistance, especially if the gas is heavy enough to lodge in the lungs for extended periods. Even completely inert gases, such as argon, can have this effect if oxygen is largely excluded.

Antipyretics

Antipyretics are substances that reduce fever. Antipyretics cause the hypothalamus to override a prostaglandin-induced increase in temperature. The body then works to lower the temperature, which results in a reduction in fever.

Most antipyretic medications have other purposes. The most common antipyretics in the United States are ibuprofen and aspirin, which are nonsteroidal anti-inflammatory drugs (NSAIDs) used primarily as analgesics (pain relievers), but which also have antipyretic properties; and acetaminophen (paracetamol), an analgesic with weak anti-inflammatory properties.

There is some debate over the appropriate use of such medications, as fever is part of the body's immune response to infection. A study published by the Royal Society claims fever suppression causes at least 1% or more influenza cases of death in the United States, which results in at least 700 extra deaths per year.

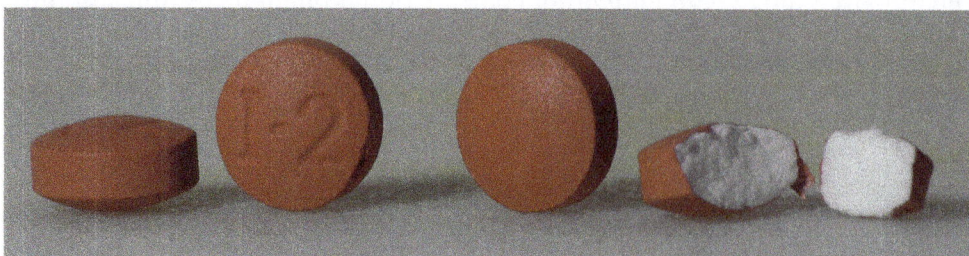

Coated 200 m g tablets of ibuprofen, a common antipyretic.

Non-pharmacological Treatment

Bathing or sponging with lukewarm or cool water can effectively reduce body temperature in those with heat illness, but not usually in those with fever. The use of alcohol baths is not an appropriate cooling method, because there have been reported adverse events associated with systemic absorption of alcohol.

Medications

Many medications have antipyretic effects and thus are useful for fever but not in treating illness, including:

- NSAIDs such as ibuprofen, naproxen, ketoprofen, and nimesulide
- Aspirin, and related salicylates such as choline salicylate, magnesium salicylate, and sodium salicylate
- Paracetamol (USAN and JAN: acetaminophen)
- Metamizole, banned in over 30 countries for causing agranulocytosis
- Nabumetone
- Phenazone (antipyrine), available in combination with benzocaine as an ear drop in the US.

Children

The U.S. Food and Drug Administration (FDA) notes that improper dosing is one of the biggest problems in giving acetaminophen (paracetamol) to children. The effectiveness of acetaminophen alone as an antipyretic in children is uncertain, with some evidence showing it is no better than physical methods. Therapies involving alternating doses of acetaminophen and ibuprofen have shown greater antipyretic effect than either drug alone. One meta-analysis indicated that ibuprofen is more effective than acetaminophen in children at similar doses when both are given alone.

Due to concerns about Reye syndrome, it is recommend that aspirin and combination products containing aspirin not be given to children or teenagers during episodes of fever-causing illnesses.

Plants

Traditional use of higher plants with antipyretic properties is a common worldwide feature of many ethnobotanical cultural systems. In ethnobotany, plants with naturally occurring antipyretic properties are commonly referred to as *febrifuge*.

Analgesics

An analgesic or painkiller is any member of the group of drugs used to achieve analgesia, relief from pain.

Analgesic drugs act in various ways on the peripheral and central nervous systems. They are distinct from anesthetics, which temporarily affect, and in some instances completely eliminate, sensation. Analgesics include paracetamol (known in North America as acetaminophen or simply APAP), the nonsteroidal anti-inflammatory drugs (NSAIDs) such as the salicylates, and opioid drugs such as morphine and oxycodone.

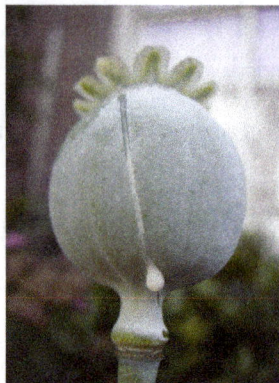

Opium poppies such as this one provide ingredients for the class of analgesics called opiates.

When choosing analgesics, the severity and response to other medication determines the choice of agent; the World Health Organization (WHO) pain ladder specifies mild analgesics as its first step.

Analgesic choice is also determined by the type of pain: For neuropathic pain, traditional analgesics are less effective, and there is often benefit from classes of drugs that are not normally considered analgesics, such as tricyclic antidepressants and anticonvulsants.

Uses

Topical nonsteroidal anti-inflammatory drugs provide pain relief in common conditions such as muscle sprains and overuse injuries. Since the side effects are also lesser, topical preparations could be preferred over oral medications in these conditions.

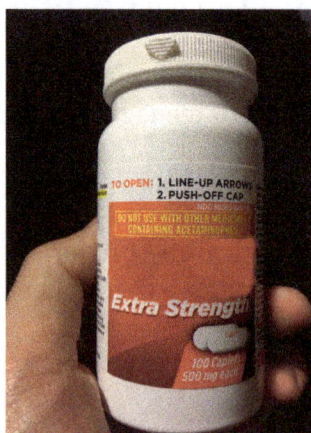

A bottle of acetaminophen.

Contraindications

Each different type of analgesic has its own associated side effects.

Classification

Analgesics are typically classified based on their mechanism of action.

Paracetamol (Acetaminophen)

Paracetamol, also known as acetaminophen or APAP, is a medication used to treat pain and fever. It is typically used for mild to moderate pain. In combination with opioid pain medication, paracetamol is now used for more severe pain such as cancer pain and after surgery. It is typically used either by mouth or rectally but is also available intravenously. Effects last between two and four hours. Paracetamol is classified as a mild analgesic. Paracetamol is generally safe at recommended doses.

NSAIDs

Nonsteroidal anti-inflammatory drugs (usually abbreviated to NSAIDs), are a drug class that groups together drugs that decrease pain and lower fever, and, in higher doses decrease inflammation. The most prominent members of this group of drugs, aspirin, ibuprofen and naproxen, are all available over the counter in most countries.

COX-2 Inhibitors

These drugs have been derived from NSAIDs. The cyclooxygenase enzyme inhibited by NSAIDs was discovered to have at least 2 different versions: COX1 and COX2. Research suggested most of the adverse effects of NSAIDs to be mediated by blocking the COX1 (constitutive) enzyme, with the analgesic effects being mediated by the COX2 (inducible) enzyme. Thus, the COX2 inhibitors were developed to inhibit only the COX2 enzyme (traditional NSAIDs block both versions in general). These drugs (such as rofecoxib, celecoxib, and etoricoxib) are equally effective analgesics when compared with NSAIDs, but cause less gastrointestinal hemorrhage in particular.

After widespread adoption of the COX-2 inhibitors, it was discovered that most of the drugs in this class increase the risk of cardiovascular events by 40% on average. This led to the withdrawal of rofecoxib and valdecoxib, and warnings on others. Etoricoxib seems relatively safe, with the risk of thrombotic events similar to that of non-coxib NSAID diclofenac.

Alcohol

Describing the effects of using alcohol to treat pain is difficult. Alcohol has biological, mental, and social effects which influence the consequences of using alcohol for pain. Moderate use of alcohol can lessen certain types of pain in certain circumstances. Attempting to use alcohol to treat pain has also been observed to lead to negative outcomes including excessive drinking and alcohol use disorder.

Medical Cannabis

Medical cannabis, or medical marijuana, refers to cannabis or its cannabinoids used to treat disease or improve symptoms. There is evidence suggesting that cannabis can be used to treat chronic pain and muscle spasms, with some trials indicating improved relief of neuropathic pain over opioids.

Combinations

Analgesics are frequently used in combination, such as the paracetamol and codeine preparations found in many non-prescription pain relievers. They can also be found in combination with vaso-constrictor drugs such as pseudoephedrine for sinus-related preparations, or with antihistamine drugs for allergy sufferers.

While the use of paracetamol, aspirin, ibuprofen, naproxen, and other NSAIDS concurrently with weak to mid-range opiates (up to about the hydrocodone level) has been said to show beneficial synergistic effects by combatting pain at multiple sites of action, several combination analgesic products have been shown to have few efficacy benefits when compared to similar doses of their individual components. Moreover, these combination analgesics can often result in significant adverse events, including accidental overdoses, most often due to confusion that arises from the multiple (and often non-acting) components of these combinations.

Alternative Medicine

Many people use alternative medicine treatments including drugs for pain relief. There is some evidence that some treatments using alternative medicine can relieve some types of pain more effectively than placebo. The available research concludes that more research would be necessary to better understand the use of alternative medicine.

Psychotropic Agents

Other psychotropic analgesic agents include ketamine (an NMDA receptor antagonist), clonidine and other α_2-adrenoreceptor agonists, and mexiletine and other local anaesthetic analogues.

Other Drugs

Drugs that have been introduced for uses other than analgesics are also used in pain management. Both first-generation (such as amitriptyline) and newer anti-depressants (such as duloxetine) are used alongside NSAIDs and opioids for pain involving nerve damage and similar problems. Other agents directly potentiate the effects of analgesics, such as using hydroxyzine, promethazine, cari-soprodol, or tripelennamine to increase the pain-killing ability of a given dose of opioid analgesic.

Adjuvant analgesics, also called atypical analgesics, include nefopam, orphenadrine, pregabalin, gabapentin, cyclobenzaprine, hyoscine (scopolamine), and other drugs possessing anticonvulsant, anticholinergic, and/or antispasmodic properties, as well as many other drugs with CNS actions. These drugs are used along with analgesics to modulate and/or modify the action of opioids when used against pain, especially of neuropathic origin.

Dextromethorphan has been noted to slow the development of tolerance to opioids and exert additional analgesia by acting upon the NMDA receptors; some analgesics such as methadone and ketobemidone and perhaps piritramide have intrinsic NMDA action.

High-alcohol liquor, two forms of which were found in the US Pharmacopoeia up until 1916 and in common use by physicians well into the 1930s, has been used in the past as an agent for dulling pain, due to the CNS depressant effects of ethyl alcohol, a notable example being the American

Civil War. However, the ability of alcohol to relieve severe pain is likely inferior to many analgesics used today (e.g., morphine, codeine). As such, in general, the idea of alcohol for analgesia is considered a primitive practice in virtually all industrialized countries today.

The use of adjuvant analgesics is an important and growing part of the pain-control field and new discoveries are made practically every year. Many of these drugs combat the side-effects of opioid analgesics, an added bonus. For example, antihistamines including orphenadrine combat the release of histamine caused by many opioids. Stimulants such as methylphenidate, caffeine, ephedrine, dextroamphetamine, methamphetamine, and cocaine work against heavy sedation and may elevate mood in distressed patients as do the antidepressants. The use of medicinal cannabis remains a debated issue.

In patients with chronic or neuropathic pain, various other substances may have analgesic properties. Tricyclic antidepressants, especially clomipramine and amitriptyline, have been shown to improve pain in what appears to be a central manner. Nefopam is used in Europe for pain relief with concurrent opioids. The exact mechanism of carbamazepine, gabapentin, and pregabalin is similarly unclear, but these anticonvulsants are used to treat neuropathic pain with differing degrees of success. Anticonvulsants are most commonly used for neuropathic pain as their mechanism of action tends to inhibit pain sensation.

Flupirtine is a centrally acting K+ channel opener with weak NMDA antagonist properties. It is used in Europe for moderate to strong pain and migraine and its muscle-relaxant properties. It has no anticholinergic properties and is believed to be devoid of any activity on dopamine, serotonin, or histamine receptors. It is not addictive, and tolerance usually does not develop. However, tolerance may develop in single cases.

Other Uses

Topical analgesia is generally recommended to avoid systemic side-effects. Painful joints, for example, may be treated with an ibuprofen- or diclofenac-containing gel (The labeling for topical diclofenac has been updated to warn about drug-induced hepatotoxicity.); capsaicin also is used topically. Lidocaine, an anesthetic, and steroids may be injected into joints for longer-term pain relief. Lidocaine is also used for painful mouth sores and to numb areas for dental work and minor medical procedures. In February 2007 the FDA notified consumers and healthcare professionals of the potential hazards of topical anesthetics entering the bloodstream when applied in large doses to the skin without medical supervision. These topical anesthetics contain anesthetic drugs such as lidocaine, tetracaine, benzocaine, and prilocaine in a cream, ointment, or gel.

Antibiotic

An antibiotic is a type of antimicrobial substance active against bacteria and is the most important type of antibacterial agent for fighting bacterial infections. Antibiotic medications are widely used in the treatment and prevention of such infections. They may either kill or inhibit the growth of bacteria. A limited number of antibiotics also possess antiprotozoal activity. Antibiotics are not effective against viruses such as the common cold or influenza; drugs which inhibit viruses are termed antiviral drugs or antivirals rather than antibiotics.

Sometimes, the term *antibiotic* which means "opposing life", is broadly used to refer to any substance used against microbes, but in the usual medical usage, antibiotics (such as penicillin) are those produced naturally (by one microorganism fighting another), whereas nonantibiotic antibacterials (such as sulfonamides and antiseptics) are fully synthetic. However, both classes have the same goal of killing or preventing the growth of microorganisms, and both are included in antimicrobial chemotherapy. "Antibacterials" include antiseptic drugs, antibacterial soaps, and chemical disinfectants, whereas antibiotics are an important class of antibacterials used more specifically in medicine and sometimes in livestock feed.

Antibiotics have been used since ancient times. Many civilizations used topical application of mouldy bread, with many references to its beneficial effects arising from ancient Egypt, China, Serbia, Greece and Rome. The first person to directly document the use of moulds to treat infections was John Parkinson. Antibiotics revolutionized medicine in the 20th century. Alexander Fleming discovered modern day penicillin in 1928. After realizing the great potential there was in penicillin, Fleming pursued the challenge of how to market it and translate it to commercial use. With help from other biochemists, penicillin was finally available for widespread use. This was significantly beneficial during wartime. Unfortunately, it didn't take long for resistance to begin. Effectiveness and easy access have also led to their overuse and some bacteria have developed resistance. This has led to widespread problems, and the World Health Organization has classified antimicrobial resistance as a "serious threat [that] is no longer a prediction for the future, it is happening right now in every region of the world and has the potential to affect anyone, of any age, in any country".

Medical uses

Antibiotics are used to treat or prevent bacterial infections, and sometimes protozoan infections. (Metronidazole is effective against a number of parasitic diseases). When an infection is suspected of being responsible for an illness but the responsible pathogen has not been identified, an empiric therapy is adopted. This involves the administration of a broad-spectrum antibiotic based on the signs and symptoms presented and is initiated pending laboratory results that can take several days.

When the responsible pathogenic microorganism is already known or has been identified, definitive therapy can be started. This will usually involve the use of a narrow-spectrum antibiotic. The choice of antibiotic given will also be based on its cost. Identification is critically important as it can reduce the cost and toxicity of the antibiotic therapy and also reduce the possibility of the emergence of antimicrobial resistance. To avoid surgery, antibiotics may be given for non-complicated acute appendicitis.

Antibiotics may be given as a preventive measure and this is usually limited to at-risk populations such as those with a weakened immune system (particularly in HIV cases to prevent pneumonia), those taking immunosuppressive drugs, cancer patients, and those having surgery. Their use in surgical procedures is to help prevent infection of incisions. They have an important role in dental antibiotic prophylaxis where their use may prevent bacteremia and consequent infective endocarditis. Antibiotics are also used to prevent infection in cases of neutropenia particularly cancer-related.

Administration

There are many different routes of administration for antibiotic treatment. Antibiotics are usually taken by mouth. In more severe cases, particularly deep-seated systemic infections, antibiotics can be given intravenously or by injection. Where the site of infection is easily accessed, antibiotics may be given topically in the form of eye drops onto the conjunctiva for conjunctivitis or ear drops for ear infections and acute cases of swimmer's ear. Topical use is also one of the treatment options for some skin conditions including acne and cellulitis. Advantages of topical application include achieving high and sustained concentration of antibiotic at the site of infection; reducing the potential for systemic absorption and toxicity, and total volumes of antibiotic required are reduced, thereby also reducing the risk of antibiotic misuse. Topical antibiotics applied over certain types of surgical wounds have been reported to reduce the risk of surgical site infections. However, there are certain general causes for concern with topical administration of antibiotics. Some systemic absorption of the antibiotic may occur; the quantity of antibiotic applied is difficult to accurately dose, and there is also the possibility of local hypersensitivity reactions or contact dermatitis occurring.

Prevalence

Antibiotic consumption varies widely between countries. The 'WHO report on surveillance of antibiotic consumption' published in 2018 analysed 2015 data from 65 countries. As measured in defined daily doses per 1,000 inhabitants per day. Mongolia had the highest consumption with a rate of 64.4. Burundi had the lowest at 4.4. Amoxicillin and Amoxicillin/clavulanic acid were the most frequently consumed.

Side Effects

Antibiotics are screened for any negative effects before their approval for clinical use, and are usually considered safe and well tolerated. However, some antibiotics have been associated with a wide extent of adverse side effects ranging from mild to very severe depending on the type of antibiotic used, the microbes targeted, and the individual patient. Side effects may reflect the pharmacological or toxicological properties of the antibiotic or may involve hypersensitivity or allergic reactions. Adverse effects range from fever and nausea to major allergic reactions, including photodermatitis and anaphylaxis. Safety profiles of newer drugs are often not as well established as for those that have a long history of use.

Common side-effects include diarrhea, resulting from disruption of the species composition in the intestinal flora, resulting, for example, in overgrowth of pathogenic bacteria, such as *Clostridium difficile*. Antibacterials can also affect the vaginal flora, and may lead to overgrowth of yeast species of the genus *Candida* in the vulvo-vaginal area. Additional side effects can result from interaction with other drugs, such as the possibility of tendon damage from the administration of a quinolone antibiotic with a systemic corticosteroid.

Correlation with Obesity

Exposure to antibiotics early in life is associated with increased body mass in humans and mouse models. Early life is a critical period for the establishment of the intestinal microbiota and for metabolic development. Mice exposed to subtherapeutic antibiotic treatment (STAT)– with either penicillin, vancomycin, or chlortetracycline had altered composition of the gut microbiota as well as its metabolic capabilities. One study has reported that mice given low-dose penicillin (1 μg/g body weight) around birth and throughout the weaning process had an increased body mass and fat mass, accelerated growth, and increased hepatic expression of genes involved in adipogenesis, compared to control mice. In addition, penicillin in combination with a high-fat diet increased fasting insulin levels in mice. However, it is unclear whether or not antibiotics cause obesity in humans. Studies have found a correlation between early exposure of antibiotics (<6 months) and increased body mass (at 10 and 20 months). Another study found that the type of antibiotic exposure was also significant with the highest risk of being overweight in those given macrolides compared to penicillin and cephalosporin. Therefore, there is correlation between antibiotic exposure in early life and obesity in humans, but whether or not there is a causal relationship remains unclear. Although there is a correlation between antibiotic use in early life and obesity, the effect of antibiotics on obesity in humans needs to be weighed against the beneficial effects of clinically indicated treatment with antibiotics in infancy.

Interactions

Birth Control Pills

There are few well-controlled studies on whether antibiotic use increases the risk of oral contraceptive failure. The majority of studies indicate antibiotics do not interfere with birth control pills, such as clinical studies that suggest the failure rate of contraceptive pills caused by antibiotics is very low (about 1%). Situations that may increase the risk of oral contraceptive failure include non-compliance (missing taking the pill), vomiting, or diarrhea. Gastrointestinal disorders or interpatient variability in oral contraceptive absorption affecting ethinylestradiol serum levels in the blood. Women with menstrual irregularities may be at higher risk of failure and should be advised to use backup contraception during antibiotic treatment and for one week after its completion. If patient-specific risk factors for reduced oral contraceptive efficacy are suspected, backup contraception is recommended.

In cases where antibiotics have been suggested to affect the efficiency of birth control pills, such as for the broad-spectrum antibiotic rifampicin, these cases may be due to an increase in the activities of hepatic liver enzymes' causing increased breakdown of the pill's active ingredients. Effects on the intestinal flora, which might result in reduced absorption of estrogens in the colon, have also been suggested, but such suggestions have been inconclusive and controversial. Clinicians have recommended that extra contraceptive measures be applied during therapies using antibiotics that are suspected to interact with oral contraceptives. More studies on the possible interactions between antibiotics and birth control pills (oral contraceptives) are required as well as careful assessment of patient-specific risk factors for potential oral contractive pill failure prior to dismissing the need for backup contraception.

Alcohol

Interactions between alcohol and certain antibiotics may occur and may cause side effects and decreased effectiveness of antibiotic therapy. While moderate alcohol consumption is unlikely to interfere with many common antibiotics, there are specific types of antibiotics, with which alcohol consumption may cause serious side effects. Therefore, potential risks of side effects and effectiveness depend on the type of antibiotic administered.

Antibiotics such as metronidazole, tinidazole, cephamandole, latamoxef, cefoperazone, cefmenoxime, and furazolidone, cause a disulfiram-like chemical reaction with alcohol by inhibiting its breakdown by acetaldehyde dehydrogenase, which may result in vomiting, nausea, and shortness of breath. In addition, the efficacy of doxycycline and erythromycin succinate may be reduced by alcohol consumption. Other effects of alcohol on antibiotic activity include altered activity of the liver enzymes that break down the antibiotic compound.

Pharmacodynamics

The successful outcome of antimicrobial therapy with antibacterial compounds depends on several factors. These include host defense mechanisms, the location of infection, and the pharmacokinetic and pharmacodynamic properties of the antibacterial. A bactericidal activity of antibacterials may depend on the bacterial growth phase, and it often requires ongoing metabolic activity and division of bacterial cells. These findings are based on laboratory studies, and in clinical settings have also been shown to eliminate bacterial infection. Since the activity of antibacterials depends frequently on its concentration, *in vitro* characterization of antibacterial activity commonly includes the determination of the minimum inhibitory concentration and minimum bactericidal concentration of an antibacterial. To predict clinical outcome, the antimicrobial activity of an antibacterial is usually combined with its pharmacokinetic profile, and several pharmacological parameters are used as markers of drug efficacy.

Combination Therapy

In important infectious diseases, including tuberculosis, combination therapy (i.e., the concurrent application of two or more antibiotics) has been used to delay or prevent the emergence of resistance. In acute bacterial infections, antibiotics as part of combination therapy are prescribed for their synergistic effects to improve treatment outcome as the combined effect of both antibiotics is better than their individual effect. Methicillin-resistant Staphylococcus aureus infections may be treated with a combination therapy of fusidic acid and rifampicin. Antibiotics used in combination may also be antagonistic and the combined effects of the two antibiotics may be less than if the individual antibiotic was given as part of a monotherapy. For example, chloramphenicol and tetracyclines are antagonists to penicillins and U.S.s. However, this can vary depending on the species of bacteria. In general, combinations of a bacteriostatic antibiotic and bactericidal antibiotic are antagonistic.

Classes

Antibiotics are commonly classified based on their mechanism of action, chemical structure, or spectrum of activity. Most target bacterial functions or growth processes. Those that target the bacterial cell wall (penicillins and cephalosporins) or the cell membrane (polymyxins), or interfere with essential bacterial enzymes (rifamycins, lipiarmycins, quinolones, and sulfonamides) have bactericidal activities. Protein synthesis inhibitors (macrolides, lincosamides, and tetracyclines) are usually bacteriostatic (with the exception of bactericidal aminoglycosides). Further categorization is based on their target specificity. "Narrow-spectrum" antibiotics target specific types of bacteria, such as gram-negative or gram-positive, whereas broad-spectrum antibiotics affect a wide range of bacteria. Following a 40-year break in discovering new classes of antibacterial compounds, four new classes of antibiotics have been brought into clinical use in the late 2000s and early 2010s: cyclic lipopeptides (such as daptomycin), glycylcyclines (such as tigecycline), oxazolidinones (such as linezolid), and lipiarmycins (such as fidaxomicin).

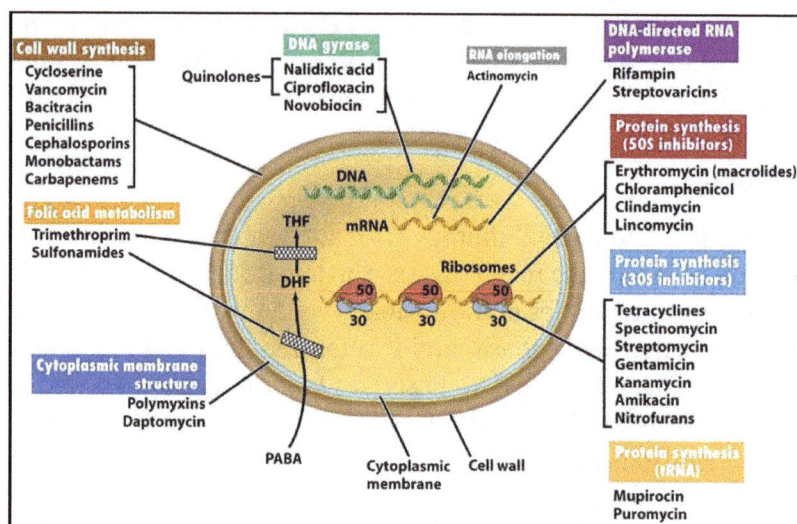

Molecular targets of antibiotics on the bacteria cell.

Production

With advances in medicinal chemistry, most modern antibacterials are semisynthetic modifications of various natural compounds. These include, for example, the beta-lactam antibiotics, which include the penicillins (produced by fungi in the genus *Penicillium*), the cephalosporins, and the carbapenems. Compounds that are still isolated from living organisms are the aminoglycosides, whereas other antibacterials—for example, the sulfonamides, the quinolones, and the oxazolidinones—are produced solely by chemical synthesis. Many antibacterial compounds are relatively small molecules with a molecular weight of less than 1000 daltons.

Since the first pioneering efforts of Howard Florey and Chain in 1939, the importance of antibiotics, including antibacterials, to medicine has led to intense research into producing antibacterials at large scales. Following screening of antibacterials against a wide range of bacteria, production of the active compounds is carried out using fermentation, usually in strongly aerobic conditions.

The use of antibiotics in modern medicine began with the discovery of synthetic antibiotics derived from dyes.

Synthetic Antibiotics Derived from Dyes

Synthetic antibiotic chemotherapy as a science and development of antibacterials began in Germany with Paul Ehrlich in the late 1880s. Ehrlich noted certain dyes would color human, animal, or bacterial cells, whereas others did not. He then proposed the idea that it might be possible to create chemicals that would act as a selective drug that would bind to and kill bacteria without harming the human host. After screening hundreds of dyes against various organisms, in 1907, he discovered a medicinally useful drug, the first synthetic antibacterial organoarsenic compound salvarsan, now called arsphenamine.

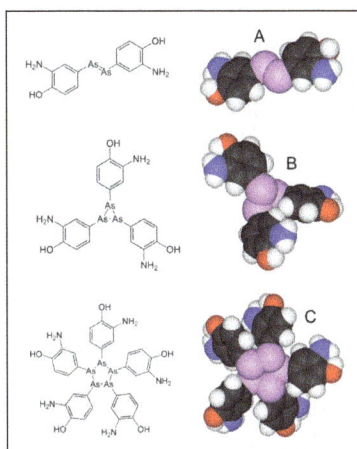

Arsphenamine, also known as salvarsan, discovered in 1907 by Paul Ehrlich.

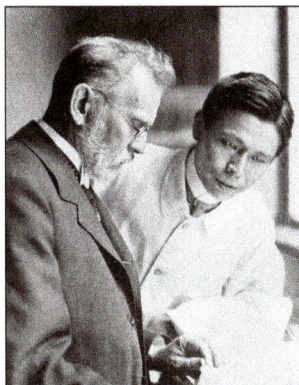

Paul Ehrlich and Sahachiro Hata.

This heralded the era of antibacterial treatment that was begun with the discovery of a series of arsenic-derived synthetic antibiotics by both Alfred Bertheim and Ehrlich in 1907. Ehrlich and Bertheim had experimented with various chemicals derived from dyes to treat trypanosomiasis in mice and spirochaeta infection in rabbits. While their early compounds were too toxic, Ehrlich and Sahachiro Hata, a Japanese bacteriologist working with Erlich in the quest for a drug to treat syphilis, achieved success with the 606th compound in their series of experiments. In 1910 Ehrlich and Hata announced their discovery, which they called drug "606", at the Congress for Internal Medicine at Wiesbaden. The Hoechst company began to market the compound toward the end of 1910 under the name Salvarsan, now known as arsphenamine. The drug was used to treat syphilis in the first half of the 20th century. In 1908, Ehrlich received the Nobel Prize in Physiology or Medicine for his contributions to immunology. Hata was nominated for the Nobel Prize in Chemistry in 1911 and for the Nobel Prize in Physiology or Medicine in 1912 and 1913.

The first sulfonamide and the first systemically active antibacterial drug, Prontosil, was developed by a research team led by Gerhard Domagk in 1932 or 1933 at the Bayer Laboratories of the IG Farben conglomerate in Germany, for which Domagk received the 1939 Nobel Prize in Physiology or Medicine. Sulfanilamide, the active drug of Prontosil, was not patentable as it had already been in use in the dye industry for some years. Prontosil had a relatively broad effect against

Gram-positive cocci, but not against enterobacteria. Research was stimulated apace by its success. The discovery and development of this sulfonamide drug opened the era of antibacterials.

Penicillin and other Natural Antibiotics

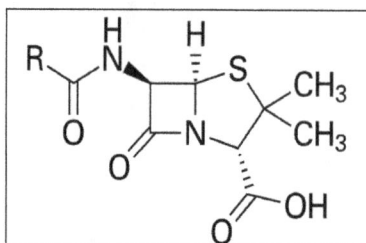

Penicillin, discovered by Alexander Fleming.

Observations about the growth of some microorganisms inhibiting the growth of other microorganisms have been reported since the late 19th century. These observations of antibiosis between microorganisms led to the discovery of natural antibacterials. Louis Pasteur observed, "if we could intervene in the antagonism observed between some bacteria, it would offer perhaps the greatest hopes for therapeutics".

In 1874, physician Sir William Roberts noted that cultures of the mold *Penicillium glaucum* that is used in the making of some types of blue cheese did not display bacterial contamination. In 1876, physicist John Tyndall also contributed to this field. Pasteur conducted research showing that *Bacillus anthracis* would not grow in the presence of the related mold *Penicillium notatum*.

In 1895 Vincenzo Tiberio, Italian physician, published a paper on the antibacterial power of some extracts of mold.

In 1897, doctoral student Ernest Duchesne submitted a dissertation, "*Contribution à l'étude de la concurrence vitale chez les micro-organismes: antagonisme entre les moisissures et les microbes*" (Contribution to the study of vital competition in micro-organisms: antagonism between molds and microbes), the first known scholarly work to consider the therapeutic capabilities of molds resulting from their anti-microbial activity. In his thesis, Duchesne proposed that bacteria and molds engage in a perpetual battle for survival. Duchesne observed that *E. coli* was eliminated by *Penicillium glaucum* when they were both grown in the same culture. He also observed that when he inoculated laboratory animals with lethal doses of typhoid bacilli together with *Penicillium glaucum*, the animals did not contract typhoid. Unfortunately Duchesne's army service after getting his degree prevented him from doing any further research. Duchesne died of tuberculosis, a disease now treated by antibiotics.

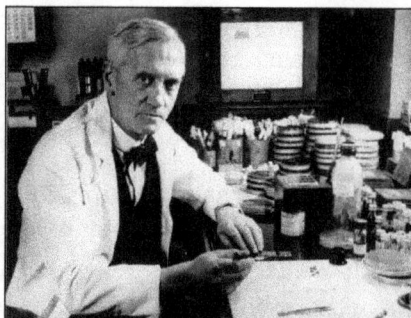

Alexander Fleming was awarded a Nobel prize for his role in the discovery of penicillin.

In 1928, Sir Alexander Fleming postulated the existence of penicillin, a molecule produced by certain molds that kills or stops the growth of certain kinds of bacteria. Fleming was working on a culture of disease-causing bacteria when he noticed the spores of a green mold, *Penicillium chrysogenum*, in one of his culture plates. He observed that the presence of the mold killed or prevented the growth of the bacteria. Fleming postulated that the mold must secrete an antibacterial substance, which he named penicillin in 1928. Fleming believed that its antibacterial properties could be exploited for chemotherapy. He initially characterized some of its biological properties, and attempted to use a crude preparation to treat some infections, but he was unable to pursue its further development without the aid of trained chemists.

Ernst Chain, Howard Florey and Edward Abraham succeeded in purifying the first penicillin, penicillin G, in 1942, but it did not become widely available outside the Allied military before 1945. Later, Norman Heatley developed the back extraction technique for efficiently purifying penicillin in bulk. The chemical structure of penicillin was first proposed by Abraham in 1942 and then later confirmed by Dorothy Crowfoot Hodgkin in 1945. Purified penicillin displayed potent antibacterial activity against a wide range of bacteria and had low toxicity in humans. Furthermore, its activity was not inhibited by biological constituents such as pus, unlike the synthetic sulfonamides. The development of penicillin led to renewed interest in the search for antibiotic compounds with similar efficacy and safety. For their successful development of penicillin, which Fleming had accidentally discovered but could not develop himself, as a therapeutic drug, Chain and Florey shared the 1945 Nobel Prize in Medicine with Fleming.

Florey credited Rene Dubos with pioneering the approach of deliberately and systematically searching for antibacterial compounds, which had led to the discovery of gramicidin and had revived Florey's research in penicillin. In 1939, coinciding with the start of World War II, Dubos had reported the discovery of the first naturally derived antibiotic, tyrothricin, a compound of 20% gramicidin and 80% tyrocidine, from *B. brevis*. It was one of the first commercially manufactured antibiotics and was very effective in treating wounds and ulcers during World War II. Gramicidin, however, could not be used systemically because of toxicity. Tyrocidine also proved too toxic for systemic usage. Research results obtained during that period were not shared between the Axis and the Allied powers during World War II and limited access during the Cold War.

Late 20th Century

During the mid-20th century, the number of new antibiotic substances introduced for medical use increased significantly. From 1935 to 1968, 12 new classes were launched. However, after this, the number of new classes dropped markedly, with only 2 new classes introduced between 1969 and 2003.

The term 'antibiosis', meaning "against life", was introduced by the French bacteriologist Jean Paul Vuillemin as a descriptive name of the phenomenon exhibited by these early antibacterial drugs. Antibiosis was first described in 1877 in bacteria when Louis Pasteur and Robert Koch observed that an airborne bacillus could inhibit the growth of *Bacillus anthracis*. These drugs were later renamed antibiotics by Selman Waksman, an American microbiologist, in 1942.

The term *antibiotic* was first used in 1942 by Selman Waksman and his collaborators in journal articles to describe any substance produced by a microorganism that is antagonistic to the growth of other microorganisms in high dilution. This definition excluded substances that kill bacteria but that are not produced by microorganisms (such as gastric juices and hydrogen peroxide). It also excluded synthetic antibacterial compounds such as the sulfonamides. In current usage, the term "antibiotic" is applied to any medication that kills bacteria or inhibits their growth, regardless of whether that medication is produced by a microorganism or not.

Alternatives

The increase in bacterial strains that are resistant to conventional antibacterial therapies together with decreasing number of new antibiotics currently being developed in the drug pipeline has prompted the development of bacterial disease treatment strategies that are alternatives to conventional antibacterials. Non-compound approaches (that is, products other than classical antibacterial agents) that target bacteria or approaches that target the host including phage therapy and vaccines are also being investigated to combat the problem.

Resistance and Modifying Agents

One strategy to address bacterial drug resistance is the discovery and application of compounds that modify resistance to common antibacterials. Resistance modifying agents are capable of partly or completely suppressing bacterial resistance mechanisms. For example, some resistance-modifying agents may inhibit multidrug resistance mechanisms, such as drug efflux from the cell, thus increasing the susceptibility of bacteria to an antibacterial. Targets include:

- The efflux inhibitor Phe-Arg-β-naphthylamide.

- Beta-lactamase inhibitors, such as clavulanic acid and sulbactam.

Metabolic stimuli such as sugar can help eradicate a certain type of antibiotic-tolerant bacteria by keeping their metabolism active.

Vaccines

Vaccines rely on immune modulation or augmentation. Vaccination either excites or reinforces the immune competence of a host to ward off infection, leading to the activation of macrophages, the production of antibodies, inflammation, and other classic immune reactions. Antibacterial vaccines have been responsible for a drastic reduction in global bacterial diseases. Vaccines made from attenuated whole cells or lysates have been replaced largely by less reactogenic, cell-free vaccines consisting of purified components, including capsular polysaccharides and their conjugates, to protein carriers, as well as inactivated toxins (toxoids) and proteins.

Phage Therapy

Phage therapy is another method for treating antibiotic-resistant strains of bacteria. Phage therapy infects pathogenic bacteria with their own viruses. Bacteriophages and their host ranges are extremely specific for certain bacteria, thus, unlike antibiotics, they do not disturb the host organism and intestinal microflora. Bacteriophages, also known simply as phages, infect and can kill bacteria and affect bacterial growth primarily during lytic cycles. Phages insert their DNA into the bacterium, where it is transcribed and used to make new phages, after which the cell will lyse, releasing new phage that are able to infect and destroy further bacteria of the same strain. The high specificity of phage protects "good" bacteria from destruction.

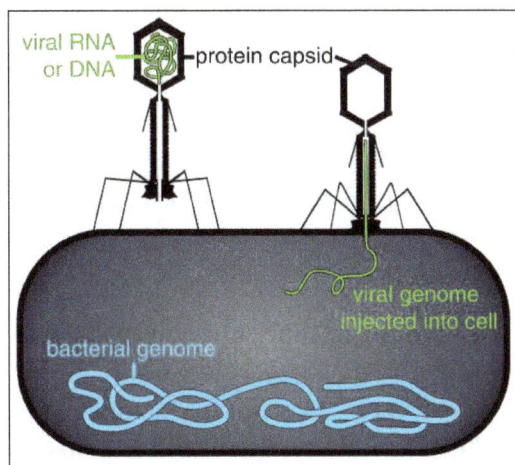

Phage injecting its genome into bacterial cell.

Some disadvantages to the use of bacteriophages also exist, however. Bacteriophages may harbour virulence factors or toxic genes in their genomes and, prior to use, it may be prudent to identify genes with similarity to known virulence factors or toxins by genomic sequencing. In addition, the oral and IV administration of phages for the eradication of bacterial infections poses a much higher safety risk than topical application. Also, there is the additional concern of uncertain immune responses to these large antigenic cocktails.

There are considerable regulatory hurdles that must be cleared for such therapies. Despite numerous challenges, the use of bacteriophages as a replacement for antimicrobial agents against MDR pathogens that no longer respond to conventional antibiotics, remains an attractive option.

Phytochemicals

Plants are an important source of antimicrobial compounds and traditional healers have long used plants to prevent or cure infectious diseases. There is a recent renewed interest into the use of natural products for the identification of new members of the 'antibiotic-ome' (defined as natural products with antibiotic activity), and their application in antibacterial drug discovery in the genomics era. Phytochemicals are the active biological component of plants and some phytochemicals including tannins, alkaloids, terpenoids, and flavonoids possess antimicrobial activity. Some antioxidant dietary supplements also contain phytochemicals (polyphenols), such as grape seed extract, and demonstrate *in vitro* anti-bacterial properties. Phytochemicals are able to inhibit peptidoglycan synthesis, damage microbial membrane structures, modify bacterial membrane surface hydrophobicity and also modulate quorum sensing. With increasing antibiotic resistance in recent years, the potential of new plant-derived antibiotics is under investigation.

New Antibiotics Development

Both the WHO and the Infectious Disease Society of America (IDSA) reported that the weak antibiotic pipeline does not match bacteria's increasing ability to develop resistance. The IDSA report noted that the number of new antibiotics approved for marketing per year had been declining and identified seven antibiotics against the Gram-negative bacilli (GNB) currently in phase 2 or phase 3 clinical trials. These drugs however, did not address the entire spectrum of resistance of GNB. According to the WHO fifty one new therapeutic entities (NTEs) - antibiotics (including combinations), are in phase 1-3 clinical trials as of May 2017. Recent entries in the clinical pipeline targeting multidrug-resistant Gram-positive pathogens has improved the treatment options due to marketing approval of new antibiotic classes, the oxazolidinones and cyclic lipopeptides. However, resistance to these antibiotics is certainly likely to occur, the need for the development new antibiotics against those pathogens still remains a high priority. Recent drugs in development that target Gram-negative bacteria have focused on re-working existing drugs to target specific micro-organisms or specific types of resistance.

A few antibiotics have received marketing authorization in the last seven years. The cephalosporin ceftaroline and the lipoglycopeptides oritavancin and telavancin for the treatment of acute bacterial skin and skin structure infection and community-acquired bacterial pneumonia. The lipoglycopeptide dalbavancin and the oxazolidinone tedizolid has also been approved for use for the treatment of acute bacterial skin and skin structure infection. The first in a new class of narrow spectrum macrocyclic antibiotics, fidaxomicin, has been approved for the treatment of *C. difficile* colitis. New cephalosporin-lactamase inhibitor combinations also approved include ceftazidime-avibactam and ceftolozane-avibactam for complicated urinary tract infection and intra-abdominal infection.

- Ceftolozane/tazobactam (CXA-201; CXA-101/tazobactam): Antipseudomonal cephalosporin/β-lactamase inhibitor combination (cell wall synthesis inhibitor). FDA approved on 19 December 2014.

- Ceftazidime/avibactam (ceftazidime/NXL104): Antipseudomonal cephalosporin/β-lactamase inhibitor combination (cell wall synthesis inhibitor). In phase 3.

- Ceftaroline/avibactam (CPT-avibactam; ceftaroline/NXL104): Anti-MRSA cephalosporin/β-lactamase inhibitor combination (cell wall synthesis inhibitor).

- Imipenem/MK-7655: Carbapenem/ β-lactamase inhibitor combination (cell wall synthesis inhibitor). In phase 2.

- Plazomicin (ACHN-490): Aminoglycoside (protein synthesis inhibitor). New Drug Application is under Priority Review by U.S. FDA.

- Eravacycline (TP-434): Synthetic tetracycline derivative / protein synthesis inhibitor targeting the ribosome. Development by Tetraphase, Phase 2 trials complete.

- Brilacidin (PMX-30063): Peptide defense protein mimetic (cell membrane disruption). In phase 2.

Streptomyces research is expected to provide new antibiotics, including treatment against MRSA and infections resistant to commonly used medication. Efforts of John Innes Centre and universities in the UK, supported by BBSRC, resulted in the creation of spin-out companies, for example Novacta Biosystems, which has designed the type-b lantibiotic-based compound NVB302 (in phase 1) to treat *Clostridium difficile* infections.

Possible improvements include clarification of clinical trial regulations by FDA. Furthermore, appropriate economic incentives could persuade pharmaceutical companies to invest in this endeavor. In the US, the Antibiotic Development to Advance Patient Treatment (ADAPT) Act was introduced with the aim of fast tracking the drug development of antibiotics to combat the growing threat of 'superbugs'. Under this Act, FDA can approve antibiotics and antifungals treating life-threatening infections based on smaller clinical trials. The CDC will monitor the use of antibiotics and the emerging resistance, and publish the data. The FDA antibiotics labeling process, 'Susceptibility Test Interpretive Criteria for Microbial Organisms' or 'breakpoints', will provide accurate data to healthcare professionals. According to Allan Coukell, senior director for health programs at The Pew Charitable Trusts, "By allowing drug developers to rely on smaller datasets, and clarifying FDA's authority to tolerate a higher level of uncertainty for these drugs when making a risk/benefit calculation, ADAPT would make the clinical trials more feasible."

Antiviral Drug

Antiviral drugs are a class of medication used specifically for treating viral infections rather than bacterial ones. Most antivirals are used for specific viral infections, while a broad-spectrum antiviral is effective against a wide range of viruses. Unlike most antibiotics, antiviral drugs do not destroy their target pathogen; instead they inhibit their development.

Antiviral drugs are one class of antimicrobials, a larger group which also includes antibiotic (also termed antibacterial), antifungal and antiparasitic drugs, or antiviral drugs based on monoclonal antibodies. Most antivirals are considered relatively harmless to the host, and therefore can be used to treat infections. They should be distinguished from viricides, which are not medication but deactivate or destroy virus particles, either inside or outside the body. Natural antivirals are produced by some plants such as eucalyptus and Australian tea trees.

Medical uses

Most of the antiviral drugs now available are designed to help deal with HIV, herpes viruses, the hepatitis B and C viruses, and influenza A and B viruses. Researchers are working to extend the range of antivirals to other families of pathogens.

Designing safe and effective antiviral drugs is difficult, because viruses use the host's cells to replicate. This makes it difficult to find targets for the drug that would interfere with the virus without also harming the host organism's cells. Moreover, the major difficulty in developing vaccines and anti-viral drugs is due to viral variation.

The emergence of antivirals is the product of a greatly expanded knowledge of the genetic and molecular function of organisms, allowing biomedical researchers to understand the structure and function of viruses, major advances in the techniques for finding new drugs, and the pressure placed on the medical profession to deal with the human immunodeficiency virus (HIV), the cause of acquired immunodeficiency syndrome (AIDS).

The first experimental antivirals were developed in the 1960s, mostly to deal with herpes viruses, and were found using traditional trial-and-error drug discovery methods. Researchers grew cultures of cells and infected them with the target virus. They then introduced into the cultures chemicals which they thought might inhibit viral activity, and observed whether the level of virus in the cultures rose or fell. Chemicals that seemed to have an effect were selected for closer study.

This was a very time-consuming, hit-or-miss procedure, and in the absence of a good knowledge of how the target virus worked, it was not efficient in discovering effective antivirals which had few side effects. Only in the 1980s, when the full genetic sequences of viruses began to be unraveled, did researchers begin to learn how viruses worked in detail, and exactly what chemicals were needed to thwart their reproductive cycle.

Virus Life Cycle

Viruses consist of a genome and sometimes a few enzymes stored in a capsule made of protein (called a capsid), and sometimes covered with a lipid layer (sometimes called an 'envelope'). Viruses cannot reproduce on their own, and instead propagate by subjugating a host cell to produce copies of themselves, thus producing the next generation.

Researchers working on such "rational drug design" strategies for developing antivirals have tried to attack viruses at every stage of their life cycles. Some species of mushrooms have been found to contain multiple antiviral chemicals with similar synergistic effects. Compounds Isolated from fruiting bodies and filtrates of various mushrooms have broad spectrum antiviral activities, but successful production and availability of such compounds as frontline antiviral is a long way away. Viral life cycles vary in their precise details depending on the type of virus, but they all share a general pattern:

- Attachment to a host cell.
- Release of viral genes and possibly enzymes into the host cell.
- Replication of viral components using host-cell machinery.
- Assembly of viral components into complete viral particles.
- Release of viral particles to infect new host cells.

Society and Culture

Several factors including cost, vaccination stigma, and acquired resistance limit the effectiveness of antiviral therapies. These issues are explored via a health policy perspective.

Costs

Cost is an important factor that limits access to antivirals therapies in the United States and internationally. The recommended treatment regimen for hepatitis C virus infection, for example, includes sofosbuvir-velpatasvir (Epclusa) and ledipasvir-sofosbuvir (Harrvoni). A twelve-week supply of these drugs amount to $113,400 and $89,712, respectively. These drugs can be manufactured generically at a cost of $100 - $250 per 12 week treatment. Pharmaceutical companies attribute the majority of these costs to research and development expenses. However, critics point to monopolistic market conditions that allow manufacturers to increase prices without facing a reduction in sales, leading to higher profits at patient's expense. Intellectual property laws, anti-importation policies, and the slow pace of FDA review limit alternative options. Recently, private-public research partnerships have been established to promote expedited, cost-effective research.

Vaccinations

Population Health

While most antivirals treat viral infection, vaccines are a preemptive first line of defense against pathogens. Vaccination involves the introduction (i.e. via injection) of a small amount of typically inactivated or attenuated antigenic material to stimulate an individual's immune system. The immune system responds by developing white blood cells to specifically combat the introduced pathogen, resulting in adaptive immunity. Vaccination in a population results in herd immunity and greatly improved population health, with significant reductions in viral infection and disease.

Vaccination Policy

Vaccination policy in the United States consists of public and private vaccination requirements. For instance, public schools require students to receive vaccinations (termed "vaccination schedule") for viruses and bacteria such as diphtheria, pertussis, and tetanus (DTaP), measles, mumps, rubella (MMR), varicella (chickenpox), hepatitis B, rotavirus, polio, and more. Private institutions might require annual influenza vaccination. The Center for Disease Control and Prevention has estimated that routine immunization of newborns prevents about 42,000 deaths and 20 million cases of disease each year, saving about $13.6 billion.

Vaccination Controversy

Despite their successes, there is plenty of stigma surrounding vaccines that cause people to be incompletely vaccinated. These "gaps" in vaccination result in unnecessary infection, death, and costs. There are two major reasons for incomplete vaccination:

- Vaccines, like other medical treatments, have a risk of causing serious complications in some individuals (i.e. severe allergic reactions). While these complications are less common than the risks faced when not vaccinated, negative media coverage can instill fear in a population. Other controversies involve the association of autism with vaccines, although this link has been thoroughly discredited by the medical community, including the Center for Disease Control and Prevention, Institute of Medicine, and National Health Service.

- Low vaccine-preventable disease rates as a result of herd immunity also make vaccines seem unnecessary and leave many unvaccinated.

Although the American Academy of Pediatrics endorses universal immunization, they note that physicians should respect parents' refusal to vaccinate their children after sufficient advising and provided the child does not face a significant risk of infection. Parents can also cite religious reasons to avoid public school vaccination mandates, but this reduces herd immunity and increases risk of viral infection.

Limitations of Vaccines

Vaccines bolster the body's immune system to better attack viruses in the "complete particle" stage, outside of the organism's cells. They traditionally consist of an attenuated (a live weakened) or inactivated (killed) version of the virus. These vaccines can, in very rare cases, harm the host by inadvertently infecting the host with a full-blown viral occupancy. Recently "subunit" vaccines have been devised that consist strictly of protein targets from the pathogen. They stimulate the immune system without doing serious harm to the host. In either case, when the real pathogen attacks the subject, the immune system responds to it quickly and blocks it.

Vaccines are very effective on stable viruses, but are of limited use in treating a patient who has already been infected. They are also difficult to successfully deploy against rapidly mutating viruses, such as influenza (the vaccine for which is updated every year) and HIV. Antiviral drugs are particularly useful in these cases.

Antiretroviral Therapy as HIV Prevention

There is significant evidence to demonstrate that antiretroviral drugs inhibit transmission when the person living with HIV has been undetectable for 6 months or longer.

Public Policy

Use and Distribution

Guidelines regarding viral diagnoses and treatments change frequently and limit quality care. Even when physicians diagnose older patients with influenza, use of antiviral treatment can be low. Provider knowledge of antiviral therapies can improve patient care, especially in geriatric medicine. Furthermore, in local health departments (LHDs) with access to antivirals, guidelines may be unclear, causing delays in treatment. With time-sensitive therapies, delays could lead to lack of treatment. Overall, national guidelines regarding infection control and management standardize care and improve patient and health care worker safety. Guidelines such as those provided by the Centers for Disease Control and Prevention (CDC) during the 2009 flu pandemic caused by the H1N1 virus, recommend antiviral treatment regimens, clinical assessment algorithms for coordination of care, and antiviral chemoprophylaxis guidelines for exposed persons, among others. Roles of pharmacists and pharmacies have also expanded to meet the needs of public during public health emergencies.

Stockpiling

Public Health Emergency Preparedness initiatives are managed by the CDC via the Office of Public Health Preparedness and Response. Funds aim to support communities in preparing for public health emergencies, including pandemic influenza. Also managed by the CDC, the Strategic National Stockpile (SNS) consists of bulk quantities of medicines and supplies for use during such emergencies. Antiviral stockpiles prepare for shortages of antiviral medications in cases of public health emergencies. During the H1N1 pandemic in 2009-2010, guidelines for SNS use by local health departments was unclear, revealing gaps in antiviral planning. For example, local health departments that received antivirals from the SNS did not have transparent guidance on the use of the treatments. The gap made it difficult to create plans and policies for their use and future availabilities, causing delays in treatment.

Anti-viral Targeting

The general idea behind modern antiviral drug design is to identify viral proteins, or parts of proteins, that can be disabled. These "targets" should generally be as unlike any proteins or parts of proteins in humans as possible, to reduce the likelihood of side effects. The targets should also be common across many strains of a virus, or even among different species of virus in the same family, so a single drug will have broad effectiveness. For example, a researcher might target a critical enzyme synthesized by the virus, but not the patient, that is common across strains, and see what can be done to interfere with its operation.

Once targets are identified, candidate drugs can be selected, either from drugs already known to have appropriate effects, or by actually designing the candidate at the molecular level with a computer-aided design program.

The target proteins can be manufactured in the lab for testing with candidate treatments by inserting the gene that synthesizes the target protein into bacteria or other kinds of cells. The cells are then cultured for mass production of the protein, which can then be exposed to various treatment candidates and evaluated with "rapid screening" technologies.

Approaches by Life Cycle Stage

Before Cell Entry

One anti-viral strategy is to interfere with the ability of a virus to infiltrate a target cell. The virus must go through a sequence of steps to do this, beginning with binding to a specific "receptor" molecule on the surface of the host cell and ending with the virus "uncoating" inside the cell and releasing its contents. Viruses that have a lipid envelope must also fuse their envelope with the target cell, or with a vesicle that transports them into the cell, before they can uncoat.

This stage of viral replication can be inhibited in two ways:

- Using agents which mimic the virus-associated protein (VAP) and bind to the cellular receptors. This may include VAP anti-idiotypic antibodies, natural ligands of the receptor and anti-receptor antibodies.

- Using agents which mimic the cellular receptor and bind to the VAP. This includes anti-VAP antibodies, receptor anti-idiotypic antibodies, extraneous receptor and synthetic receptor mimics.

This strategy of designing drugs can be very expensive, and since the process of generating anti-idiotypic antibodies is partly trial and error, it can be a relatively slow process until an adequate molecule is produced.

Entry Inhibitor

A very early stage of viral infection is viral entry, when the virus attaches to and enters the host cell. A number of "entry-inhibiting" or "entry-blocking" drugs are being developed to fight HIV. HIV most heavily targets the immune system's white blood cells known as "helper T cells", and identifies these target cells through T-cell surface receptors designated "CD4" and "CCR5". Attempts to interfere with the binding of HIV with the CD4 receptor have failed to stop HIV from infecting helper T cells, but research continues on trying to interfere with the binding of HIV to the CCR5 receptor in hopes that it will be more effective.

HIV infects a cell through fusion with the cell membrane, which requires two different cellular molecular participants, CD4 and a chemokine receptor (differing depending on the cell type). Approaches to blocking this virus/cell fusion have shown some promise in preventing entry of the virus into a cell. At least one of these entry inhibitors—a biomimetic peptide called Enfuvirtide, or the brand name Fuzeon—has received FDA approval and has been in use for some time. Potentially, one of the benefits from the use of an effective entry-blocking or entry-inhibiting agent is that it potentially may not only prevent the spread of the virus within an infected individual but also the spread from an infected to an uninfected individual.

One possible advantage of the therapeutic approach of blocking viral entry (as opposed to the currently dominant approach of viral enzyme inhibition) is that it may prove more difficult for the virus to develop resistance to this therapy than for the virus to mutate or evolve its enzymatic protocols.

Uncoating Inhibitor

Inhibitors of uncoating have also been investigated. Amantadine and rimantadine have been introduced to combat influenza. These agents act on penetration and uncoating.

Pleconaril works against rhinoviruses, which cause the common cold, by blocking a pocket on the surface of the virus that controls the uncoating process. This pocket is similar in most strains of rhinoviruses and enteroviruses, which can cause diarrhea, meningitis, conjunctivitis, and encephalitis.

Some scientists are making the case that a vaccine against rhinoviruses, the predominant cause of the common cold, is achievable. Vaccines that combine dozens of varieties of rhinovirus at once are effective in stimulating antiviral antibodies in mice and monkeys, researchers have reported in Nature Communications in 2016.

Rhinoviruses are the most common cause of the common cold; other viruses such as respiratory syncytial virus, parainfluenza virus and adenoviruses can cause them too. Rhinoviruses also exacerbate asthma attacks. Although rhinoviruses come in many varieties, they do not drift to the same degree that influenza viruses do. A mixture of 50 inactivated rhinovirus types should be able to stimulate neutralizing antibodies against all of them to some degree.

During Viral Synthesis

A second approach is to target the processes that synthesize virus components after a virus invades a cell.

Reverse Transcription

One way of doing this is to develop nucleotide or nucleoside analogues that look like the building blocks of RNA or DNA, but deactivate the enzymes that synthesize the RNA or DNA once the analogue is incorporated. This approach is more commonly associated with the inhibition of reverse transcriptase (RNA to DNA) than with "normal" transcriptase (DNA to RNA).

The first successful antiviral, aciclovir, is a nucleoside analogue, and is effective against herpesvirus infections. The first antiviral drug to be approved for treating HIV, zidovudine (AZT), is also a nucleoside analogue.

An improved knowledge of the action of reverse transcriptase has led to better nucleoside analogues to treat HIV infections. One of these drugs, lamivudine, has been approved to treat hepatitis B, which uses reverse transcriptase as part of its replication process. Researchers have gone further and developed inhibitors that do not look like nucleosides, but can still block reverse transcriptase.

Another target being considered for HIV antivirals include RNase H – which is a component of reverse transcriptase that splits the synthesized DNA from the original viral RNA.

Integrase

Another target is integrase, which integrate the synthesized DNA into the host cell genome.

Transcription

Once a virus genome becomes operational in a host cell, it then generates messenger RNA (mRNA) molecules that direct the synthesis of viral proteins. Production of mRNA is initiated by proteins known as transcription factors. Several antivirals are now being designed to block attachment of transcription factors to viral DNA.

Translation/Antisense

Genomics has not only helped find targets for many antivirals, it has provided the basis for an entirely new type of drug, based on "antisense" molecules. These are segments of DNA or RNA that are designed as complementary molecule to critical sections of viral genomes, and the binding of these antisense segments to these target sections blocks the operation of those genomes. A phosphorothioate antisense drug named fomivirsen has been introduced, used to treat opportunistic eye infections in AIDS patients caused by cytomegalovirus, and other antisense antivirals are in development. An antisense structural type that has proven especially valuable in research is morpholino antisense.

Morpholino oligos have been used to experimentally suppress many viral types:

- Caliciviruses

- Flaviviruses (including WNV)

- Dengue

- HCV

- Coronaviruses

Translation/Ribozymes

Yet another antiviral technique inspired by genomics is a set of drugs based on ribozymes, which are enzymes that will cut apart viral RNA or DNA at selected sites. In their natural course, ribozymes are used as part of the viral manufacturing sequence, but these synthetic ribozymes are designed to cut RNA and DNA at sites that will disable them.

A ribozyme antiviral to deal with hepatitis C has been suggested, and ribozyme antivirals are being developed to deal with HIV. An interesting variation of this idea is the use of genetically modified cells that can produce custom-tailored ribozymes. This is part of a broader effort to create genetically modified cells that can be injected into a host to attack pathogens by generating specialized proteins that block viral replication at various phases of the viral life cycle.

Protein Processing and Targeting

Interference with post translational modifications or with targeting of viral proteins in the cell is also possible.

Protease Inhibitors

Some viruses include an enzyme known as a protease that cuts viral protein chains apart so they can be assembled into their final configuration. HIV includes a protease, and so considerable research has been performed to find "protease inhibitors" to attack HIV at that phase of its life cycle. Protease inhibitors became available in the 1990s and have proven effective, though they can have unusual side effects, for example causing fat to build up in unusual places. Improved protease inhibitors are now in development.

Protease inhibitors have also been seen in nature. A protease inhibitor was isolated from the Shiitake mushroom (*Lentinus edodes*). The presence of this may explain the Shiitake mushroom's noted antiviral activity *in vitro*.

Assembly

Rifampicin acts at the assembly phase.

Release Phase

The final stage in the life cycle of a virus is the release of completed viruses from the host cell, and this step has also been targeted by antiviral drug developers. Two drugs named zanamivir (Relenza) and oseltamivir (Tamiflu) that have been recently introduced to treat influenza prevent the release of viral particles by blocking a molecule named neuraminidase that is found on the surface of flu viruses, and also seems to be constant across a wide range of flu strains.

Immune System Stimulation

A second category of tactics for fighting viruses involves encouraging the body's immune system to attack them, rather than attacking them directly. Some antivirals of this sort do not focus on a specific pathogen, instead stimulating the immune system to attack a range of pathogens.

One of the best-known of this class of drugs are interferons, which inhibit viral synthesis in infected cells. One form of human interferon named "interferon alpha" is well-established as part of the standard treatment for hepatitis B and C, and other interferons are also being investigated as treatments for various diseases.

A more specific approach is to synthesize antibodies, protein molecules that can bind to a pathogen and mark it for attack by other elements of the immune system. Once researchers identify a particular target on the pathogen, they can synthesize quantities of identical "monoclonal" antibodies to link up that target. A monoclonal drug is now being sold to help fight respiratory syncytial virus in babies, and antibodies purified from infected individuals are also used as a treatment for hepatitis B.

Acquired Resistance

Antiviral resistance can be defined by a decreased susceptibility to a drug caused by changes in viral genotypes. In cases of antiviral resistance, drugs have either diminished or no effectiveness against their target virus. The issue inevitably remains a major obstacle to antiviral therapy as it has developed to almost all specific and effective antimicrobials, including antiviral agents.

The Centers for Disease Control and Prevention (CDC) inclusively recommends those six months and older to get a yearly vaccination to protect from influenza A viruses (H1N1) and (H3N2) and up to two influenza B viruses (depending on the vaccination). Comprehensive protection starts by ensuring vaccinations are current and complete. However, vaccines are preventative and are not generally used once a patient has been infected with a virus. Additionally, the availability of these vaccines can be limited based on financial or locational reasons which can prevent the effectiveness of herd immunity, making effective antivirals a necessity.

The three FDA-approved neuraminidase antiviral flu drugs available in the United States, recommended by the CDC, include: oseltamivir (Tamiflu), zanamivir (Relenza), and peramivir (Rapivab). Influenza antiviral resistance often results from changes occurring in neuraminidase and hemagglutinin proteins on the viral surface. Currently, neuraminidase inhibitors (NAIs) are the most frequently prescribed antivirals because they are effective against both influenza A and B. However, antiviral resistance is known to develop if mutations to the neuraminidase proteins prevent NAI binding. This was seen in the H257Y mutation, which was responsible for oseltamivir resistance to H1N1 strains in 2009. The inability of NA inhibitors to bind to the virus allowed this strain of virus with the resistance mutation to spread due to natural selection. Furthermore, a study published in 2009 in Nature Biotechnology emphasized the urgent need for augmentation of oseltamivir (Tamiflu) stockpiles with additional antiviral drugs including zanamivir (Relenza). This finding was based on a performance evaluation of these drugs supposing the 2009 H1N1 'Swine Flu' neuraminidase (NA) were to acquire the Tamiflu-resistance (His274Tyr) mutation which is currently widespread in seasonal H1N1 strains.

Origin of Antiviral Resistance

The genetic makeup of viruses is constantly changing, which can cause a virus to become resistant to currently available treatments. Viruses can become resistant through spontaneous or intermittent mechanisms throughout the course of an antiviral treatment. Immunocompromised patients, more often than immunocompetent patients, hospitalized with pneumonia are at the highest risk of developing oseltamivir resistance during treatment. Subsequent to exposure to someone else with the flu, those who received oseltamivir for "post-exposure prophylaxis" are also at higher risk of resistance.

The mechanisms for antiviral resistance development depend on the type of virus in question. RNA viruses such as hepatitis C and influenza A have high error rates during genome replication because RNA polymerases lack proofreading activity. RNA viruses also have small genome sizes that are typically less than 30 kb, which allow them to sustain a high frequency of mutations. DNA viruses, such as HPV and herpesvirus, hijack host cell replication machinery, which gives them proofreading capabilities during replication. DNA viruses are therefore less error prone, are generally less diverse, and are more slowly evolving than RNA viruses. In both cases, the likelihood of mutations is exacerbated by the speed with which viruses reproduce, which provides more opportunities for mutations to occur in successive replications. Billions of viruses are produced every day during the course of an infection, with each replication giving another chance for mutations that encode for resistance to occur.

Multiple strains of one virus can be present in the body at one time, and some of these strains may contain mutations that cause antibiotic resistance. This effect, called the quasispecies model, results in immense variation in any given sample of virus, and gives the opportunity for natural selection to favor viral strains with the highest fitness every time the virus is spread to a new host. Also, recombination, the joining of two different viral variants, and reassortment, the swapping of viral gene segments among viruses in the same cell, play a role in resistance, especially in influenza.

Antiviral resistance has been reported in antivirals for herpes, HIV, hepatitis B and C, and influenza, but antiviral resistance is a possibility for all viruses. Mechanisms of antiviral resistance vary between virus types.

Detection of Antiviral Resistance

National and international surveillance is performed by the CDC to determine effectiveness of the current FDA-approved antiviral flu drugs. Public health officials use this information to make current recommendations about the use of flu antiviral medications. WHO further recommends in-depth epidemiological investigations to control potential transmission of the resistant virus and prevent future progression. As novel treatments and detection techniques to antiviral resistance are enhanced so can the establishment of strategies to combat the inevitable emergence of antiviral resistance.

Treatment Options for Antiviral Resistant Pathogens

If a virus is not fully wiped out during a regimen of antivirals, treatment creates a bottleneck in the viral population that selects for resistance, and there is a chance that a resistant strain may repopulate the host. Viral treatment mechanisms must therefore account for the selection of resistant viruses.

The most commonly used method for treating resistant viruses is combination therapy, which uses multiple antivirals in one treatment regimen. This is thought to decrease the likelihood that one mutation could cause antiviral resistance, as the antivirals in the cocktail target different stages of the viral life cycle. This is frequently used in retroviruses like HIV, but a number of studies have demonstrated its effectiveness against influenza A, as well. Viruses can also be screened for resistance to drugs before treatment is started. This minimizes exposure to unnecessary antivirals and ensures that an effective medication is being used. This may improve patient outcomes and could help detect new resistance mutations during routine scanning for known mutants. However, this has not been consistently implemented in treatment facilities at this time.

Antiseptics

Antiseptics are antimicrobial substances that are applied to living tissue/skin to reduce the possibility of infection, sepsis, or putrefaction. Antiseptics are generally distinguished from *antibiotics* by the latter's ability to safely destroy bacteria within the body, and from *disinfectants*, which destroy microorganisms found on non-living objects.

Some antiseptics are true *germicides*, capable of destroying microbes (bacteriocidal), while others are bacteriostatic and only prevent or inhibit their growth.

Antibacterials include antiseptics that have the proven ability to act against bacteria. Microbicides which destroy virus particles are called viricides or antivirals. Antifungals, also known as an antimycotics, are pharmaceutical fungicides used to treat and prevent mycosis (fungal infection).

Surgery

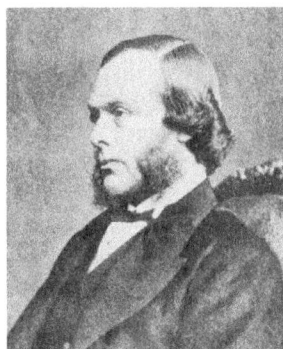
Joseph Lister.

The widespread introduction of antiseptic surgical methods was initiated by the publishing of the paper *Antiseptic Principle of the Practice of Surgery* in 1867 by Joseph Lister, which was inspired by Louis Pasteur's germ theory of putrefaction. In this paper, Lister advocated the use of carbolic acid (phenol) as a method of ensuring that any germs present were killed. Some of this work was anticipated by:

- Ancient Greek physicians Galen (*circa* 130–200) and Hippocrates (*circa* 400 BC) and Sumerian clay tablets dating from 2150 BC that advocate the use of similar techniques.

- Medieval surgeons Hugh of Lucca, Theoderic of Servia, and his pupil Henri de Mondeville were opponents of Galen's opinion that pus was important to healing, which had led ancient and medieval surgeons to let pus remain in wounds. They advocated draining and cleaning the wound edges with wine, dressing the wound after suturing, if necessary and leaving the dressing on for ten days, soaking it in warm wine all the while, before changing it. Their theories were bitterly opposed by Galenist Guy de Chauliac and others trained in the classical tradition.

- Oliver Wendell Holmes, Sr., who published *The Contagiousness of Puerperal Fever* in 1843.

- Florence Nightingale, who contributed substantially to the report of the Royal Commission on the Health of the Army (1856–1857), based on her earlier work.

- Ignaz Semmelweis, who published his work *The Cause, Concept and Prophylaxis of Childbed Fever* in 1861, summarizing experiments and observations since 1847.

Some Common Antiseptics

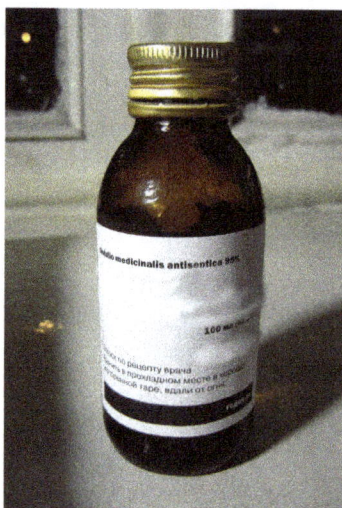

A bottle of ethanol (95%) – an antiseptic.

- Alcohols, including ethanol and 2-propanol/isopropanol are sometimes referred to as *surgical spirit*. They are used to disinfect the skin before injections are given, among other uses.

- Chlorhexidine gluconate is used as a skin antiseptic and to treat inflammation of the gums (gingivitis).

- Chloroxylenol is an antiseptic and disinfectant which is used for skin disinfection and cleaning surgical instruments. It is also used within a number of household disinfectants and wound cleaners.

- Hydrogen peroxide is used as a 6% (20 Vols) solution to clean and deodorize wounds and ulcers. More commonly, 3% solutions of hydrogen peroxide have been used in household first aid for scrapes, etc. However, the strong oxidization causes scar formation and increases healing time during fetal development.

- Iodine is usually used in an alcohol solution (called tincture of iodine) or as Lugol's iodine solution as a pre- and postoperative antiseptic. Some studies do not recommend disinfecting minor wounds with iodine because of concern that it may induce scar tissue formation and increase healing time. However, concentrations of 1% iodine or less have not been shown to increase healing time and are not otherwise distinguishable from treatment with saline. Novel iodine antiseptics containing povidone-iodine (an iodophor, complex of povidone, a water-soluble polymer, with triiodide anions I_3^-, containing about 10% of active iodine) are far better tolerated, do not negatively affect wound healing, and leave a deposit of active iodine, thereby creating the so-called "remnant", or persistent, effect. The great advantage of iodine antiseptics is their wide scope of antimicrobial activity, killing all principal pathogens and, given enough time, even spores, which are considered to be the most difficult form of microorganisms to be inactivated by disinfectants and antiseptics.

- Octenidine dihydrochloride, currently increasingly used in continental Europe, often as a chlorhexidine substitute.

- Polyhexanide (polyhexamethylene biguanide, PHMB) is an antimicrobial compound suitable for clinical use in critically colonized or infected acute and chronic wounds. The physicochemical action on the bacterial envelope prevents or impedes the development of resistant bacterial strains.

- Balsam of Peru is a mild antiseptic.

- Dakin's solution is a sodium hypochlorite solution, originally also containing boric acid to lower pH. It is mostly used on live tissues for cleaning wounds of bacteria, fungi and viruses. Because of practicality of preparation and lower cost, it is largely used in Veterinary Medicine treatments. It is colourless and does not stain the animal's fur or affect its aesthetic or commercial value.

- Super-oxidized solutions (SOS) contain hypochlorous acid (HClO) (<0.005%) and are stabilised at a neutral pH. SOS are rapidly acting (30s-5m), broad spectrum antiseptics that are clinically effective at non-cytotoxic concentrations that in contrast to many cytotoxic antiseptics, support wound healing There is now growing consensus that modern SOS are more effective for healing wounds faster.

Evolved Resistance

After continued exposure to antiseptics, bacteria may evolve to the point where they are no longer harmed by these compounds. Bacteria can also develop a resistance to antiseptics, but the effect is generally less pronounced.

The mechanisms by which bacteria evolve may vary in response to different antiseptics. Low concentrations of an antiseptic may encourage growth of a bacterial strain that is resistant to the antiseptic, where a higher concentration of the antiseptic would simply kill the bacteria. In addition, use of an excessively high concentration of an antiseptic may cause tissue damage or slow the process of wound healing. Consequently, antiseptics are most effective when used at the correct concentration—a high enough concentration to kill harmful bacteria, fungi or viruses, but a low enough concentration to avoid damage to the tissue.

Tranquilizer

Tranquilizer is also called Tranquillizer drug that is used to reduce anxiety, fear, tension, agitation, and related states of mental disturbance. Tranquilizers fall into two main classes, major and minor. Major tranquilizers, which are also known as antipsychotic agents, or neuroleptics, are so called because they are used to treat major states of mental disturbance in schizophrenics and other psychotic patients. By contrast, minor tranquilizers, which are also known as antianxiety agents, or anxiolytics, are used to treat milder states of anxiety and tension in healthy individuals or people with less serious mental disorders. The major and minor tranquilizers bear only a superficial resemblance to each other, and the trend has been to drop the use of the word tranquilizer altogether in reference to such drugs, though the term persists in popular usage.

Major tranquilizers are highly selective in alleviating the delusions, hallucinations, and disordered thinking of schizophrenics and other psychotic patients. The drugs return agitated, excited, and irrational patients to a state of rational calm, and they have enabled many seriously ill people who would otherwise be hospitalized to live at home and engage in productive work. Major tranquilizers do not cure schizophrenia but merely suppress its symptoms, and they are usually prescribed on a long-term basis. The basic types are the phenothiazines, thioxanthines, butyrophenones, clozapine, and rauwolfia alkaloids. The phenothiazines are the most widely used of these and include the drug chlorpromazine (q.v.). They are thought to work by blocking the neurotransmitter dopamine in the brain. This leads to a reduction of psychotic symptoms but can also result in such unwanted side effects as tremors of the limbs, rigidity, restlessness, and involuntary spasms of the facial muscles, tongue, and lips. The thioxanthines and the butyrophenones, chief among which is haloperidol (Haldol), are similar to the phenothiazines. Another drug, clozapine, whose exact mode of action remains unclear relieves schizophrenic symptoms in some patients who are not helped by phenothiazines. Clozapine lacks the side effects of the phenothiazines but tends to induce an infectious disease known as agranulocytosis. The rauwolfia alkaloids, such as reserpine, are no longer in common use.

The principal minor tranquilizers are the benzodiazepines, among which are diazepam(Valium), chlordiazepoxide (Librium), and alprazolam (Xanax). These drugs have a calming effect and eliminate both the physical and psychological effects of anxiety or fear. Besides the treatment of anxiety disorders, they are widely used to relieve the strain and worry arising from stressful circumstances in daily life. Because of this, benzodiazepines are among the most widely prescribed drugs in the world. Benzodiazepines work by enhancing the action of the neurotransmitter gamma-aminobutyric acid (GABA), which inhibits anxiety by reducing certain nerve-impulse transmissions within the brain. Benzodiazepines resemble barbiturates in their side effects: sleepiness, drowsiness, reduced alertness, and unsteadiness of gait. Though less dangerous than barbiturates, they can produce physical dependency even in moderate dosages, and the body develops a tolerance to them, necessitating the use of progressively larger doses. The drugs are thus intended for short- and medium-term use. Other, less commonly used minor tranquilizers include meprobamate (Equanil, Miltown) and buspirone (BuSpar).

References

- "FDA requires strong warnings for opioid analgesics, prescription opioid cough products, and benzodiazepine labeling related to serious risks and death from combined use". FDA. August 31, 2016. Retrieved 1 September 2016

- Classifications, drug-abuse: luxury.rehabs.com, Retrieved 1June, 2019

- Löscher, W.; Rogawski, M. A. (2012). "How theories evolved concerning the mechanism of action of barbiturates". Epilepsia. 53: 12–25. Doi:10.1111/epi.12025. PMID 23205959

- Drug-categories-and-their-effects: newbeginningsdrugrehab.org, Retrieved 2July, 2019

- "Bulletin on Narcotics – 1962 Issue 3 – 004". UNODC (United Nations Office of Drugs and Crime). 1962-01-01. Retrieved 2014-01-15

- Olkkola KT, Ahonen J (2008). "Midazolam and other benzodiazepines". In Schüttler J, Schwilden H (eds.). Modern Anesthetics. Handbook of Experimental Pharmacology. 182. Pp. 335–60. Doi:10.1007/978-3-540-74806-9_16. ISBN 978-3-540-72813-9. PMID 18175099

- Central-nervous-system-agents, drug-class: drugs.com, Retrieved 3 August, 2019

- Hájos, N.; Katona, I.; Naiem, S. S.; Mackie, K.; Ledent, C.; Mody, I.; Freund, T. F. (2000). "Cannabinoids inhibit hippocampal gabaergic transmission and network oscillations". European Journal of Neuroscience. 12 (9): 3239–3249. Doi:10.1046/j.1460-9568.2000.00217.x. PMID 10998107

- "Minimum Legal Age Limits". IARD.org. International Alliance for Responsible Drinking. Retrieved 23 June 2016

- Tranquilizer, science; britannica.com, Retrieved 4 January, 2019

- Gould, K (2016). "Antibiotics: From prehistory to the present day". Journal of Antimicrobial Chemotherapy. 71 (3): 572–575. Doi:10.1093/jac/dkv484. PMID 26851273

- "Funding and Guidance for State and Local Health Departments". Centers for Disease Control and Prevention. Retrieved 21 October 2016

Drug Discovery, Design and Development

- **Drug Synthesis**
- **Drug Discovery**
- **Drug Design**
- **Structure-Activity Relationships**
- **Quantitative Structure Activity Relationship**
- **Drug Development**

Drug discovery refers to the process by which new candidate medications are discovered. The inventive process of finding new medications based on the knowledge of a biological target is referred to as drug design. Drug development is the process of bringing new pharmaceutical drugs to the market. The topics elaborated in this chapter will help in gaining a better perspective about drug discovery, design and development.

Drug Synthesis

Chemical synthesis is the construction of complex chemical compounds from simpler ones. It is the process by which many substances important to daily life are obtained. It is applied to all types of chemical compounds, but most syntheses are of organic molecules.

Chemists synthesize chemical compounds that occur in nature in order to gain a better understanding of their structures. Synthesis also enables chemists to produce compounds that do not form naturally for research purposes. In industry, synthesis is used to make products in large quantity.

Chemical compounds are made up of atoms of different elements, joined together by chemical bonds. A chemical synthesis usually involves the breaking of existing bonds and the formation of new ones. Synthesis of a complex molecule may involve a considerable number of individual reactions leading in sequence from available starting materials to the desired end product. Each step usually involves reaction at only one chemical bond in the molecule.

In planning the route of chemical synthesis, chemists usually visualize the end product and work backward toward increasingly simpler compounds. For many compounds, it is possible to establish alternative synthetic routes. The ones actually used depend on many factors, such as cost and availability of starting materials, the amount of energy needed to make the reaction proceed at a satisfactory rate, and the cost of separating and purifying the end products. Moreover, knowledge of the reaction mechanism and the function of the chemical structure (or behaviour of the functional groups) helps to accurately determine the most-favoured pathway that leads to the desired reaction product.

A goal in planning a chemical synthesis is to find reactions that will affect only one part of the molecule, leaving other parts unchanged. Another goal is to produce high yields of the desired product in as short a time as possible. Often, reactions in a synthesis compete, reducing the yield of a desired product. Competition can also lead to the formation of side products which can be difficult to separate from the main one. In some industrial syntheses, by-product formation can be welcome if the by-products are commercially useful. Diethyl ether, for example, is a by-product of the large-scale synthesis of ethanol (ethyl alcohol) from ethylene. Both the alcohol and ether are valuable and can be separated easily.

The reactions involved in chemical syntheses usually, but not always, involve at least two different substances. Some molecules will change into others solely under the effect of heat, for example, while others react on exposure to radiation (e.g., ultraviolet light) or to electric current. However, where two or more different substances interact, they need to be brought into close proximity with one another. This is usually done by carrying out the syntheses with the elements or compounds in their liquid or gaseous states. Where the reactants are involatile solids, reaction is often carried out in solution.

The rate of a chemical reaction generally increases with temperature; chemical syntheses are thus often carried out at elevated temperatures. The industrial synthesis of nitric acid from ammonia and oxygen, for instance, is carried out at about 900 °C (1,650 °F). Frequently, heating will increase the rate of a reaction insufficiently or the instability of one or more reactants prevents application. In such cases catalysts—substances that speed up or slow down a reaction—are used. Most industrial processes involve the use of catalysts.

Some substances react so rapidly and violently that only careful control of the conditions will lead to the desired product. When ethylene gas is synthesized to polyethylene, one of the most common plastics, a large amount of heat is released. If this release is not controlled in some way—e.g., by cooling the reactor vessel—the ethylene molecules decompose to carbon and hydrogen.

Many techniques have been developed to separate the products of chemical synthesis. These often involve a phase change. For example, the product of a synthetic reaction may not dissolve in a particular solvent, while the starting materials do. In this case, the product will precipitate out as a solid and can be separated from the mixture by filtration. Alternatively, if both starting materials and products are volatile, it may be possible to separate them by distillation.

Certain chemical syntheses lend themselves readily to the use of automated techniques. Automatic DNA (deoxyribonucleic acid) synthesizers, for example, are widely used to produce specific protein sequences.

Drug Discovery

Historically, drugs were discovered by identifying the active ingredient from traditional remedies or by serendipitous discovery, as with penicillin. More recently, chemical libraries of synthetic small molecules, natural products or extracts were screened in intact cells or whole organisms to identify substances that had a desirable therapeutic effect in a process known as classical pharmacology. After sequencing of the human genome allowed rapid cloning and synthesis of large quantities of purified proteins, it has become common practice to use high throughput screening of large compounds libraries against isolated biological targets which are hypothesized to be disease-modifying in a process known as reverse pharmacology. Hits from these screens are then tested in cells and then in animals for efficacy.

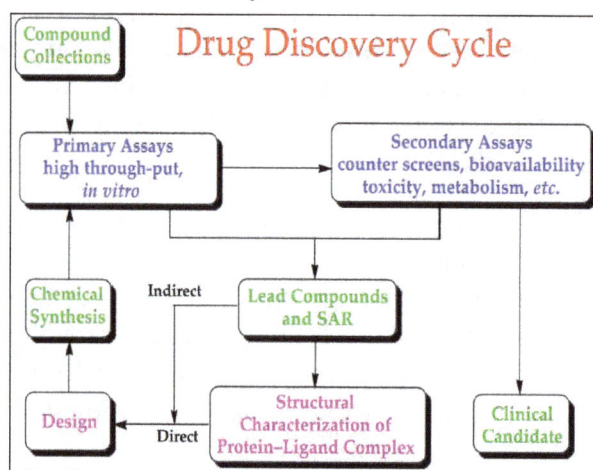

In the fields of medicine, biotechnology and pharmacology, drug discovery is the process by which new candidate medications are discovered.

Modern drug discovery involves the identification of screening hits, medicinal chemistry and optimization of those hits to increase the affinity, selectivity (to reduce the potential of side effects), efficacy/potency, metabolic stability (to increase the half-life), and oral bioavailability. Once a compound that fulfills all of these requirements has been identified, the process of drug development can continue, and, if successful, clinical trials. One or more of these steps may, but not necessarily, involve computer-aided drug design.

Modern drug discovery is thus usually a capital-intensive process that involves large investments by pharmaceutical industry corporations as well as national governments (who provide grants and loan guarantees). Despite advances in technology and understanding of biological systems, drug discovery is still a lengthy, "expensive, difficult, and inefficient process" with low rate of new therapeutic discovery. In 2010, the research and development cost of each new molecular entity was about US$1.8 billion. Currently, basic discovery research is funded primarily by governments and by philanthropic organizations, while late-stage development is funded primarily by pharmaceutical companies or venture capitalists. To be allowed to come to market, drugs must undergo several phases of clinical trials, and most drugs fail. Small companies have a critical role, often then selling the rights to larger companies that have the resources to run the clinical trials.

Discovering drugs that may be a commercial success, or a public health success, involves a complex interaction between investors, industry, academia, patent laws, regulatory exclusivity, marketing and the need to balance secrecy with communication. Meanwhile, for disorders whose rarity means that no large commercial success or public health effect can be expected, the orphan drug funding process ensures that people who experience those disorders can have some hope of pharmacotherapeutic advances.

The idea that the effect of a drug in the human body is mediated by specific interactions of the drug molecule with biological macromolecules, (proteins or nucleic acids in most cases) led scientists to the conclusion that individual chemicals are required for the biological activity of the drug. This made for the beginning of the modern era in pharmacology, as pure chemicals, instead of crude extracts of medicinal plants, became the standard drugs. Examples of drug compounds isolated from crude preparations are morphine, the active agent in opium, and digoxin, a heart stimulant originating from Digitalis lanata. Organic chemistry also led to the synthesis of many of the natural products isolated from biological sources.

Historically, substances, whether crude extracts or purified chemicals, were screened for biological activity without knowledge of the biological target. Only after an active substance was identified was an effort made to identify the target. This approach is known as classical pharmacology, forward pharmacology, or phenotypic drug discovery.

Later, small molecules were synthesized to specifically target a known physiological/pathological pathway, avoiding the mass screening of banks of stored compounds. This led to great success, such as the work of Gertrude Elion and George H. Hitchings on purine metabolism, the work of James Black on beta blockers and cimetidine, and the discovery of statins by Akira Endo. Another champion of the approach of developing chemical analogues of known active substances was Sir David Jack at Allen and Hanbury's, later Glaxo, who pioneered the first inhaled selective beta2-adrenergic agonist for asthma, the first inhaled steroid for asthma, ranitidine as a successor to cimetidine, and supported the development of the triptans.

Gertrude Elion, working mostly with a group of fewer than 50 people on purine analogues, contributed to the discovery of the first anti-viral; the first immunosuppressant (azathioprine) that allowed human organ transplantation; the first drug to induce remission of childhood leukaemia; pivotal anti-cancer treatments; an anti-malarial; an anti-bacterial; and a treatment for gout.

Cloning of human proteins made possible the screening of large libraries of compounds against specific targets thought to be linked to specific diseases. This approach is known as reverse pharmacology and is the most frequently used approach today.

Targets

The definition of "target" itself is something argued within the pharmaceutical industry. Generally, the "target" is the naturally existing cellular or molecular structure involved in the pathology of interest that the drug-in-development is meant to act on. However, the distinction between a "new" and "established" target can be made without a full understanding of just what a "target" is. This distinction is typically made by pharmaceutical companies engaged in discovery and development of therapeutics. In an estimate from 2011, 435 human genome products were identified as therapeutic drug targets of FDA-approved drugs.

"Established targets" are those for which there is a good scientific understanding, supported by a lengthy publication history, of both how the target functions in normal physiology and how it is involved in human pathology. This does not imply that the mechanism of action of drugs that are thought to act through a particular established target is fully understood. Rather, "established" relates directly to the amount of background information available on a target, in particular functional information. The more such information is available, the less investment is (generally) required to develop a therapeutic directed against the target. The process of gathering such functional information is called "target validation" in pharmaceutical industry parlance. Established targets also include those that the pharmaceutical industry has had experience mounting drug discovery campaigns against in the past; such a history provides information on the chemical feasibility of developing a small molecular therapeutic against the target and can provide licensing opportunities and freedom-to-operate indicators with respect to small-molecule therapeutic candidates.

In general, "new targets" are all those targets that are not "established targets" but which have been or are the subject of drug discovery campaigns. These typically include newly discovered proteins, or proteins whose function has now become clear as a result of basic scientific research.

The majority of targets currently selected for drug discovery efforts are proteins. Two classes predominate: G-protein-coupled receptors (or GPCRs) and protein kinases.

Screening and Design

The process of finding a new drug against a chosen target for a particular disease usually involves high-throughput screening (HTS), wherein large libraries of chemicals are tested for their ability to modify the target. For example, if the target is a novel GPCR, compounds will be screened for their ability to inhibit or stimulate that receptor: if the target is a protein kinase, the chemicals will be tested for their ability to inhibit that kinase.

Another important function of HTS is to show how selective the compounds are for the chosen target, as one wants to find a molecule which will interfere with only the chosen target, but not other, related targets. To this end, other screening runs will be made to see whether the "hits" against the chosen target will interfere with other related targets – this is the process of cross-screening. Cross-screening is important, because the more unrelated targets a compound hits, the more likely that off-target toxicity will occur with that compound once it reaches the clinic.

It is very unlikely that a perfect drug candidate will emerge from these early screening runs. One of the first steps is to screen for compounds that are unlikely to be developed into drugs; for example compounds that are hits in almost every assay, classified by medicinal chemists as "pan-assay interference compounds", are removed at this stage, if they were not already removed from the chemical library. It is often observed that several compounds are found to have some degree of activity, and if these compounds share common chemical features, one or more pharmacophores can then be developed. At this point, medicinal chemists will attempt to use structure-activity relationships (SAR) to improve certain features of the lead compound:

- Increase activity against the chosen target.

- Reduce activity against unrelated targets.

- Improve the druglikeness or ADME properties of the molecule.

This process will require several iterative screening runs, during which, it is hoped, the properties of the new molecular entities will improve, and allow the favoured compounds to go forward to in vitro and in vivo testing for activity in the disease model of choice.

Amongst the physico-chemical properties associated with drug absorption include ionization (pKa), and solubility; permeability can be determined by PAMPA and Caco-2. PAMPA is attractive as an early screen due to the low consumption of drug and the low cost compared to tests such as Caco-2, gastrointestinal tract (GIT) and Blood–brain barrier (BBB) with which there is a high correlation.

A range of parameters can be used to assess the quality of a compound, or a series of compounds, as proposed in the Lipinski's Rule of Five. Such parameters include calculated properties such as cLogP to estimate lipophilicity, molecular weight, polar surface area and measured properties, such as potency, in-vitro measurement of enzymatic clearance etc. Some descriptors such as ligand efficiency (LE) and lipophilic efficiency (LiPE) combine such parameters to assess druglikeness.

While HTS is a commonly used method for novel drug discovery, it is not the only method. It is often possible to start from a molecule which already has some of the desired properties. Such a molecule might be extracted from a natural product or even be a drug on the market which could be improved upon (so-called "me too" drugs). Other methods, such as virtual high throughput screening, where screening is done using computer-generated models and attempting to "dock" virtual libraries to a target, are also often used.

Another important method for drug discovery is *de novo* drug design, in which a prediction is made of the sorts of chemicals that might (e.g.) fit into an active site of the target enzyme. For example, virtual screening and computer-aided drug design are often used to identify new chemical moieties that may interact with a target protein. Molecular modelling and molecular dynamics simulations can be used as a guide to improve the potency and properties of new drug leads.

There is also a paradigm shift in the drug discovery community to shift away from HTS, which is expensive and may only cover limited chemical space, to the screening of smaller libraries (maximum a few thousand compounds). These include fragment-based lead discovery (FBDD) and protein-directed dynamic combinatorial chemistry. The ligands in these approaches are usually much smaller, and they bind to the target protein with weaker binding affinity than those hits that are identified from HTS. Further modified through organic synthesis into lead compounds are often required. Such modifications are often guided by protein X-ray crystallography of the protein-fragment complex. The advantages of these approaches are that they allow more efficient screening and the compound library, although small, typically covers a large chemical space when compared to HTS.

Phenotypic screens have also provided new chemical starting points in drug discovery. A variety of models have been used including yeast, zebrafish, worms, immortalized cell lines, primary cell lines, patient-derived cell lines and whole animal models. These screens are designed to find compounds which reverse a disease phenotype such as death, protein aggregation, mutant protein expression, or cell proliferation as examples in a more holistic cell model or organism. Smaller screening sets are often used for these screens, especially when the models are expensive or time-consuming to run. In many cases, the exact mechanism of action of hits from these screens is unknown and may require extensive target deconvolution experiments to ascertain.

Once a lead compound series has been established with sufficient target potency and selectivity and favourable drug-like properties, one or two compounds will then be proposed for drug development. The best of these is generally called the lead compound, while the other will be designated as the "backup".

Traditionally many drugs and other chemicals with biological activity have been discovered by studying allelopathy – chemicals that organisms create that affect the activity of other organisms in the fight for survival.

Despite the rise of combinatorial chemistry as an integral part of lead discovery process, natural products still play a major role as starting material for drug discovery. A 2007 report found that of the 974 small molecule new chemical entities developed between 1981 and 2006, 63% were natural derived or semisynthetic derivatives of natural products. For certain therapy areas, such as antimicrobials, antineoplastics, antihypertensive and anti-inflammatory drugs, the numbers were higher. In many cases, these products have been used traditionally for many years.

Natural products may be useful as a source of novel chemical structures for modern techniques of development of antibacterial therapies. Despite the implied potential, only a fraction of Earth's living species has been tested for bioactivity.

Plant-derived

Many secondary metabolites produced by plants have potential therapeutic medicinal properties. These secondary metabolites contain bind to and modify the function of proteins (receptors, enzymes, etc.). Consequently, plant derived natural products have often been used as the starting point for drug discovery.

Until the Renaissance, the vast majority of drugs in Western medicine were plant-derived extracts. This has resulted in a pool of information about the potential of plant species as important sources of starting materials for drug discovery. Botanical knowledge about different metabolites and hormones that are produced in different anatomical parts of the plant (e.g. roots, leaves, and flowers) are crucial for correctly identifying bioactive and pharmacological plant properties. Identifying new drugs and getting them approved for market has proved to be a stringent process due to regulations set by national drug regulatory agencies.

Jasmonates

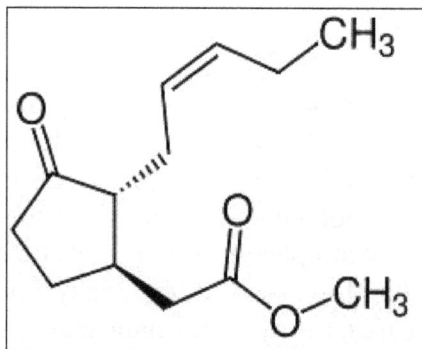

Chemical structure of methyl jasmonate (JA).

Jasmonates are important in responses to injury and intracellular signals. They induce apoptosis and protein cascade via proteinase inhibitor, have defense functions, and regulate plant responses to different biotic and abiotic stresses. Jasmonates also have the ability to directly act on mitochondrial membranes by inducing membrane depolarization via release of metabolites.

Jasmonate derivatives (JAD) are also important in wound response and tissue regeneration in plant cells. They have also been identified to have anti-aging effects on human epidermal layer. It is suspected that interact with proteoglycans (PG) and glycosaminoglycan (GAG) polysaccharides, which are essential extracellular matrix (ECM) components to help remodel the ECM. The discovery of JADs on skin repair has introduced newfound interest in the effects of these plant hormones in therapeutic medicinal application.

Salicylates

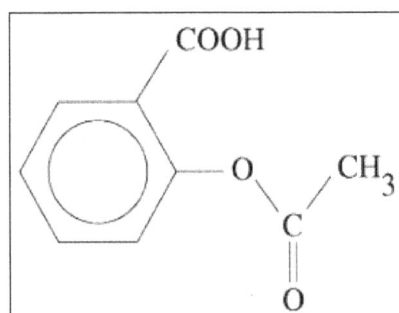

Chemical structure of acetylsalicylic acid, more commonly known as Aspirin.

Salicylic acid (SA), a phytohormone, was initially derived from willow bark and has since been identified in many species. It is an important player in plant immunity, although its role is still not fully understood by scientists. They are involved in disease and immunity responses in plant and animal tissues. They have salicylic acid binding proteins (SABPs) that have shown to affect multiple animal tissues. The first discovered medicinal properties of the isolated compound was involved in pain and fever management. They also play an active role in the suppression of cell proliferation. They have the ability to induce death in lymphoblastic leukemia and other human cancer cells. One of the most common drugs derived from salicylates is aspirin, also known as acetylsalicylic acid, with anti-inflammatory and anti-pyretic properties.

Microbial Metabolites

Microbes compete for living space and nutrients. To survive in these conditions, many microbes have developed abilities to prevent competing species from proliferating. Microbes are the main source of antimicrobial drugs. Streptomyces isolates have been such a valuable source of antibiotics, that they have been called medicinal molds. The classic example of an antibiotic discovered as a defense mechanism against another microbe is penicillin in bacterial cultures contaminated by *Penicillium* fungi in 1928.

Marine Invertebrates

Marine environments are potential sources for new bioactive agents. Arabinose nucleosides discovered from marine invertebrates in 1950s, demonstrated for the first time that sugar moieties other than ribose and deoxyribose can yield bioactive nucleoside structures. It took until 2004 when the first marine-derived drug was approved. For example, the cone snail toxin ziconotide, also known as Prialt treats severe neuropathic pain. Several other marine-derived agents are now in clinical trials for indications such as cancer, anti-inflammatory use and pain. One class of these agents are bryostatin-like compounds, under investigation as anti-cancer therapy.

Chemical Diversity

Combinatorial chemistry was a key technology enabling the efficient generation of large screening libraries for the needs of high-throughput screening. However, now, after two decades of combinatorial chemistry, it has been pointed out that despite the increased efficiency in chemical synthesis, no increase in lead or drug candidates has been reached. This has led to analysis of chemical characteristics of combinatorial chemistry products, compared to existing drugs or natural products. The chemoinformatics concept chemical diversity, depicted as distribution of compounds in the chemical space based on their physicochemical characteristics, is often used to describe the difference between the combinatorial chemistry libraries and natural products. The synthetic, combinatorial library compounds seem to cover only a limited and quite uniform chemical space, whereas existing drugs and particularly natural products, exhibit much greater chemical diversity, distributing more evenly to the chemical space. The most prominent differences between natural products and compounds in combinatorial chemistry libraries is the number of chiral centers (much higher in natural compounds), structure rigidity (higher in natural compounds) and number of aromatic moieties (higher in combinatorial chemistry libraries). Other chemical differences between these two groups include the nature of heteroatoms (O and N enriched in natural products, and S and halogen atoms more often present in synthetic compounds), as well as level of non-aromatic unsaturation (higher in natural products). As both structure rigidity and chirality are well-established factors in medicinal chemistry known to enhance compounds specificity and efficacy as a drug, it has been suggested that natural products compare favourably to today's combinatorial chemistry libraries as potential lead molecules.

Screening

Two main approaches exist for the finding of new bioactive chemical entities from natural sources.

The first is sometimes referred to as random collection and screening of material, but the collection is far from random. Biological (often botanical) knowledge is often used to identify families that show promise. This approach is effective because only a small part of earth's biodiversity has ever been tested for pharmaceutical activity. Also, organisms living in a species-rich environment need to evolve defensive and competitive mechanisms to survive. Those mechanisms might be exploited in the development of beneficial drugs.

A collection of plant, animal and microbial samples from rich ecosystems can potentially give rise to novel biological activities worth exploiting in the drug development process. One example of a successful use of this strategy is the screening for antitumour agents by the National Cancer Institute, started in the 1960s. Paclitaxel was identified from Pacific yew tree *Taxus brevifolia*. Paclitaxel showed anti-tumour activity by a previously undescribed mechanism (stabilization of microtubules) and is now approved for clinical use for the treatment of lung, breast and ovarian cancer, as well as for Kaposi's sarcoma. Early in the 21st century, Cabazitaxel (made by Sanofi, a

French firm), another relative of taxol has been shown effective against prostate cancer, also because it works by preventing the formation of microtubules, which pull the chromosomes apart in dividing cells (such as cancer cells). Other examples are: 1. Camptotheca (Camptothecin · Topotecan · Irinotecan · Rubitecan · Belotecan); 2. Podophyllum (Etoposide · Teniposide); 3a. Anthracyclines (Aclarubicin · Daunorubicin · Doxorubicin · Epirubicin · Idarubicin · Amrubicin · Pirarubicin · Valrubicin · Zorubicin); 3b. Anthracenediones (Mitoxantrone · Pixantrone).

The second main approach involves ethnobotany, the study of the general use of plants in society, and ethnopharmacology, an area inside ethnobotany, which is focused specifically on medicinal uses.

Artemisinin, an antimalarial agent from sweet wormtree *Artemisia annua*, used in Chinese medicine since 200BC is one drug used as part of combination therapy for multiresistant *Plasmodium falciparum*.

Structural Elucidation

The elucidation of the chemical structure is critical to avoid the re-discovery of a chemical agent that is already known for its structure and chemical activity. Mass spectrometry is a method in which individual compounds are identified based on their mass/charge ratio, after ionization. Chemical compounds exist in nature as mixtures, so the combination of liquid chromatography and mass spectrometry (LC-MS) is often used to separate the individual chemicals. Databases of mass spectras for known compounds are available, and can be used to assign a structure to an unknown mass spectrum. Nuclear magnetic resonance spectroscopy is the primary technique for determining chemical structures of natural products. NMR yields information about individual hydrogen and carbon atoms in the structure, allowing detailed reconstruction of the molecule's architecture.

Drug Design

Drug design, often referred to as rational drug design or simply rational design, is the inventive process of finding new medications based on the knowledge of a biological target. The drug is most commonly an organic small molecule that activates or inhibits the function of a biomolecule such as a protein, which in turn results in a therapeutic benefit to the patient. In the most basic sense, drug design involves the design of molecules that are complementary in shape and charge to the biomolecular target with which they interact and therefore will bind to it. Drug design frequently but not necessarily relies on computer modeling techniques. This type of modeling is sometimes referred to as computer-aided drug design. Finally, drug design that relies on the knowledge of the three-dimensional structure of the biomolecular target is known as structure-based drug design. In addition to small molecules, biopharmaceuticals including peptides and especially therapeutic antibodies are an increasingly important class of drugs and computational methods for improving the affinity, selectivity, and stability of these protein-based therapeutics have also been developed.

The phrase "drug design" is to some extent a misnomer. A more accurate term is ligand design (i.e., design of a molecule that will bind tightly to its target). Although design techniques for prediction of binding affinity are reasonably successful, there are many other properties, such as bioavailability, metabolic half-life, side effects, etc., that first must be optimized before a ligand can become a safe and efficacious drug. These other characteristics are often difficult to predict with rational design techniques. Nevertheless, due to high attrition rates, especially during clinical phases of drug development, more attention is being focused early in the drug design process on selecting candidate drugs whose physicochemical properties are predicted to result in fewer complications during development and hence more likely to lead to an approved, marketed drug. Furthermore, in vitro experiments complemented with computation methods are increasingly used in early drug discovery to select compounds with more favorable ADME (absorption, distribution, metabolism, and excretion) and toxicological profiles.

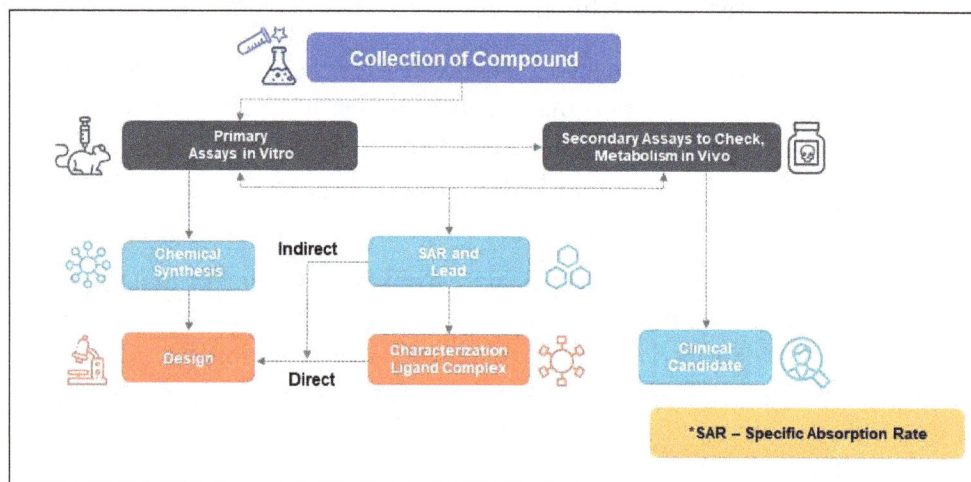

Drug Targets

A biomolecular target (most commonly a protein or nucleic acid) is a key molecule involved in a particular metabolic or signaling pathway that is associated with a specific disease condition or pathology or to the infectivity or survival of a microbial pathogen. Potential drug targets are not necessarily disease causing but must by definition be disease modifying. In some cases, small molecules will be designed to enhance or inhibit the target function in the specific disease modifying pathway. Small molecules (for example receptor agonists, antagonists, inverse agonists, or modulators; enzyme activators or inhibitors; or ion channel openers or blockers) will be designed that are complementary to the binding site of target. Small molecules (drugs) can be designed so as not to affect any other important "off-target" molecules (often referred to as antitargets) since drug interactions with off-target molecules may lead to undesirable side effects. Due to similarities in binding sites, closely related targets identified through sequence homology have the highest chance of cross reactivity and hence highest side effect potential.

Most commonly, drugs are organic small molecules produced through chemical synthesis, but biopolymer-based drugs (also known as biopharmaceuticals) produced through biological processes are becoming increasingly more common. In addition, mRNA-based gene silencing technologies may have therapeutic applications.

Rational Drug Discovery

In contrast to traditional methods of drug discovery (known as forward pharmacology), which rely on trial-and-error testing of chemical substances on cultured cells or animals, and matching the apparent effects to treatments, rational drug design (also called reverse pharmacology) begins with a hypothesis that modulation of a specific biological target may have therapeutic value. In order for a biomolecule to be selected as a drug target, two essential pieces of information are required. The first is evidence that modulation of the target will be disease modifying. This knowledge may come from, for example, disease linkage studies that show an association between mutations in the biological target and certain disease states. The second is that the target is "druggable". This means that it is capable of binding to a small molecule and that its activity can be modulated by the small molecule.

Once a suitable target has been identified, the target is normally cloned and produced and purified. The purified protein is then used to establish a screening assay. In addition, the three-dimensional structure of the target may be determined.

The search for small molecules that bind to the target is begun by screening libraries of potential drug compounds. This may be done by using the screening assay (a "wet screen"). In addition, if the structure of the target is available, a virtual screen may be performed of candidate drugs. Ideally the candidate drug compounds should be "drug-like", that is they should possess properties that are predicted to lead to oral bioavailability, adequate chemical and metabolic stability, and minimal toxic effects. Several methods are available to estimate druglikeness such as Lipinski's Rule of Five and a range of scoring methods such as lipophilic efficiency. Several methods for predicting drug metabolism have also been proposed in the scientific literature.

Due to the large number of drug properties that must be simultaneously optimized during the design process, multi-objective optimization techniques are sometimes employed. Finally because of the limitations in the current methods for prediction of activity, drug design is still very much reliant on serendipity and bounded rationality.

Computer-aided Drug Design

The most fundamental goal in drug design is to predict whether a given molecule will bind to a target and if so how strongly. Molecular mechanics or molecular dynamics is most often used to estimate the strength of the intermolecular interaction between the small molecule and its biological target. These methods are also used to predict the conformation of the small molecule and to model conformational changes in the target that may occur when the small molecule binds to it. Semi-empirical, ab initio quantum chemistry methods, or density functional theory are often used to provide optimized parameters for the molecular mechanics calculations and also provide an estimate of the electronic properties (electrostatic potential, polarizability, etc.) of the drug candidate that will influence binding affinity.

Molecular mechanics methods may also be used to provide semi-quantitative prediction of the binding affinity. Also, knowledge-based scoring function may be used to provide binding affinity estimates. These methods use linear regression, machine learning, neural nets or other statistical techniques to derive predictive binding affinity equations by fitting experimental affinities to computationally derived interaction energies between the small molecule and the target.

Ideally, the computational method will be able to predict affinity before a compound is synthesized and hence in theory only one compound needs to be synthesized, saving enormous time and cost. The reality is that present computational methods are imperfect and provide, at best, only qualitatively accurate estimates of affinity. In practice it still takes several iterations of design, synthesis, and testing before an optimal drug is discovered. Computational methods have accelerated discovery by reducing the number of iterations required and have often provided novel structures.

Drug design with the help of computers may be used at any of the following stages of drug discovery:

- Hit identification using virtual screening (structure- or ligand-based design)

- Hit-to-lead optimization of affinity and selectivity (structure-based design, QSAR, etc.)

- Lead optimization of other pharmaceutical properties while maintaining affinity

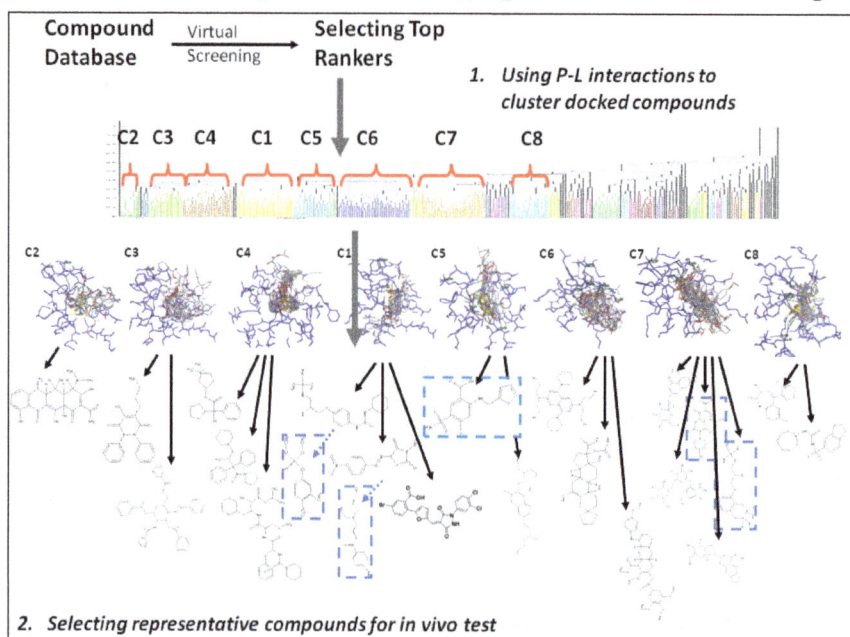

Flowchart of a Usual Clustering Analysis for Structure-Based Drug Design

In order to overcome the insufficient prediction of binding affinity calculated by recent scoring functions, the protein-ligand interaction and compound 3D structure information are used for analysis. For structure-based drug design, several post-screening analyses focusing on protein-ligand interaction have been developed for improving enrichment and effectively mining potential candidates:

- Consensus scoring:

  ○ Selecting candidates by voting of multiple scoring functions.

  ○ May lose the relationship between protein-ligand structural information and scoring criterion.

- Cluster analysis:

  ○ Represent and cluster candidates according to protein-ligand 3D information.

  ○ Needs meaningful representation of protein-ligand interactions.

Types

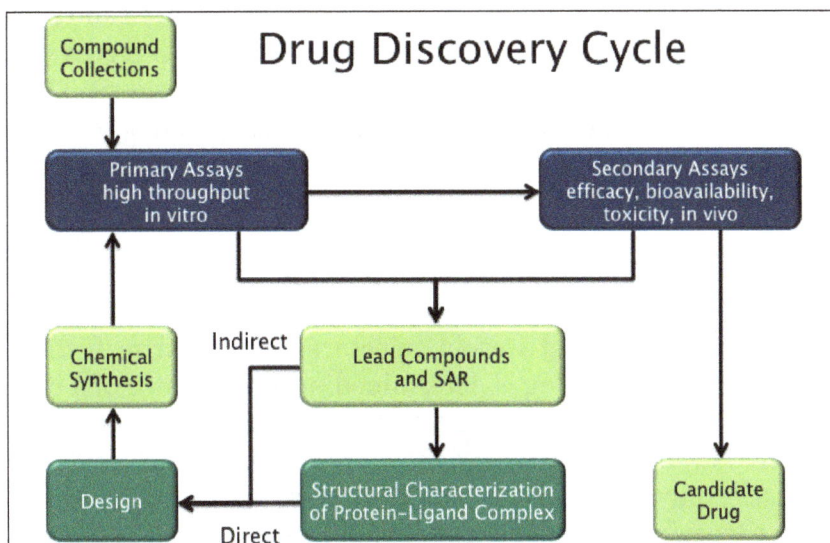

Drug discovery cycle highlighting both ligand-based (indirect) and structure-based (direct) drug design strategies.

There are two major types of drug design. The first is referred to as ligand-based drug design and the second, structure-based drug design.

Ligand-based

Ligand-based drug design (or indirect drug design) relies on knowledge of other molecules that bind to the biological target of interest. These other molecules may be used to derive a pharmacophore model that defines the minimum necessary structural characteristics a molecule must possess in order to bind to the target. In other words, a model of the biological target may be built based on the knowledge of what binds to it, and this model in turn may be used to design new molecular entities that interact with the target. Alternatively, a quantitative structure-activity relationship (QSAR), in which a correlation between calculated properties of molecules and their experimentally determined biological activity, may be derived. These QSAR relationships in turn may be used to predict the activity of new analogs.

Structure-based

Structure-based drug design (or direct drug design) relies on knowledge of the three dimensional structure of the biological target obtained through methods such as x-ray crystallography or NMR spectroscopy. If an experimental structure of a target is not available, it may be possible to create a homology model of the target based on the experimental structure of a related protein. Using the structure of the biological target, candidate drugs that are predicted to bind with high affinity and selectivity to the target may be designed using interactive graphics and the intuition of a medicinal chemist. Alternatively various automated computational procedures may be used to suggest new drug candidates.

Current methods for structure-based drug design can be divided roughly into three main categories. The first method is identification of new ligands for a given receptor by searching large databases of 3D structures of small molecules to find those fitting the binding pocket of the receptor using fast approximate docking programs. This method is known as virtual screening. A second category is de novo design of new ligands. In this method, ligand molecules are built up within the constraints of the binding pocket by assembling small pieces in a stepwise manner. These pieces can be either individual atoms or molecular fragments. The key advantage of such a method is that novel structures, not contained in any database, can be suggested. A third method is the optimization of known ligands by evaluating proposed analogs within the binding cavity.

Binding Site Identification

Binding site identification is the first step in structure based design. If the structure of the target or a sufficiently similar homolog is determined in the presence of a bound ligand, then the ligand should be observable in the structure in which case location of the binding site is trivial. However, there may be unoccupied allosteric binding sites that may be of interest. Furthermore, it may be that only apoprotein (protein without ligand) structures are available and the reliable identification of unoccupied sites that have the potential to bind ligands with high affinity is non-trivial. In brief, binding site identification usually relies on identification of concave surfaces on the protein that can accommodate drug sized molecules that also possess appropriate "hot spots" (hydrophobic surfaces, hydrogen bonding sites, etc.) that drive ligand binding.

Scoring Functions

Structure-based drug design attempts to use the structure of proteins as a basis for designing new ligands by applying the principles of molecular recognition. Selective high affinity binding to the target is generally desirable since it leads to more efficacious drugs with fewer side effects. Thus, one of the most important principles for designing or obtaining potential new ligands is to predict the binding affinity of a certain ligand to its target (and known antitargets) and use the predicted affinity as a criterion for selection.

One early general-purposed empirical scoring function to describe the binding energy of ligands to receptors was developed by Böhm. This empirical scoring function took the form:

$$\Delta G_{bind} = \Delta G_0 + \Delta G_{hb} \sum_{h-bonds} + \Delta G_{ionic-int} + \Delta G_{lipophilic} |A| + \Delta G_{rot} NROT$$

where:

- ΔG_0 – empirically derived offset that in part corresponds to the overall loss of translational and rotational entropy of the ligand upon binding.

- ΔG_{hb} – contribution from hydrogen bonding.

- ΔG_{ionic} – contribution from ionic interactions.

- ΔG_{lip} – contribution from lipophilic interactions where $|A_{lipo}|$ is surface area of lipophilic contact between the ligand and receptor.

- ΔG_{rot} – entropy penalty due to freezing a rotatable in the ligand bond upon binding.

A more general thermodynamic "master" equation is as follows:

$$\Delta G_{bind} = -RT \; In \; K_d$$

$$K_d = \frac{[Ligand][Receptor]}{[Complex]}$$

$$\Delta G_{bind} = \Delta G_{desolvation} + \Delta G_{motion} + \Delta G_{configuration} + \Delta G_{interaction}$$

where:

- Desolvation – enthalpic penalty for removing the ligand from solvent.

- Motion – entropic penalty for reducing the degrees of freedom when a ligand binds to its receptor.

- Configuration – conformational strain energy required to put the ligand in its "active" conformation.

- Interaction – enthalpic gain for "resolvating" the ligand with its receptor.

The basic idea is that the overall binding free energy can be decomposed into independent components that are known to be important for the binding process. Each component reflects a certain kind of free energy alteration during the binding process between a ligand and its target receptor. The Master Equation is the linear combination of these components. According to Gibbs free energy equation, the relation between dissociation equilibrium constant, K_d, and the components of free energy was built.

Various computational methods are used to estimate each of the components of the master equation. For example, the change in polar surface area upon ligand binding can be used to estimate the desolvation energy. The number of rotatable bonds frozen upon ligand binding is proportional to the motion term. The configurational or strain energy can be estimated using molecular mechanics calculations. Finally the interaction energy can be estimated using methods such as the change in non polar surface, statistically derived potentials of mean force, the number of hydrogen bonds formed, etc. In practice, the components of the master equation are fit to experimental data using multiple linear regression. This can be done with a diverse training set including many types of ligands and receptors to produce a less accurate but more general "global" model or a more restricted set of ligands and receptors to produce a more accurate but less general "local" model.

Examples:

A particular example of rational drug design involves the use of three-dimensional information about biomolecules obtained from such techniques as X-ray crystallography and NMR spectroscopy. Computer-aided drug design in particular becomes much more tractable when there is a high-resolution structure of a target protein bound to a potent ligand. This approach to drug discovery is sometimes referred to as structure-based drug design. The first unequivocal example of the application of structure-based drug design leading to an approved drug is the carbonic anhydrase inhibitor dorzolamide, which was approved in 1995.

Another important case study in rational drug design is imatinib, a tyrosine kinase inhibitor designed specifically for the *bcr-abl* fusion protein that is characteristic for Philadelphia chromosome-positive leukemias (chronic myelogenous leukemia and occasionally acute lymphocytic leukemia). Imatinib is substantially different from previous drugs for cancer, as most agents of chemotherapy simply target rapidly dividing cells, not differentiating between cancer cells and other tissues.

Additional examples include:

- Many of the atypical antipsychotics.

- Cimetidine, the prototypical H$_2$-receptor antagonist from which the later members of the class were developed.

Druglikeness

Druglikeness is a qualitative concept used in drug design for how "druglike" a substance is with respect to factors like bioavailability. It is estimated from the molecular structure before the substance is even synthesized and tested. A druglike molecule has properties such as:

- Solubility in both water and fat, as an orally administered drug needs to pass through the intestinal lining after it is consumed, be carried in aqueous blood and penetrate the lipid-based cell membrane to reach the inside of a cell. A model compound for the lipophilic cellular membrane is 1-octanol (a lipophilic hydrocarbon), so the logarithm of the octanol/water partition coefficient, known as LogP, is used to predict the solubility of a potential oral drug. This coefficient can be experimentally measured or predicted computationally, in which case it is sometimes called "cLogP".

- Potency at the biological target. High potency (high value of pIC$_{50}$) is a desirable attribute in drug candidates, as it reduces the risk of non-specific, off-target pharmacology at a given concentration. When associated with low clearance, high potency also allows for low total dose, which lowers the risk of idiosyncratic drug reactions.

- Ligand efficiency and lipophilic efficiency.

- Molecular weight: The smaller the better, because diffusion is directly affected. The great majority of drugs on the market have molecular weights between 200 and 600 Daltons, and particularly <500; they belong to the group of small molecules.

A traditional method to evaluate druglikeness is to check compliance of Lipinski's Rule of Five, which covers the numbers of hydrophilic groups, molecular weight and hydrophobicity.

Since the drug is transported in aqueous media like blood and intracellular fluid, it has to be sufficiently water-soluble in the absolute sense (i.e. must have a minimum chemical solubility in order to be effective). Solubility in water can be estimated from the number of hydrogen bond donors vs. alkyl sidechains in the molecule. Low water solubility translates to slow absorption and action. Too many hydrogen bond donors, on the other hand, lead to low fat solubility, so that the drug cannot penetrate the cell membrane to reach the inside of the cell.

Based on one definition, a drug-like molecule has a logarithm of partition coefficient (log P) between -0.4 and 5.6, molecular weight 160-480 g/mol, molar refractivity of 40-130, which is related to the volume and molecular weight of the molecule and has 20-70 atoms.

Substructures with known toxic, mutagenic or teratogenic properties affect the usefulness of a designed molecule. However, several poisons have a good druglikeness. Natural toxins are used in pharmacological research to find out their mechanism of action, and if it could be exploited for beneficial purposes. Alkylnitro compounds tend to be irritants, and Michael acceptors, such as enones, are alkylating agents and thus potentially mutagenic and carcinogenic.

Druglikeness indices are inherently limited tools. Druglikeness can be estimated for any molecule, and does not evaluate the actual specific effect that the drug achieves (biological activity). Simple rules are not always accurate and may unnecessarily limit the chemical space to search: many best-selling drugs have features that cause them to score low on various druglikeness indices. Furthermore, first-pass metabolism, which is biochemically selective, can destroy the pharmacological activity of a compound despite good druglikeness.

Druglikeness is not relevant for most biologics, since they are usually proteins that need to be injected, because proteins are digested if eaten.

Structure-Activity Relationships

The structure–activity relationship (SAR) is the relationship between the chemical structure of a molecule and its biological activity. This idea was first presented by Crum-Brown and Fraser in 1865. The analysis of SAR enables the determination of the chemical group responsible for evoking a target biological effect in the organism. This allows modification of the effect or the potency of a bioactive compound (typically a drug) by changing its chemical structure. Medicinal chemists use the techniques of chemical synthesis to insert new chemical groups into the biomedical compound and test the modifications for their biological effects.

This method was refined to build mathematical relationships between the chemical structure and the biological activity, known as quantitative structure–activity relationships (QSAR). A related term is structure affinity relationship (SAFIR).

Structure-biodegradability Relationship

The large number of synthetic organic chemicals currently in production presents a huge challenge for timely collection of detailed environmental data on each compound. The concept of structure biodegradability relationships (SBR) has been applied to explain variability in persistence among organic chemicals in the environment. Early attempts generally consisted of examining the degradation of a homologous series of structurally related compounds under identical conditions with a complex "universal" inoculum, typically derived from numerous sources. This approach revealed that the nature and positions of substituents affected the apparent biodegradability of several chemical classes, with resulting general themes, such as halogens generally conferring persistence under aerobic conditions. Subsequently, more quantitative approaches have been developed using principles of QSAR and often accounting for the role of sorption (bioavailability) in chemical fate.

Structure Activity Relationships Analysis

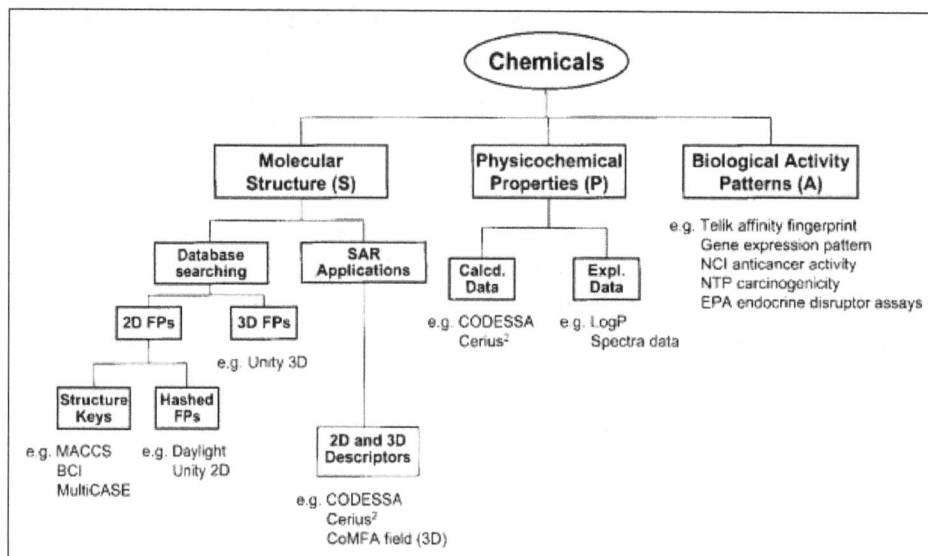

Three level of approach to characterize chemical compounds.

Structure Activity Relationship techniques are currently employed in a wide range of applications, including: In-silico design of virtual chemical libraries that explore molecular diversity for subsequent synthesis and screening; screening proprietary, commercially available, and public databases for lead discovery; and, mining gene expression data from microarray experiments for target identification. It is obvious from these examples that SAR technology now fulfills expanding roles in handling large and expanding sources of data. The analysis of SAR allows the detection of the functional group which has biological effect on the organism, which facilitates the modification of a bioactive compound by changing its chemical structure. Chemists use advanced techniques of chemical synthesis to introduce new chemical groups into the biomedical compound and test the effect of modifications on their biological functions. This method was refined to build mathematical relationships between the chemical structure and the biological activity, known as quantitative structure activity relationships (QSAR). The basic assumption underlying SAR analysis is that similar molecules have identical functions. The underlying problem is therefore how to define small difference on molecular level, since each kind of activity, e.g. reaction ability, solubility, target activity, and may also related to another difference.

Statistical Methods for SAR Analysis

- Multiple Linear Regression (MLR).

- Principal Component Analysis.

- Artificial Neural Networks (ANN).

- Support Vector Machine (SVM).

Quantitative Structure Activity Relationship

Quantitative structure–activity relationship models (QSAR models) are regression or classification models used in the chemical and biological sciences and engineering. Like other regression models, QSAR regression models relate a set of "predictor" variables (X) to the potency of the response variable (Y), while classification QSAR models relate the predictor variables to a categorical value of the response variable.

In QSAR modeling, the predictors consist of physico-chemical properties or theoretical molecular descriptors of chemicals; the QSAR response-variable could be a biological activity of the chemicals. QSAR models first summarize a supposed relationship between chemical structures and biological activity in a data-set of chemicals. Second, QSAR models predict the activities of new chemicals.

Related terms include quantitative structure–property relationships (QSPR) when a chemical property is modeled as the response variable. "Different properties or behaviors of chemical molecules have been investigated in the field of QSPR. Some examples are quantitative structure–reactivity relationships (QSRRs), quantitative structure–chromatography relationships (QSCRs) and, quantitative structure–toxicity relationships (QSTRs), quantitative structure–electrochemistry relationships (QSERs), and quantitative structure–biodegradability relationships (QSBRs)."

As an example, biological activity can be expressed quantitatively as the concentration of a substance required to give a certain biological response. Additionally, when physicochemical properties or structures are expressed by numbers, one can find a mathematical relationship, or quantitative structure-activity relationship, between the two. The mathematical expression, if carefully validated can then be used to predict the modeled response of other chemical structures.

A QSAR has the form of a mathematical model:

Activity = f(physiochemical properties and/or structural properties) + error.

The error includes model error (bias) and observational variability, that is, the variability in observations even on a correct model.

Essential Steps in QSAR Studies

Principal steps of QSAR/QSPR including (i) Selection of Data set and extraction of structural/empirical descriptors (ii) variable selection, (iii) model construction and (iv) validation evaluation."

SAR and the SAR Paradox

The basic assumption for all molecule based hypotheses is that similar molecules have similar activities. This principle is also called Structure–Activity Relationship (SAR). The underlying problem is therefore how to define a *small* difference on a molecular level, since each kind of activity, e.g. reaction ability, biotransformation ability, solubility, target activity, and so on, might depend on another difference. Good examples were given in the bioisosterism reviews by Patanie/LaVoie and Brown.

In general, one is more interested in finding strong trends. Created hypotheses usually rely on a finite number of chemical data. Thus, the induction principle should be respected to avoid overfitted hypotheses and deriving overfitted and useless interpretations on structural/molecular data.

The *SAR paradox* refers to the fact that it is not the case that all similar molecules have similar activities.

Types

Fragment based (Group Contribution)

Analogously, the "partition coefficient"—a measurement of differential solubility and itself a component of QSAR predictions—can be predicted either by atomic methods (known as "XLogP" or "ALogP") or by chemical fragment methods (known as "CLogP" and other variations). It has been shown that the logP of compound can be determined by the sum of its fragments; fragment-based methods are generally accepted as better predictors than atomic-based methods. Fragmentary values have been determined statistically, based on empirical data for known logP values. This method gives mixed results and is generally not trusted to have accuracy of more than ±0.1 units.

Group or Fragment based QSAR is also known as GQSAR. GQSAR allows flexibility to study various molecular fragments of interest in relation to the variation in biological response. The molecular fragments could be substituents at various substitution sites in congeneric set of molecules or could be on the basis of pre-defined chemical rules in case of non-congeneric sets. GQSAR also considers cross-terms fragment descriptors, which could be helpful in identification of key fragment interactions in determining variation of activity. Lead discovery using Fragnomics is an emerging paradigm. In this context FB-QSAR proves to be a promising strategy for fragment library design and in fragment-to-lead identification endeavours.

An advanced approach on fragment or group-based QSAR based on the concept of pharmacophore-similarity is developed. This method, pharmacophore-similarity-based QSAR (PS-QSAR) uses topological pharmacophoric descriptors to develop QSAR models. This activity prediction may assist the contribution of certain pharmacophore features encoded by respective fragments toward activity improvement and/or detrimental effects.

3D-QSAR

The acronym 3D-QSAR or 3-D QSAR refers to the application of force field calculations requiring three-dimensional structures of a given set of small molecules with known activities (training set). The training set needs to be superimposed (aligned) by either experimental data (e.g. based on ligand-protein crystallography) or molecule superimposition software. It uses computed potentials, e.g. the Lennard-Jones potential, rather than experimental constants and is concerned with the overall molecule rather than a single substituent. The first 3-D QSAR was named Comparative Molecular Field Analysis (CoMFA) by Cramer et al. It examined the steric fields (shape of the molecule) and the electrostatic fields which were correlated by means of partial least squares regression (PLS).

The created data space is then usually reduced by a following feature extraction. The following learning method can be any of the already mentioned machine learning methods, e.g. support vector machines. An alternative approach uses multiple-instance learning by encoding molecules as sets of data instances, each of which represents a possible molecular conformation. A label or response is assigned to each set corresponding to the activity of the molecule, which is assumed to be determined by at least one instance in the set (i.e. some conformation of the molecule).

On June 18, 2011 the Comparative Molecular Field Analysis (CoMFA) patent has dropped any restriction on the use of GRID and partial least-squares (PLS) technologies.

Chemical Descriptor Based

In this approach, descriptors quantifying various electronic, geometric, or steric properties of a molecule are computed and used to develop a QSAR. This approach is different from the fragment (or group contribution) approach in that the descriptors are computed for the system as whole rather than from the properties of individual fragments. This approach is different from the 3D-QSAR approach in that the descriptors are computed from scalar quantities (e.g., energies, geometric parameters) rather than from 3D fields.

An example of this approach is the QSARs developed for olefin polymerization by half sandwich compounds.

Modeling

In the literature it can be often found that chemists have a preference for partial least squares (PLS) methods, since it applies the feature extraction and induction in one step.

Data Mining Approach

Computer SAR models typically calculate a relatively large number of features. Because those lack structural interpretation ability, the preprocessing steps face a feature selection problem (i.e., which structural features should be interpreted to determine the structure-activity relationship). Feature selection can be accomplished by visual inspection (qualitative selection by a human); by data mining; or by molecule mining.

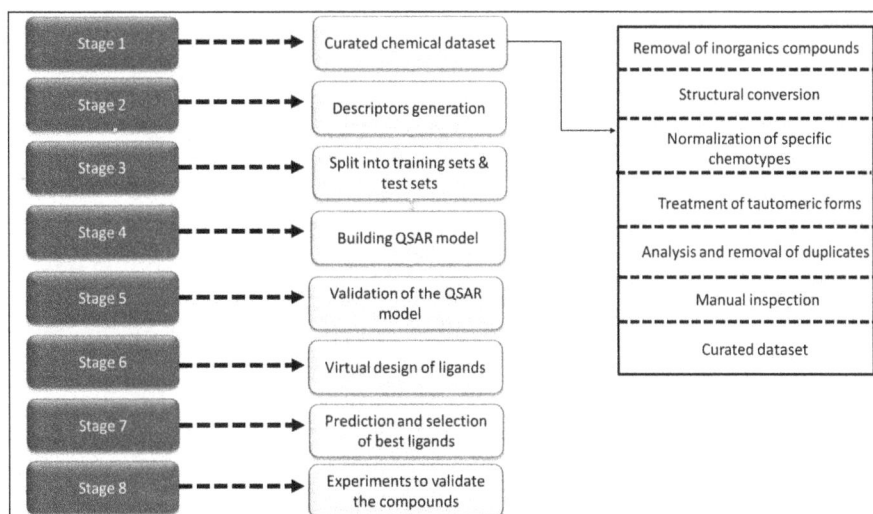

QSAR protocol: Matched Molecular Pair Analysis.

A typical data mining based prediction uses e.g. support vector machines, decision trees, artificial neural networks for inducing a predictive learning model.

Molecule mining approaches, a special case of structured data mining approaches, apply a similarity matrix based prediction or an automatic fragmentation scheme into molecular substructures. Furthermore, there exist also approaches using maximum common subgraph searches or graph kernels.

Typically QSAR models derived from non linear machine learning is seen as a "black box", which fails to guide medicinal chemists. Recently there is a relatively new concept of matched molecular pair analysis or prediction driven MMPA which is coupled with QSAR model in order to identify activity cliffs.

Evaluation of the Quality of QSAR Models

QSAR modeling produces predictive models derived from application of statistical tools correlating biological activity (including desirable therapeutic effect and undesirable side effects) or physico-chemical properties in QSPR models of chemicals (drugs/toxicants/environmental pollutants) with descriptors representative of molecular structure or properties. QSARs are being applied in many disciplines, for example: risk assessment, toxicity prediction, and regulatory decisions in addition to drug discovery and lead optimization. Obtaining a good quality QSAR model depends on many factors, such as the quality of input data, the choice of descriptors and statistical methods for modeling and for validation. Any QSAR modeling should ultimately lead to statistically robust and predictive models capable of making accurate and reliable predictions of the modeled response of new compounds.

For validation of QSAR models, usually various strategies are adopted:

- Internal validation or cross-validation (actually, while extracting data, cross validation is a measure of model robustness, the more a model is robust (higher q2) the less data extraction perturb the original model).

- External validation by splitting the available data set into training set for model development and prediction set for model predictivity check.

- Blind external validation by application of model on new external data.

- Data randomization or Y-scrambling for verifying the absence of chance correlation between the response and the modeling descriptors.

The success of any QSAR model depends on accuracy of the input data, selection of appropriate descriptors and statistical tools, and most importantly validation of the developed model. Validation is the process by which the reliability and relevance of a procedure are established for a specific purpose; for QSAR models validation must be mainly for robustness, prediction performances and applicability domain (AD) of the models.

Some validation methodologies can be problematic. For example, *leave one-out* cross-validation generally leads to an overestimation of predictive capacity. Even with external validation, it is difficult to determine whether the selection of training and test sets was manipulated to maximize the predictive capacity of the model being published.

Different aspects of validation of QSAR models that need attention include methods of selection of training set compounds, setting training set size and impact of variable selection for training set models for determining the quality of prediction. Development of novel validation parameters for judging quality of QSAR models is also important.

Application

Chemical

One of the first historical QSAR applications was to predict boiling points.

It is well known for instance that within a particular family of chemical compounds, especially of organic chemistry, that there are strong correlations between structure and observed properties. A simple example is the relationship between the number of carbons in alkanes and their boiling points. There is a clear trend in the increase of boiling point with an increase in the number carbons, and this serves as a means for predicting the boiling points of higher alkanes.

A still very interesting application is the Hammett equation, Taft equation and pKa prediction methods.

Biological

The biological activity of molecules is usually measured in assays to establish the level of inhibition of particular signal transduction or metabolic pathways. Drug discovery often involves the use of QSAR to identify chemical structures that could have good inhibitory effects on specific targets and have low toxicity (non-specific activity). Of special interest is the prediction of partition coefficient log P, which is an important measure used in identifying "druglikeness" according to Lipinski's Rule of Five.

While many quantitative structure activity relationship analyses involve the interactions of a family of molecules with an enzyme or receptor binding site, QSAR can also be used to study the interactions between the structural domains of proteins. Protein-protein interactions can be quantitatively analyzed for structural variations resulted from site-directed mutagenesis.

It is part of the machine learning method to reduce the risk for a SAR paradox, especially taking into account that only a finite amount of data is available. In general, all QSAR problems can be divided into coding and learning.

Applications

(Q)SAR models have been used for risk management. QSARS are suggested by regulatory authorities; in the European Union, QSARs are suggested by the REACH regulation, where "REACH" abbreviates "Registration, Evaluation, Authorisation and Restriction of Chemicals".

The chemical descriptor space whose convex hull is generated by a particular training set of chemicals is called the training set's applicability domain. Prediction of properties of novel chemicals that are located outside the applicability domain uses extrapolation, and so is less reliable (on average) than prediction within the applicability domain. The assessment of the reliability of QSAR predictions remains a research topic.

The QSAR equations can be used to predict biological activities of newer molecules before their synthesis.

Drug Development

Drug development is the process of bringing a new pharmaceutical drug to the market once a lead compound has been identified through the process of drug discovery. It includes preclinical research on microorganisms and animals, filing for regulatory status, such as via the United States Food and Drug Administration for an investigational new drug to initiate clinical trials on humans, and may include the step of obtaining regulatory approval with a new drug application to market the drug.

New Chemical Entity Development

Broadly, the process of drug development can be divided into preclinical and clinical work.

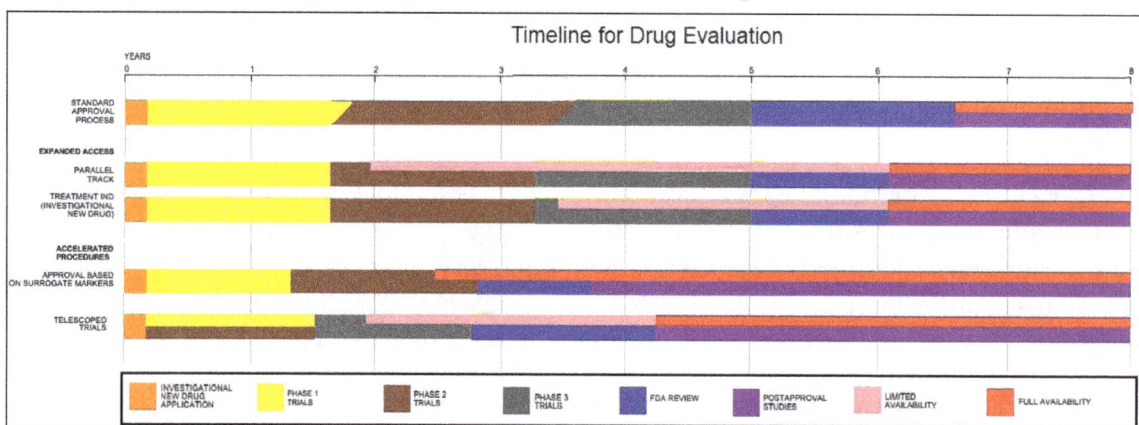

Timeline showing the various drug approval tracks and research phases.

Pre-clinical

New chemical entities (NCEs, also known as new molecular entities or NMEs) are compounds that emerge from the process of drug discovery. These have promising activity against a particular biological target that is important in disease. However, little is known about the safety, toxicity, pharmacokinetics, and metabolism of this NCE in humans. It is the function of drug development to assess all of these parameters prior to human clinical trials. A further major objective of drug development is to recommend the dose and schedule for the first use in a human clinical trial ("first-in-man" [FIM] or First Human Dose [FHD]).

In addition, drug development must establish the physicochemical properties of the NCE: its chemical makeup, stability, and solubility. Manufacturers must optimize the process they use to make the chemical so they can scale up from a medicinal chemist producing milligrams, to manufacturing on the kilogram and ton scale. They further examine the product for suitability to package as capsules, tablets, aerosol, intramuscular injectable, subcutaneous injectable, or intravenous formulations. Together, these processes are known in preclinical and clinical development as *chemistry, manufacturing, and control* (CMC).

Many aspects of drug development focus on satisfying the regulatory requirements of drug licensing authorities. These generally constitute a number of tests designed to determine the major toxicities of a novel compound prior to first use in humans. It is a legal requirement that an assessment of major organ toxicity be performed (effects on the heart and lungs, brain, kidney, liver and digestive system), as well as effects on other parts of the body that might be affected by the drug (e.g., the skin if the new drug is to be delivered through the skin). Increasingly, these tests are made using *in vitro* methods (e.g., with isolated cells), but many tests can only be made by using experimental animals to demonstrate the complex interplay of metabolism and drug exposure on toxicity.

The information is gathered from this preclinical testing, as well as information on CMC, and submitted to regulatory authorities (in the US, to the FDA), as an Investigational New Drug (IND) application. If the IND is approved, development moves to the clinical phase.

Clinical Phase

Clinical trials involve three or four steps:

- Phase I trials, usually in healthy volunteers, determine safety and dosing.

- Phase II trials are used to get an initial reading of efficacy and further explore safety in small numbers of patients having the disease targeted by the NCE.

- Phase III trials are large, pivotal trials to determine safety and efficacy in sufficiently large numbers of patients with the targeted disease. If safety and efficacy are adequately proved, clinical testing may stop at this step and the NCE advances to the new drug application (NDA) stage.

- Phase IV trials are post-approval trials that are sometimes a condition attached by the FDA, also called post-market surveillance studies.

The process of defining characteristics of the drug does not stop once an NCE begins human clinical trials. In addition to the tests required to move a novel drug into the clinic for the first time, manufacturers must ensure that any long-term or chronic toxicities are well-defined, including effects on systems not previously monitored (fertility, reproduction, immune system, among others). They must also test the compound for its potential to cause cancer (carcinogenicity testing).

If a compound emerges from these tests with an acceptable toxicity and safety profile, and the company can further show it has the desired effect in clinical trials, then the NCE portfolio of evidence can be submitted for marketing approval in the various countries where the manufacturer plans to sell it. In the United States, this process is called a "new drug application" or NDA.

Most NCEs fail during drug development, either because they have unacceptable toxicity or because they simply do not have the intended effect on the targeted disease as shown in clinical trials.

A trend toward the collection of biomarker and genetic information from clinical trial participants, and increasing investment by companies in this area, led by 2018 to fully half of all drug trials collecting this information, the prevalence reaching above 80% among oncology trials.

Drug development in the past has mostly been a hit or a miss affair with a large number of compounds being synthesized at random. Luck has played a great part, but we can now recognize strategies which have evolved over the years:

- Variation of substituents.

- Extension of the structure.

- Chain extensions/contractions.

- Ring expansions/contractions.

- Ring variations.

- Isosteres.

- Simplification of the structure.

- Rigidification of the structure.

Variation of Substituents

Once the essential groups for biological activity have been identified, substituents are varied since this is usually quite easy to do synthetically. The aim here is to fine tune the molecule and to optimize its activity. Biological activity may depend not only on how well the compound interacts with its receptor, but also on a whole range of physical features such as basicity, lipophilicity, electronic distribution, and size. The idea of varying substituents is to attach a series of substituents such that these physical features are varied one by one. In reality, it is rarely possible to change one physical feature without affecting another. For example, replacing a methyl group on a nitrogen with an ethyl group could affect the basicity of the nitrogen atom, but the size of the molecule is also increased. Either of these changes might have an effect on the activity of a drug and it would be difficult to know which was more important without more results. The following are routine variations which can be carried out.

Alkyl Substituents

If the molecule has an easily accessible functional group such as an alcohol, phenol, or amino group, then alkyl chains of various lengths and bulks such as methyl, ethyl, propyl, butyl, isopropyl, isobutyl or rm-butyl can be attached.

Different alkyl groups on a nitrogen atom may alter the basicity and/or lipophilicity of the drug and thus affect how strongly the drug binds to its binding site or how easily the compound crosses membrane barriers.

Larger alkyl groups, however, increase the bulk of the compound and this may confer selectivity on the drug. For example, in the case of a compound which interacts with two different receptors, a bulkier alkyl substituent may prevent the drug from binding to one of those receptors and so cut down side-effects.

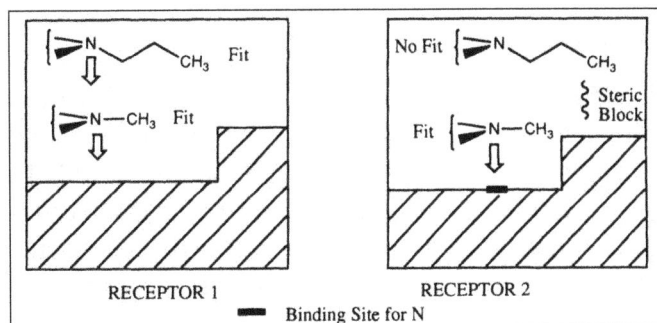

Use of a larger alkyl group to confer selectivity on a drug.

Aromatic Substitutions

A favourite approach for aromatic compounds is to vary the substitution pattern. This may give increased activity if the relevant binding groups are not already in the ideal positions for bonding.

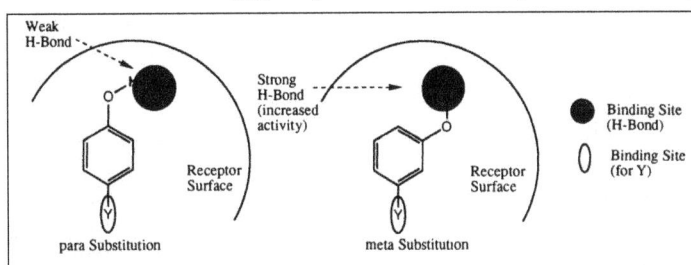

Aromatic substitutions.

Electronic effects may also be involved. For example, an electron withdrawing nitro group will affect the basicity of an aromatic amine more significantly if it is in the para position rather than the meta position. We have noted already that varying the basicity of a nitrogen atom may have a biological effect.

If the substitution pattern is ideal, then we can try varying the substituents themselves. Substituents of different sizes and electronic properties are usually tried to see if steric and electronic factors have any effect on activity. It may be that activity is improved by having a more electron withdrawing substituent, in which case a nitro substituent might be tried in place of a chloro substituent.

The chemistry involved in these procedures is usually straightforward and so these analogues are made as a matter of course whenever a novel drug structure is discovered or developed. Furthermore, the variation of aromatic or aliphatic substituents is open to quantitative structure-activity studies (QSARs) as described in Chapter.

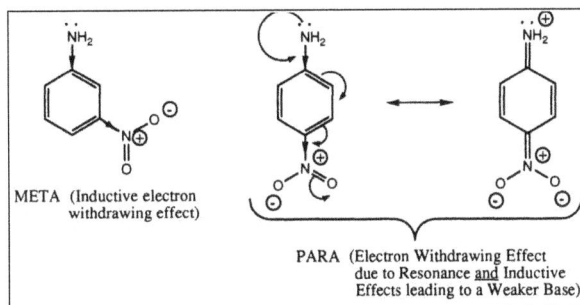

Electronic effects of aromatic substitutions.

Extension of the Structure

This strategy has been used successfully on natural products such as morphine. It might seem strange that a natural product which is produced in a plant or a fungus should have important biological effects in the human body. One possible explanation for this could be that the natural product is present in the body as well. However, this seems unlikely. Therefore, we have to conclude that it is a happy coincidence that morphine has the right shape and binding groups to interact with a painkilling receptor in the body. This leads to some interesting conclusions.

Since there is a painkilling receptor in the body we have to accept that there is a neurotransmitter (or hormone) which switches on that receptor. We already know that it cannot be morphine, so the painkilling molecule has to have a different shape and possibly different binding groups. Assuming that the body's own painkiller is the ideal molecule for its receptor, then we must also conclude that morphine is not the ideal molecule. For example, it is perfectly possible that the natural painkiller has four important binding interactions with its receptor, whereas morphine has only three. Therefore, why not add binding groups to the morphine skeleton to search for that fourth binding site? This tactic has been employed successfully to produce compounds such as the phenethyl analogue of morphine which has 14 times greater activity. Such a result suggests that the extra binding site on the receptor is hydrophobic, interacting with the aromatic ring by van der Waals interactions.

Frequently, this extension tactic has resulted in a compound which acts as an antagonist rather than as an agonist. In this case, the extra binding site is not one used by the natural agonist or substrate. The binding interaction is different and no biological response results.

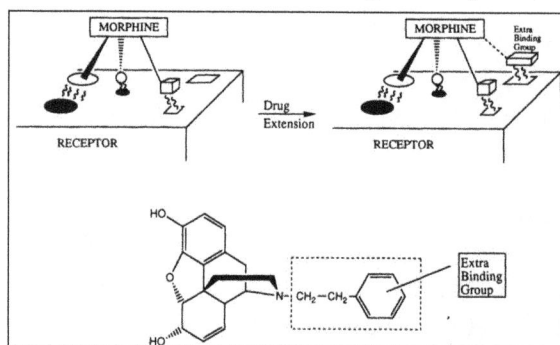

Extension of morphine to provide a fourth binding group.

Chain Extensions/Contractions

Some drugs have two important binding groups linked together by a chain. Many of the natural neurotransmitters are like this. It is possible that the chain length is not ideal for the best interaction. Therefore, shortening or lengthening the chain length is a useful tactic to try.

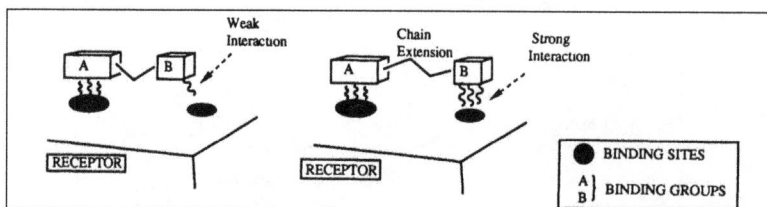

Chain extension.

Ring Expansions/Contractions

If a drug has a ring, it is generally worth synthesizing analogues where one of these rings is expanded or contracted by one unit. The principle behind this approach is much the same as varying the substitution pattern of an aromatic ring. Expanding or contracting the ring puts the binding groups in different positions relative to each other and, with luck, may lead to better interactions with the binding site.

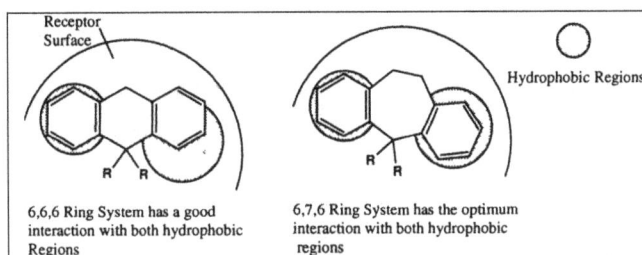

Ring expansion.

Ring Variations

A further popular approach for compounds containing an aromatic ring is to try replacing the aromatic ring with a range of heteroaromatic rings of different ring size and heteroatom positions. Admittedly, a lot of these changes are merely ways of avoiding patent restrictions and do not result in significant improvements, but sometimes there are significant advantages in changing a ring system.

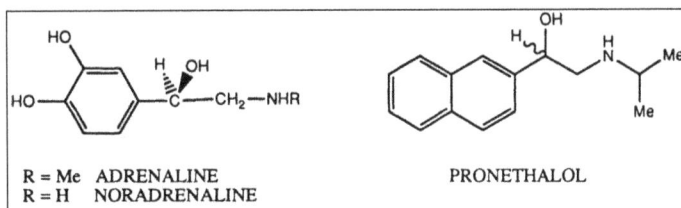

Ring variation of adrenaline.

One of the major advances in the development of the selective beta blockers was the replacement of the aromatic ring in adrenaline with a naphthalene ring system (pronethalol). This resulted in a compound which was able to distinguish between two very similar receptors, the alpha and beta receptors for adrenaline. One possible explanation for this could be that the beta receptor has a larger van der Waals binding area for the aromatic system than the alpha receptor and can interact more strongly with pronethalol than with adrenaline. Another possible explanation is that the naphthalene ring system is sterically too big for the alpha receptor but is just right for the beta receptor.

Isosteres

Isosteres are atoms or groups of atoms which have the same valency (or number of outer shell electrons). For example, SH, NH_2, and CH_3 are isosteres of OH, while S, NH, and CH_2 are isosteres of O. Isosteres have often been used to design an inhibitor or to increase metabolic stability. The idea is to alter the character of the molecule in as subtle a way as possible. Replacing O with CH_2, for example, will make little difference to the size of the analogue, but will have a marked effect on its polarity, electronic distribution, and bonding. Replacing OH with the larger SH may not have such an influence on the electronic character, but steric factors become more significant. Isosteric groups could be used to determine whether a particular group is involved in hydrogen bonding. For example, replacing OH and CH_3 would completely destroy hydrogen bonding, whereas replacing OH with NH_2 would not the beta blocker propranolol has an ether linkage. Replacement of the OCH_2 segment with the isosteres CH=CH, SCH_2, or CH_2CH_2 eliminates activity, whereas replacement with $NHCH_2$ retains activity (though reduced). These results show that the ether oxygen is important to the activity of the drug and suggests that it is involved in hydrogen bonding with the receptor.

Replacing the methyl of a methyl ester group with NH_2 has been a useful tactic in stabilizing esters which are susceptible to enzymatic hydrolysis. The NH_2 group is the same size as the methyl and therefore has no steric effect. However, it has totally different electronic properties, and as such can feed electrons into the carboxyl group and stabilize it from hydrolysis.

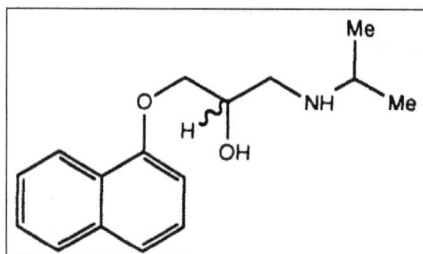

Propranolol.

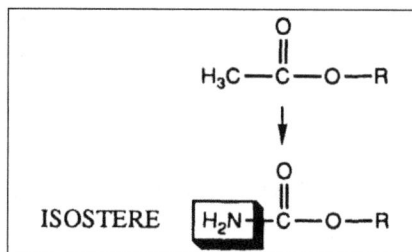

Isosteric replacement of a methyl with an amino group.

Although fluorine does not have the same valency as hydrogen, it is often considered an isostere of that atom since it is virtually the same size. Replacement of a hydrogen atom with a fluorine atom will therefore have little steric effect, but since the fluorine is strongly electronegative, the electronic effect may be dramatic.

The use of fluorine as an isostere for hydrogen has been highly successful in recent years. One example is the antitumour drug 5-fluorouracil described in Section. The drug is accepted by the target enzyme since it appears little different from the normal substrate (uracil). However, the mechanism of the enzyme-catalysed reaction is totally disrupted. Fluorine has replaced a hydrogen atom which must be lost as a proton during the mechanism. There is no chance of fluorine departing as a positively charged species.

Simplification of the Structure

If the essential groups of a drug have been identified, then by implication, it might be possible to discard non-essential parts of the structure without losing activity. The advantage would be in gaining a far simpler compound which would be much easier and cheaper to synthesize in the laboratory. For example, let us consider our hypothetical natural product Glipine. The essential groups have been marked and so we might aim to synthesize compounds such as those shown in Fig. These have simpler structures, but still retain the groups which we have identified as being essential.

This tactic was used successfully with the alkaloid cocaine. It was well known that cocaine had local anaesthetic properties and it was hoped to develop a local anaesthetic based on a simplified structure of cocaine which could be easily synthesized in the laboratory. Success resulted with the discovery of procaine (or Novocaine) in 1909.

However, there is a trade-off involved when simplifying molecules. The advantage in obtaining simpler compounds may be outweighed by the disadvantage of increased side-effects and reduced selectivity. We shall see below how these undesirable properties can creep in with simpler molecules and why the opposite tactic of rigidification can be just as useful as that of simplification.

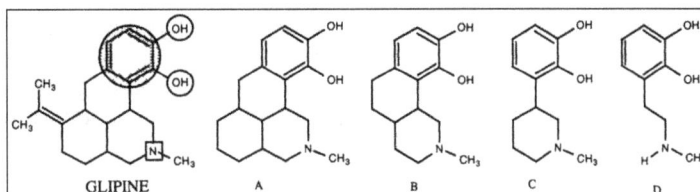

Glipine analogues.

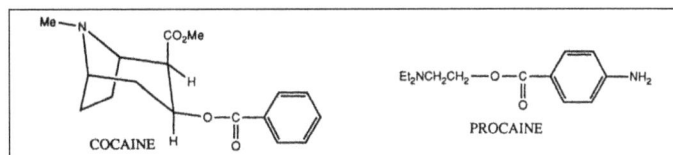

Cocaine and procaine.

Rigidification of the Structure

Rigidification has been a popular tactic used to increase the activity of a drug or to reduce its side-effects. In order to understand why, let us consider again our hypothetical neurotransmitter from Chapter. This is quite a simple molecule and highly flexible. Bond rotation can lead to a large number of conformations or shapes. However, as seen from the receptor/messenger interaction, conformation I is the conformation accepted by the receptor. Other conformations such as II have the ionized amino group too far away from the anionic centre to interact efficiently and so this is an inactive conformation for our model receptor site. However, it is quite possible that there exists a different receptor which is capable of binding conformation II. If this is the case, then our model neurotransmitter could switch on two different receptors and give two different biological responses.

References

- Ray, Amit. "7 Limitations of Molecular Docking & Computer Aided Drug Design and Discovery". Inner Light Publishers. Retrieved 21 Oct 2018

- Chemical-synthesis, science: britannica.com, Retrieved 5 February, 2019

- Erlanson DA, mcdowell RS, O'Brien T (July 2004). "Fragment-based drug discovery". Journal of Medicinal Chemistry. 47 (14): 3463–82. Doi:10.1021/jm040031v. PMID 15214773

- Structure-activity-relationship-sar-analysis, services: creative-proteomics.com, Retrieved 6 March, 2019

- Herper, Matthew (11 August 2013). "The Cost Of Creating A New Drug Now $5 Billion, Pushing Big Pharma To Change". Forbes, Pharma & Healthcare. Retrieved 17 July 2016

- Sertkaya, A; Wong, H. H.; Jessup, A; Beleche, T (2016). "Key cost drivers of pharmaceutical clinical trials in the United States". Clinical Trials. 13 (2): 117–26. Doi:10.1177/1740774515625964. PMID 26908540

INDEX

www.ingramcontent.com/pod-product-compliance
Lightning Source LLC
Chambersburg PA
CBHW061304190326
41458CB00011B/3760